Visit our website

to find out about other books from Churchill Livingstone and other imprints in Harcourt Health Sciences

Register free at
www.harcourt-international.com

and you will get

- **the latest information on new books, journals and electronic products in your chosen subject areas**

- **the choice of e-mail or post alerts or both, when there are any new books in your chosen areas**

- **news of special offers and promotions**

- **information about products from all Harcourt Health Sciences imprints including W. B. Saunders, Churchill Livingstone, and Mosby**

You will also find an easily searchable catalogue, online ordering, information on our extensive list of journals...and much more!

Visit the Harcourt Health Sciences website today!

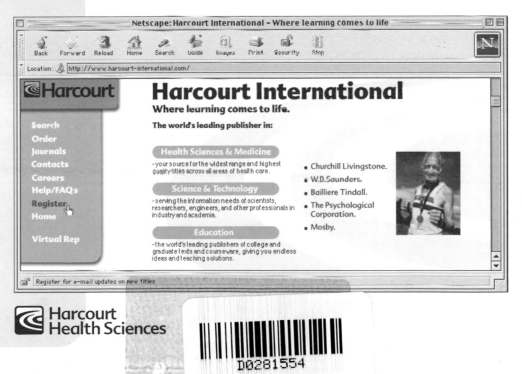

District Nursing

For Churchill Livingstone:

Senior Commissioning Editor: Ninette Premdas
Head of Project Management: Ewan Halley
Project Development Manager: Katrina Mather
Designer: George Ajayi

District Nursing

Providing Care in a Supportive Context

Edited by

Sally Lawton RGN NDNCert RCNT RDNT MA PhD
Senior Lecturer in Nursing, Robert Gordon University, Aberdeen, UK

Jane Cantrell MSc BNurs RGN RHV NDNCert CertEd
Lecturer in Nursing, University of Dundee, Dundee, UK

Jane Harris MSc BNurs RGN RHV NDNCert RDNT RM PWT
Lecturer in Nursing, University of Abertay Dundee, Dundee, UK

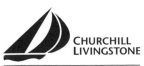
CHURCHILL
LIVINGSTONE

EDINBURGH LONDON NEW YORK PHILADELPHIA ST LOUIS SYDNEY TORONTO 2000

CHURCHILL LIVINGSTONE
An imprint of Harcourt Publishers Limited

© Harcourt Publishers Limited 2000

📖 is a registered trademark of Harcourt Publishers Limited

The right of Sally Lawton, Jane Cantrell and Jane Harris to be identified as authors of this work has been asserted by them in accordance with the Copyright, Designs and Patents Act 1988

First published 2000

ISBN 0 443 06250 1

British Library Cataloguing in Publication Data
A catalogue record for this book is available from the British Library

Library of Congress Cataloging in Publication Data
A catalog record for this book is available from the Library of Congress

Note
Medical knowledge is constantly changing. As new information becomes available, changes in treatment, procedures, equipment and the use of drugs become necessary. The editors, contributors and the publishers have taken care to ensure that the information given in this text is accurate and up to date. However, readers are strongly advised to confirm that the information, especially with regard to drug usage, complies with the latest legislation and standards of practice.

The
publisher's
policy is to use
**paper manufactured
from sustainable forests**

Printed in China

Contents

Contributors

Val Baker RGN NDNCert BSC
Head of IM & T, Lothian Primary Care NHS
Trust, Edinburgh, UK

Judith Canham RN NDNCert CPT PGDE DNT MSc
Senior Lecturer, Department of Health Care
Studies, The Manchester Metropolitan
University, Manchester, UK

Lis Cook BA(Hons) RGN RM DNCert
Nurse Director, Queen's Nursing Institute
Scotland, Edinburgh, UK

Rona Ferguson BA(Hons) MPhil
Centre for Contemporary History, Glasgow
Caledonian University, Glasgow, UK

Susan Hickie MSc Public Health DipNursing RN RM
RHV RHVT
Professional Officer, National Board for
Nursing, Midwifery and Health Visiting for
Scotland, Edinburgh, UK

Lisbeth Hockey SRN SCM HV QNS RNT BSc Econ
(Hons) PhD
Research Consultant, Formerly Director
Nursing Studies Unit, University of Edinburgh,
Edinburgh, UK

Sue Howard RGN RHC DNCert CertEd DNT, MA
Educational Advisor, Royal College of Nursing,
London, UK

Emma McIntosh BA (Hons) MSc Research Fellow
Health Economics Research Unit, University of
Aberdeen, Aberdeen, UK

Heather Marr MSC DipCNE NDNCert RGN RMN
Senior Nursing Lecturer, University of
Dundee, School of Nursing and Midwifery,
Dundee, UK

Sue Plummer MBA DMS RGN RM DN
Director of Nursing, Borders Primary Care
Trust, Melrose, UK

Fiona Redworth RGN NDNCert RNT MSc PGCE
Senior Lecturer, NEWI, Health and Community
Studies, Wrexham, UK

Graham C. Rumbold MSc BA RGN NDN CHNT RNT
DNT
Coordinator, International Affairs and
Countinuing Professional Development, Centre
for Health Care Education, University College
Northampton, Northampton, UK

Mandy Ryan BA (Hons) MSc PhD MRC Senior Fellow
Health Economics Research Unit, University of
Aberdeen, Aberdeen, UK

Helen Sweet MA BA RGN SCM
Researcher, Humanities Research Centre, School
of Humanities, Oxford Brookes University,
Oxford, UK

Dianne Watkins RGN RM HVCert RNT MSc CertEd
Lecturer in Health Visiting/Head of Primary
Care Development Unit, School of Nursing and
Midwifery Studies, University of Wales, College
of Medicine, Cardiff, UK

John Unsworth MSc BSc(Hons) BA RGN OND DPSN
PGCE
Practice Development Nurse, Northumbria
Healthcare NHS Trust, Wallsend Health Centre,
Newcastle, UK

Preface

The aim of this book is to provide a comprehensive text that explores key community healthcare issues from a district nursing perspective. The book has been targeted primarily at qualified first-level registered nurses who are undertaking the Specialist Practitioner Qualification Community Nursing in the Home (District Nursing). The book provides a resource for students which will underpin both the core and specialist modules that comprise this community specialist practitioner programme through the exploration of current issues.

We hope that the book will also be of interest to qualified district nurses and pre-registration students. The editors acknowledge that the structure and organisation of community nursing services vary according to the provision of health services within different counties of the United Kingdom and they have endeavoured to develop a general textbook that will be relevant to nurses working in a variety of settings.

In recent years there has been a growth in the number of books aiming to address issues relevant to community nurses and of use to those undertaking community pathways of specialist practitioner programmes. Some contain chapters which are specific to individual pathways but generally these are brief, lack the scope and depth required at this level of study and fail to conceptualise fully the uniqueness of individual specialist roles. Readers/students therefore need a more indepth text specific to their speciality. Although such texts exist for other pathways (e.g. practice nursing, health visiting, community mental health

nursing, school nursing), there is no single text which explores the nature of district nursing.

As experienced district nurse practitioners and educators, the editors believe that district nursing is unique in terms of its scope and the skills required to respond effectively to the needs of patients, clients, families and carers in a range of community settings.

The book is divided into four sections reflecting four themes which are relevant to specialist practitioner programmes. Many of the issues discussed are complex, relating to more than one theme, and links are highlighted and developed between chapters and sections.

Section 1 explores the context of supportive care in district nursing and introduces the reader to the Davies & Oberle model of supportive care which is used as a framework to explain the nature of district nursing. This model was developed in the early 1990s following an investigation into the work of a community-based palliative care nurse. It shows that the skills of community-based nursing develop during meeting, caring for and completion of care for individuals and their families. It addresses physical, educational and organisational aspects of care as well as discussing how such patterns of care may affect nurses themselves.

Section 2 looks at the context of care within district nursing. It has five chapters and explores demography, health trends, the political environment in which care is delivered, multiprofessional working and the historical background of district nursing.

Section 3 examines the professional context in which district nurses work. It includes chapters on research, developing roles, the impact of nurse prescribing, the education of district nurses and relevant legal and ethical issues.

The final section highlights the management context of district nursing practice. Chapters in this section detail the management of care, management of change, quality and clinical effectiveness, economics and information management.

A feature of the book is the use of vignettes, in the form of small pieces of illustrative text written by district nurses which augment and enliven the main text. We aim to give readers insight into and appreciation of real-life situations and enable them to link theory with practice in these vignettes.

The three editors are all qualified district nurses with many years' experience. Although now involved in education, two of the editors have experience in leading courses for district nurses and the third has been involved in pre-registration developments in community nursing. The contributors to the book come from a range of professions in education, research, managerial and service backgrounds and from different parts of the United Kingdom.

On behalf of the individual chapter authors we would like to express our gratitude to all colleagues who have shared their thoughts and experiences and allowed us to use them in the vignettes.

Sally Lawton
Jane Cantrell
Aberdeen 2000   Jane Harris

The Davies & Oberle model of supportive care applied to district nursing

Sally Lawton

SECTION CONTENTS

Key points

- The Davies & Oberle model of supportive care
- The application of the book's contents to the model

The aim of this opening chapter is to outline a model that can be used to describe the process of district nursing. Throughout the book, the wide-ranging nature of district nursing will be highlighted, set as it is within the complex nature of primary health care. To begin this textbook, we wanted to bring all the key issues together within a framework for practice. The Davies & Oberle (1990) model of supportive care is an ideal way to present this synthesis. The first vignette explains how Sally was introduced to this model.

Box 1   Framework for evaluation of nursing models (adapted from Fawcett 1995)

- Why was the model developed?
- What are the origins of the model?

These two questions need to be answered to gain some understanding of the potential applicability of a model developed in a different clinical setting to district nursing.

- How does the model interpret the nursing metaparadigm?
- Will the model be able to meet the philosophy of care identified by the nursing team?

These two questions enable the nursing team to discuss the similarities and differences between the model and their own philosophy of nursing care.

- How would the nurse use the model in practice in conjunction with the nursing process?
- What preparation will the nursing team need to understand and use the model?
- Will the model be able to demonstrate the breadth and depth of nursing undertaken by the district nursing team?

Vignette 1   Sally's story

Over the years that I have been involved in district nursing, both as a practitioner and as a teacher, I have often found it hard to explain the dimensions of district nursing practice. In more recent times, there has been a feeling that district nursing has been reduced to a series of tasks and, without any framework to describe its nature and complexity, it is hard to defend those less tangible aspects. However, I have always felt that the skill of district nursing lay in the relationship that the nurse built with patients or their families in the community setting whether a visit was a once-only or over a long time-frame.

I was working on the development of a palliative care unit in 1993 when a palliative care tutor introduced me to the Davies & Oberle model of supportive care. Although it is based upon work in the USA, having had a number of discussions with Kathy Oberle, one of the authors, and hearing about its use in a number of settings, I felt it was the missing framework that at last helped me explain how district nursing worked. I have already used it as an analytical framework in a small research project exploring the nursing needs of individuals with Alzheimer's disease in the home setting (Lawton 1997).

Since then, I have talked about it to district nurses who have shared my enthusiasm for it and we wanted to use it in this book to illustrate the scope of district nursing practice and the support that the district nurse gives the patient, but also needs herself when working in this often isolating area of clinical practice. The model has been discussed in relation to clinical care at home by Coles (1996), who concluded that the model may enable community nurses to interpret the changing nature of community nursing work.

The model is described below using an analytical framework adapted from Fawcett (1995). This framework may also be of use in evaluation of models of nursing care. It is presented as a series of questions as shown in Box 1.

ORIGINS AND DEVELOPMENT OF THE MODEL

The model emerged as the result of a qualitative research project (Davies & Oberle 1990) investigating, in depth, the work of a palliative home care nurse in the USA who found that her annual statistics did not reflect the full extent of her nursing care. Many district nurses would share such feelings that the wider elements of their practice remain unrecognised and this issue is raised in Chapter 13. Following a series of detailed interviews over a period of 25 hours, she explained the positive and negative challenges of her work in the community setting, using 10 of her cases.

Initially, it may be questionable how this applies to the work of a district nurse who works with a wide group of patients but despite the focus on palliative care in the study, the issues discussed were more to do with community nursing itself, rather than about the speciality of palliative care nursing.

The model also covers care as a developmental process and bears some similarity to the work of Peplau (1988) in the study of the relationship a nurse has with a patient and the concern of nursing with the 'interpersonal process'. Peplau recognises a four-stage process which begins with the meeting between the nurse and the patient as strangers, moving towards a period of the recognition of needs, the development of strategies to meet the needs and parting at the end of the relationship, in the final stage which Peplau identifies as the resolution. It is similar to district nursing practice in the development of the phases of care within the community setting as well as the acknowledgement of the various functions that the nurse may have as supporter, educator and facilitator.

This research detailed the work of one nurse but a great amount of data was gathered which subsequently allowed a deep analysis to be carried out. This is an example of a qualitative research study and this approach is discussed in more detail in Chapter 6.

The nursing metaparadigm

Before a nursing model can be applied to guide practice, the abstract framework has to be in place. This process of abstraction has been clarified by the identification of the metaparadigm of nursing, universal concepts that make up the elements of the discipline and what nursing in general is about (Fawcett 1995). Four elements of the metaparadigm have been identified.

1. *Person*. This can be an individual, a family, group or community that is receiving nursing care.
2. *Health*. The state of well-being of the person or group being cared for.
3. *Environment*. The setting for the nursing practice as well as the context of the person in his own life.
4. *Nursing*. The interventions, goals and outcomes that nurses can undertake in a systematic and measurable way.

Thibodeau (1983) has suggested that the four elements of the nursing metaparadigm have to be described precisely to understand a particular model of nursing. These four elements must be applicable to all nursing practice in any context, be neutral and show a unique aspect for the discipline of nursing.

Can these four elements be applied to district nursing practice? As district nurses work with individuals and groups, they will be seeing people at various stages of the health continuum, from short-term health problems which are fully resolvable right through to people in the final stages of life. In fact, one of the elements of district nursing practice that is so challenging is the variety of people and health conditions encountered and the need for a wide knowledge base. The environment concept is very applicable to district nursing practice in both aspects: the fact that nursing is delivered in the primary care setting and the closer understanding of the person in his own context which occurs within district nursing practice. Finally, the concept of nursing is valid for work in the district nursing setting and it is the use of a nursing model that assists in the systematic approach to care planning, delivery and evaluation of the care given.

Therefore, the nursing metaparadigm is of relevance from an individual level right through to the goals of the organisation that the district nurse is working for. The concepts of the metaparadigm link to the values and beliefs that we as district nurses hold about nursing and the people we nurse.

The Davies & Oberle model does have something to say about the nurse, the environment in which care is delivered and the development of the relationship between the nurse and the individual, so it does reflect three of the four elements which make up the metaparadigm of nursing. It does not explore the concept of health, as do other models of nursing care, however it promotes the development of a healthy care giving environment for both the patient and the nurse.

One of the strengths of the Davies & Oberle model of supportive care is that it offers the nurse a framework within which care can be planned and delivered using a relevant model of nursing.

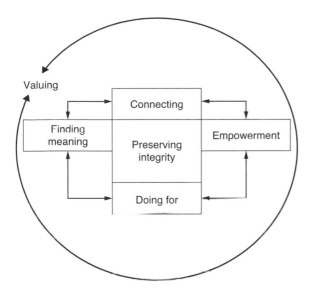

Figure 1   The Davies & Oberle model of supportive care (adapted from Davies & Oberle 1990).

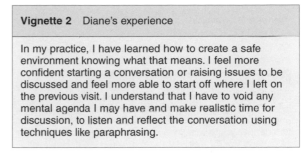

Vignette 2   Diane's experience

In my practice, I have learned how to create a safe environment knowing what that means. I feel more confident starting a conversation or raising issues to be discussed and feel more able to start off where I left on the previous visit. I understand that I have to void any mental agenda I may have and make realistic time for discussion, to listen and reflect the conversation using techniques like paraphrasing.

It could also help district nurses articulate their education and development needs as well as offering an understanding about the changes in health-care needs and the development of the work of the district nurse.

STRUCTURE OF THE MODEL

From the analysis of the data gathered in the interviews with the palliative care nurse, six dimensions emerged which form the basis of the model itself. Davies & Oberle describe the dimensions within the model as being linked but also having their own discrete qualities. The elements of the model are reflected in the SERVQUAL model of service quality mentioned in Chapter 13. Figure 1 shows a diagram of the dimensions of the model.

Preserving integrity

Two of the dimensions relate to the professional attitude and personal concerns of the nurse. In fact, the central dimension relates to the 'preservation of the integrity' of the nurse. This can be seen in the following vignette in which Dianne, a district nurse, explains how she keeps this sense of integrity.

This again illustrates the different focus of this model of nursing. Other dimensions illustrate what supportive care actually means when working with patients and their families in the home setting. There is a sense of order to the construction of the model which helps to demonstrate the nature of district nursing in terms of location, workload and range of skills. The central dimension is now described.

Valuing

This overarching concept applies to all the parts of the model. It is split into two dimensions: 'global' and 'particular'.

The 'global' values supported in the model are reflected in the UKCC (1992) *Code of professional conduct* which reminds us of the general need to respect the people that we care for regardless of cultural beliefs, race, age and gender. As will be seen in Chapter 1, the district nurse is often working in a multicultural environment.

The other part of the valuing concept is identified as being 'particular' and this refers to the respect for the actual people that form the caseload of the district nurse. This valuing takes place once a working relationship has developed between the patient and a nurse who understands and respects a patient's unique life circumstances. This implies that the district nurse will plan and ensure the delivery of care in a non-judgemental way. Chapter 13 highlights the importance of gaining the patient's perspective as part of the provision of a quality service. The study by Davy (1998) discussed in Chapter 13 alludes to the need to value patients as people and Chapter 10 explores the notion of valuing in greater detail.

> **Vignette 3** Valuing
>
> Frances, an experienced district nurse in a city practice, recalled an elderly gentleman who was living in poor circumstances. Access to the house was sporadic and the cleanliness of the home setting did not reflect her personal value of hygiene. However, the patient had lived in this house for many years and did not wish any outsiders coming in. Frances had been asked to visit this gentleman to assess a wound on his leg but more often than not, he refused to let anyone see it. However, after a few visits, the gentleman let her see his wound on the condition that she did not touch it and she left bandages.
>
> As can be seen from this, the concept of 'valuing' is closely linked to the ethical principle of respect and our own value system for nursing. It also serves to illustrate the 'connecting' dimension which is described next and reflects the challenges of access that district nurses may have to face and the importance, in this example, of continuity of care.

This vignette clearly illustrates the challenges faced by the district nurse in the 'valuing' dimension. Depending on where you work, as a district nurse you could find yourself visiting a person living in a cardboard box or a castle. Each person, regardless of his location, should have access to an equal level of care. Whether he chooses to accept that care is another matter. In Frances' situation, she was allowed to see the gentleman's wound now and again. However, he would not give access to any of the other nurses. Why did she continue to visit what might seem a futile situation? It was because she valued this gentleman's own particular circumstances and realised that he had health problems that she could help him alleviate if he learned to trust her.

Chapter 14 emphasises the notion of 'value' from another perspective – the value that is placed on the effectiveness of the district nurse's work.

Connecting

This is the first of the discrete dimensions within the model of supportive care. It has three components to it and each of these will be explored in relation to district nursing:

1. making the connection
2. sustaining the connection
3. breaking the connection.

Making the connection

One of the first challenges that the new district nurse faces is arriving at the door of a stranger following a referral, sometimes knowing little more than a name! Most district nurses will be able to recall an incident such as this. Essentially, though, you are planning care as a visitor to the household and this may be the one and only visit or the beginning of a long-term care relationship. In both situations, the first meeting is crucial in enabling you to gain access to a patient again and the skills of assessment are vital at this early stage.

Davies & Oberle discuss the importance of the nurse gaining the trust of the patient and this is most important when visiting patients in their own homes. However, as the next vignette shows, this process may take some time to achieve. Here is what Jane, a district nurse, said about building a relationship with a patient that reflects this notion of making a connection.

> **Vignette 4** Making a connection
>
> Mr McLeod had been diagnosed with prostatic cancer 2 years ago. Recently, he discovered that he had bone metastases after suffering a collapsed lumbar vertebra. With the introduction of an analgesic regime and palliative radiotherapy, I made the first connection with the family, who were naturally very anxious. For the first 2 weeks, I visited them frequently, giving information, providing equipment and discussing the plan of care with them. It took at least 8 weeks to get to a comfortable level to discuss how his wife was feeling and how the illness had affected them as a couple. I could not have asked that before as their trust of me was not complete and the family were still in denial about the seriousness of what was happening. They definitely were gauging my abilities and reaction to his illness. From that moment on we moved into a different level of conversation and the wife and daughter felt able to talk about how they were feeling.

This vignette shows the skill of the district nurse in gaining the trust of the patient and his family as well as the need to work with the family as well as the patient.

Sustaining the connection

Davies & Oberle subdivide this part of the connection process into three elements. The first element is called 'being available', both in the patient's understanding about the nature of the visits as well as the nurse being available by telephone. Then they highlight the need to spend some time with the patient, making it appear as if you had all the time in the world (when the reality may be quite different!). Over a long period of care, the investment of time with a patient at this stage may be beneficial to the trusting relationship that then develops.

The second element is called 'secret sharing' and is reflected in the original study of spouses of patients telling the nurse confidential information, knowing that it would not be divulged.

The third element of the connection is referred to as the 'giving of self' and in the study this is demonstrated by the nurse recalling how she talked with the patient, laughed and showed sadness on occasion. The ability to be open with patients is an aspect of assertiveness although it may have to be balanced with the 'preserving integrity' concept of the model.

Breaking the connection

In the study, the connection began to break when the patient died. However, in other instances the connection may be broken when the course of care has ended or the patient is admitted to a hospital or care facility. In these situations, the nurse has to learn to break the connection and this may be difficult, as shown in the following vignette. The end of the care offers an opportunity to review the care delivered and the Davies & Oberle model of supportive care could act as a framework for such reflection.

Vignette 5   Breaking a connection

I can reflect on the time that I took over a caseload from another district nurse who had found it hard to discharge patients or their families after the period of active care had ended. These visits were known as 'supervisory visits' and it was often uncomfortable for another nurse to take such visits over when you had not been involved in the 'making and sustaining' phases of the connection. In fact, I am sure it must have been difficult for the families too. In many of these instances, my first visit was the final visit – the connection had been broken, but by a stranger. That taught me a valuable lesson about the need to gently break a connection, as Davies and Oberle called it.

Empowering

Davies & Oberle identified five subcomponents of the empowering nature of the nurse's supportive role. This is possibly one of the hardest categories to measure and as, Davies & Oberle note, it can be intangible.

Facilitation

The actions that a district nurse takes may enable a family to become more empowered and these actions will be based upon knowledge and previous experience as well as the ability to set patient and family-centred goals of care. The link to the overarching valuing concept can be seen in this category as family members may be unwilling to become involved and the nurse may have to accept such limitations (if they are perceived as such). By making a connection with the family, it may be possible to identify other strategies for facilitating care.

Chapter 1 stresses that the knowledge base required by the district nurse should include a broad understanding of the community being served. The ability to influence local public policy through knowledge, helping patients to learn about a health-care issue and suppor-ting community action are a fundamental part of the Ottawa Charter discussed in Chapter 1. The knowledge of politics and social policy discussed in Chapter 3 is relevant here.

> **Vignette 6**   Gill's story
>
> Gill recalls being fully introduced to Orem's model of nursing when studying for her district nursing qualification. Her experience in district nursing enabled her to see how useful it was to have a model which encouraged self-care and which saw the patient and carers assume responsibility for care.
>
> She began to use the model in practice and recalls how useful it was with a patient with rheumatoid arthritis who had a cerebrovascular accident. This experience had left him feeling frustrated, withdrawn and depressed. Gill knew that she had to take account of this when planning his care and explained to him how the model could help his rehabilitation process. In partnership, they worked out the self-care deficits and prioritised short-, medium- and long-term goals, each with a review date. After a period of 8 weeks, he could shower by himself, dress and walk round his garden.
>
> Gill's reservation about the model were its use in a setting where another model was the norm. Orem in particular, she says, requires the commitment and dedication of all, as less experienced staff may jeopardise the care plan by intervening inappropriately from the best of intentions.

Encouraging

This subcomponent is identified in the model as promoting the patient's perspective on an issue. Davies & Oberle suggest that encouraging a patient to talk about an issue may be an empowering act in itself. It may also include teaching a patient or carer to undertake an aspect of care with support from the district nurse. The model of nursing care used by the nurse in this situation may be seen as an act of encouragement. In the following vignette, Gill discusses how she worked with a patient during his rehabilitation using Orem's model of self-care (Leddy & Pepper 1993).

Defusing

Patients and their carers may be unhappy with their own situation, with the district nurse as the 'agent of health care' or any number of other situations. The district nurse needs to have well-developed communication skills in order to help the patient deal with such feelings of frustration or anger and also to deal with her own. The importance of the development of effective communication skills will be referred to throughout this book. Nurses working on their own in potentially violent situations also need to use defusing skills.

Mending

The model recognises that as patients near the end of their lives, families may try to resolve any differences that there have been or, conversely, various 'factions' may emerge within the family. The difficulty for the district nurse in this situation is that they may find themselves in the middle of a complex and often long-standing issue. One set of family members will air their feelings about the limitations of the other set and so on.

Giving information

Having the key information is a crucial part of making any decision. The district nurse is in a position to help patients understand information that they have received from another source or to find information on the patient's behalf in an advocacy role. This will be facilitated if the nurse has made a good connection with the family and there is trust and confidence in the information that is being shared. Examples of the kinds of information include treatment schedules, how equipment works and the role of other agencies involved in the care of the patient. The onus here is on the district nurse to keep abreast of changing approaches to the care and treatment of various conditions.

However, the ethical principles of confidentiality and truth telling are important in this context. Chapter 15 will discuss the growth of computerised sources of information and the impact this may have on the patient and family.

Doing for

This component of the model is probably what people outside district nursing think the speciality is all about! It is also a limitation as it describes one element of nursing people in their homes, but not the whole picture. If the work is carried out and measured only in a quantitative way, then this category reflects how many tasks have been undertaken but leaves the wider aspects of district nursing unrecognised, a factor raised in Chapter 14 in the discussion about conjoint analysis. In addition, Chapter 14 raises the economic implications of the development of a new service. Chapter 11 will accentuate the impact of change on the 'doing for' role during the introduction of care management in the early 1980s. However, it also discusses the flexible nature of district nursing and the ability to move with the times. Furthermore, Chapter 12 offers strategies for dealing with the change process.

This category of the model has two subdivisions.

Taking charge

This first element is when the nurse intervenes to help a patient by direct care giving, choosing a specific product or planning a programme of nursing care with the patient. It may also involve delegating work to other staff and contacting other agencies to obtain additional help. A further understanding of the impact of health economics will demonstrate the importance of accurate resource allocation within this component.

An issue that will be raised throughout the book is the ever-changing nature of district nursing practice. A study undertaken by McDonald et al (1997) illustrates the changing pressures caused by higher day surgery lists, early hospital discharge policies and an increase in the number of patients at home with complex health-care needs. The demands that these pressures place on the district nurse are heavy in terms of the need for ongoing professional development. The need to provide evidence-based care is also relevant to this component and is an issue elaborated on in Chapter 6.

Team playing

This element of the 'doing for' category focuses on the relationship the nurse has with colleagues as well as with other health and social care professionals in the social and voluntary care sectors. This is set in historical perspective in Chapter 5. This role of the district nurse was explored in a study undertaken by Griffiths & Luker (1994). In this study, 16 G and H grade nurses working for two health authorities in the north west of England were interviewed and observed during 130 patient contact visits. The researchers noted some of the unspoken rules within district nursing culture within their observations. The issue of not making decisions or formulating care plans for someone else's patients was a major feature of the results. It appeared from the study that this had more to do with avoiding making commitments on behalf of other nurses and also keeping relationships 'smooth' rather than addressing the care needs of the patient in question. This also applied to a nurse changing another nurse's care, even if it was felt that the care in question was not ideal. The study recommended that a recognised system of clinical supervision would help to address these issues and remove some of the 'invisibility' of the work of the district nurse. Clinical supervision is discussed in Chapter 9.

Chapter 4 explores the impact on the district nurse of teamworking across the different primary health-care disciplines. Indeed, it will be suggested that true collaboration is yet to be achieved. Furthermore, Chapter 7 discusses the potential for conflict when the district nurse feels that she is answerable to more than one agency who may hold different values. The chapter notes the need for respect of other members in a team and the sharing of a common goal. A specific example of a nurse in a prescribing 'team' is found in Chapter 8.

Finding meaning

The final category in the model covers how the nurse may help the patient find some sense of understanding about what is happening to him within the patient's frame of reference. Focusing on living and the acknowledgement of death are how this is illustrated by Davies & Oberle. Quality care is defined later in the book as 'what is good for patients developed in partnership with professional care'. This could be assisting a

> **Vignette 7** Finding meaning
>
> After nursing a gentleman with advanced heart disease to his death, surrounded by a supportive family, I made an arrangement to visit his widow several times to discuss issues surrounding his illness and death at the request of the family. The family felt she was very vulnerable on her own and wondered if she would cope, but she had a very different agenda for discussion. Her uncomplicated grief enabled her to revel in the description of the positive side of their lives and not just the recent illness. We talked in depth about loneliness, sadness, loss of companionship and status. She slowly began to see herself as a person again, not just as a carer, and moved forward in a calm and positive way. My visits became less frequent and we both acknowledged that a healing had taken place. The bereavement side to our visits is over now and we both know that. I still go and take this lady's bloods every 4 months and we have chats about everything from politics to managing children!

patient and his family to find meaning in an illness. In the following vignette, Susan discusses the help she gave to a widow to help her find meaning about the death of her husband.

It can be seen from this category that the full role of supportive care within district nursing may be very challenging and for this reason, the preservation of personal integrity touches each of the other four caring dimensions in the model. Working in isolation can be stressful, both for the new district nurse and the more experienced person. The need for support from other colleagues may vary at different times but the need to reflect on experiences, learn from them and continue to develop is constant. Davies & Oberle identify these components as the need to look inward, to value self and acknowledge our individual reactions to the situations we encounter and the people that we meet.

In Chapter 14 the reader is reminded of the importance of self-assurance and the positive impact of district nursing on patient care. Chapter 4 highlights the need for clarity of purpose in one's own role. Chapter 12 confirms the need to preserve integrity during a process of change and the need for support. The recent development of clinical supervision, discussed in Chapter 9, may enhance this.

THE NURSING PROCESS

The Davies & Oberle model of supportive care does not fit the four recognised stages of the nursing process, but as it is a model that describes how nurses approach their work, rather than the specific details of how they carry out nursing with a particular person, this is not a criticism of the model itself. The model certainly offers an opportunity for the development of criteria that would enable it to be used in the same way as the other models of nursing care. It also offers district nursing a structure for evaluation and reflection. For example, it could be used to reflect upon the causes of stress in district nursing in relation to the 'preservation of integrity' category. It was used in this way by Davies & Oberle as a framework to understand burnout in a group of nurses working in an acute setting. This later study suggested that nurses may become disillusioned with practice when the system in which they work 'forces nurses to betray their personal values in the context of their professional practice' (Oberle & Davies 1991). The authors state that nurses may concentrate fully on the 'doing for' dimension because that is what is deemed to be quantifiable and time pressures allow for nothing more. When this situation persists, the authors suggest that this causes a division between nurses' values and the reality of practice. This leads to the 'doing for' dimension becoming separated from the remaining dimensions of the model.

The model could also be used to clarify the roles and values that are held by the nursing team. Have you ever thought about the values and beliefs that you hold about your work and in turn heard what other members of the primary care team consider to be important? When such exercises are run in a classroom, students are often amazed at the range of values and beliefs that their peers reveal. This is something to be welcomed as each person can add more knowledge and thoughts to explain what nursing is. It also confirms why there are a variety of different conceptual models of nursing. At a national level, the UKCC (1992) *Code of professional conduct* identifies the values and beliefs that are held by the profession.

Walsh (1998) provides a detailed discussion of the way a group of nurses in a ward setting developed their own approach to care planning and, with adaptation, this could be used in a primary care-based setting. The necessary requirements are to have a goal, short meetings over a period of time and the support of colleagues.

A problem-based learning approach has recently been used to facilitate the development of a philosophy of nursing for a team of eight nurses in a community hospital. This process has taken approximately 6 months with fortnightly meetings each lasting 2 hours. It has provided an opportunity for the team to sit together and share their views. Not all the members have been able to attend all the meetings, but the information is shared with everybody so that all staff can feel involved.

Initially, the group answered the question 'What do we know about this already?' This enabled the group to brainstorm their beliefs and values about their nursing practice, the environment that they worked in and the priorities for nursing that they have.

The next phase was to identify 'What information do we need to develop our philosophy of nursing?'. The group gathered information from the health trust, from the UKCC and from the literature on nursing philosophy. The material was shared and discussed which helped the group to formulate their own philosophy of nursing. A similar process could be adopted in a district nursing setting. It has given the nurses in the study an opportunity to share their views and values as well as helping them to achieve their Post-Registration Education and Practice (PREP) (UKCC 1999) requirements based on a reflection of their own practice.

APPLICATION TO PRACTICE

Discussions held with district nursing students, many of whom have been working in the community setting for considerable periods, revealed

Box 2	Summary of the Davies & Oberle model of nursing
Valuing	Global and particular
Connecting	Making
	Sustaining
	Breaking
Empowering	Facilitation
	Encouraging
	Defusing
	Mending
	Giving information
Doing for	Taking charge
	Team playing
Finding meaning	
Preserving integrity	

that they have seen an immediate applicability to their practice of the Davies & Oberle model of supportive care. It recognises the stages in the relationships that are developed with patients. One issue is the ending of a relationship that has been built up with a family over a long time and the difficulty that the nurse and family can have in 'letting go'. The pressures faced by district nurses can be alleviated to a certain extent by having an understanding of what is happening and this model of supportive care enables this understanding to be clarified. It is used in this book to show the relevance of the sections on the context of care, professional context and management context. The summary of the components of the model are shown in Box 2.

CONCLUSION

This chapter has offered the reader an introduction to the Davies & Oberle model of supportive care as applied to the district nursing setting. It has also served as an introduction to the book which is split into three further sections: the context of care, the professional context and the management context. The chapters that make up these three sections have been linked in this chapter to the relevant dimensions of the Davies & Oberle model of supportive care.

REFERENCES

Coles L 1996 Clinical care at home In: Gastrell P, Edwards J (eds) Community health nursing: frameworks for practice. Baillière Tindall, London

Davies B, Oberle K 1990 Dimensions of the supportive role of the nurse in palliative care. Oncology Nursing Forum 17(1): 87–94

Davy M 1998 Patients' views of the care given by district nurses. Professional Nurse 13(8): 498–502

Griffiths J, Luker K 1994 Intraprofessional teamwork in district nursing: whose interest? Journal of Advanced Nursing 20: 1038–1045

Fawcett J 1995 Analysis and evaluation of conceptual models of nursing, 3rd edn. F A Davis, Philadelphia

Lawton S 1997 The nursing needs of individuals in the home setting with Alzheimer's disease. Report for Alzheimer Scotland. Action on Dementia, Edinburgh

Leddy S, Pepper J M 1993 Conceptual bases of professional nursing 3e. Lippincott, Philadelphia

McDonald A, Langford A, Boldero N 1997 The future of community nursing in the United Kingdom: district nursing, health visiting and school nursing. Journal of Advanced Nursing 26: 257–265

Oberle K, Davies B 1991 An exploration of nursing disillusionment. Canadian Journal of Nursing Research 25(1): 67–76

Peplau H 1988 Interpersonal relationships in nursing. Macmillan, Basingstoke

Thibodeau J 1983 Nursing models: analysis and evaluation. Wadsworth, Belmant, California

Walsh M 1998 Models and critical pathways in clinical nursing, 3rd edn. Baillière Tindall, Oxford

UKCC 1992 The code of professional conduct for nurses, midwives and health visitors. UKCC, London

UKCC 1999 The continuing development standard. UKCC, London

District nursing within the context of care

SECTION CONTENTS

Jane Cantrell

Lis Cook

Sue Howard

Fiona Redworth, Dianne Watkins

Helen Sweet, Rona Ferguson

1

Health trends and strategies: a macro to micro approach

Jane Cantrell

Key points

- The World Health Organisation
- Health in Europe
- The UK government
- Health authorities and health boards
- Health promotion in primary care
- District nursing and health promotion
- Community profiling

INTRODUCTION

An increasing emphasis has been placed on health and health promotion in the role of nurses over the past 20 years. This has been due to various national and international strategies that have given significance to this role (DoH 1992, NHS Executive 1993). For district nurses to understand their health promotion role, it is important that they have an understanding of how world, European, government and National health service strategies interface with primary care and impact on the day-to-day work of a district nurse.

Therefore this chapter will employ a framework that takes a macro-to-micro approach (Fig. 1.1). This approach will clearly demonstrate the links between global health strategies such as Health for All and the Ottawa Charter, European health initiatives, government health targets, the National Health Service and primary health care. District nurses are a key group of community nurses who have a responsibility within primary care to assess and facilitate the health needs of the populations that they serve. This chapter is designed to explore how the various strategies

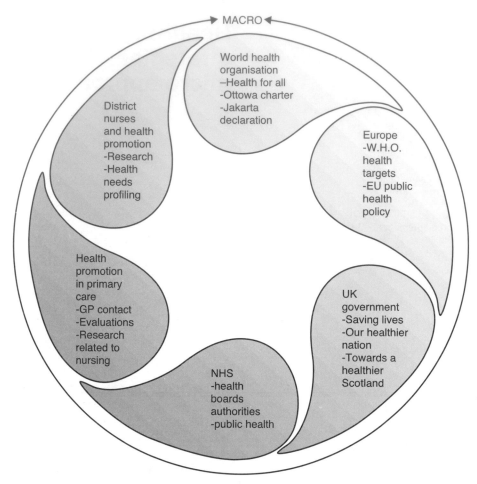

Figure 1.1 The macro-to-micro approach.

coexist and inform decisions that are made about priorities within public health and how these strategies impact on and facilitate the work of the district nurse.

THE WORLD HEALTH ORGANISATION

The World Health Organisation has impacted on 'world health' through various strategies and frameworks that have been generated and agreed through discussion in the various forums at international level.

One of the most influential of these strategies has been the Declaration of Alma-Ata which was agreed at an international conference on primary health care in 1978. This was the beginning of the Health for All movement, whereby the declaration expressed an urgent need for 'Action by all governments, all health and development workers and the world community to protect and promote the health of all people of the world …' (WHO 1979).

The declaration endorses the fundamental right of human beings to health and affirms the need for social and economic development to achieve this, alongside people's right to participate in the 'planning and implementation' of health care. The declaration goes on to pronounce that:

A main social target of governments, international organisations and the whole world community in the coming decades should be the attainment by all people of the world by the year 2000 of a level of health that will permit them to lead a socially and economically productive life. Primary health care is the key to attaining this target as part of development in the spirit of social justice. (WHO 1979)

This is a very grand statement and it could be suggested that it may be unattainable. On reflection, it must be remembered that this declaration was produced 22 years before 'the year 2000' and this must have seemed in the distant future. Today, although the principles of Health for All are still relevant, the year 2000 is here and the goal still seems daunting. It is interesting to note the importance of primary health care within the declaration and to consider the current policy context within the United Kingdom, where there is the explicit move to a primary care-led NHS. Another criticism of the declaration is the requirement to know how the governments and health-care workers of the world will achieve such a far-reaching target as well as work towards the other statements within the declaration.

There has been some criticism that Health for All is unachievable and that it has failed even in countries who potentially had the money to invest in such a strategy (Baum & Sanders 1995). These authors assert that the 'goals and targets approach to health promotion' that the European division of the WHO and many governments have adopted is reductionist and is trying to address extremely complex issues with a very 'logical, tidy and manageable approach'. They also suggest that many governments of the time had embraced the philosophies of the New Right, one of these being the issue of individualism which, it could be argued, is directly opposite to the philosophies espoused in Health for All and the Ottawa Charter.

From a more positive perspective, Health for All does give a framework and goals which can be aimed for, even if these at times appear to be unachievable.

Another important milestone in terms of health and health promotion which went some way to addressing the concerns about achieving Health for All was the Ottawa Charter, which was conceived at the First International Conference on Health Promotion in 1986 (WHO 1986) (Box 1.1). The charter considered a definition of health promotion, the prerequisites for health and the three key principles of health promotion.

The Ottawa Charter has captured the imagination of organisations interested in health promotion and has been used as a framework for planning by many conventional establishments such as the Royal College of Physicians (Catford 1996). Levin & Ziglio (1996) assert that its popularity is due to the inclusion of both traditional considerations such as personal health skills alongside the more recent impetus given to community development and participation.

Primarily this charter for action relates to national and local government but could also be applied to district nursing practice (Box 1.2).

Box 1.1 Ottawa Charter for Health Promotion framework for action (WHO 1986)

- Build healthy public policy
- Create supportive environments
- Strengthen community action
- Develop personal skills
- Reorient health services

Box 1.2 Ottawa Charter related to district nursing practice

- Influencing healthy public policy related to their communities and considering the health consequences of their actions.
- Helping to create supportive environments by using their potential knowledge of the community in which they work and the information gathered within the community health profile.
- Facilitating community action through the empowerment of local groups.

- Assisting patients/clients to learn throughout life, thereby giving them the knowledge to make informed choices.
- Fostering an awareness within primary care and communities to move increasingly towards a health-promoting philosophy.

The Ottawa Charter has been extremely influential in terms of providing a framework for health promotion activity and has been used to give structure to further WHO health promotion strategies such as healthy cities, the health-promoting hospital and healthy workplaces.

There has been some criticism of the Ottawa Charter in that it does not give priority to any one area of activity and that some of the activities may come into conflict with each other; for example, by strengthening community action, one community may have a larger voice and therefore receive more resources than another. This may cause tension in an area and militate against healthy public policy.

Subsequent WHO conferences have continued to endorse the principles of Health for All and the Ottawa Charter, the latest declaration being from the Fourth International Conference on Health Promotion held in Jakarta in 1997 (WHO 1997). This discusses the priorities for health promotion into the 21st century.

1. *Promote social responsibility for health.* This includes the need for the public and private sectors to pursue health policies and practices, such as the restriction of the production and supply of harmful substances and the protection of the environment through the use of sustainable resources.
2. *Increase investments for health development.* This asks for governments to increase investment in the prerequisites for health, such as housing and education, as well as for health services. Needs of particular groups, e.g. women, children, older people, should be taken into consideration.
3. *Consolidate and expand partnerships for health.* Skills and resources can be shared between different organisations and levels of government to enhance health and social development within a country or community.
4. *Increase community capacity and empower the individual.* Empowering communities and individuals requires resources, education and training.
5. *Secure an infrastructure for health promotion.* Funding and resources for health promotion

are vital and new innovative ways of influencing governments and other organisations to fund health promotion need to be considered.

There is some evidence of consideration of these priorities by the current British government within both the White Papers related to the National Health Service (DoH 1997, Scottish Office 1997) and the government strategies related to public health (DoH 1999, Scottish Office 1999, Welsh Office 1998). An example is the recognition of the importance of collaboration and sharing of resources between different organisations and levels of government within the health White Papers and the realisation of the importance of the prerequisites of health such as housing and education which is evident within the government strategies on health.

The World Health Report 1998 (WHO 1998a) considers the impact of Health for All and indicates that an evaluation carried out in 1997 showed notable progress worldwide in addressing issues related to 'health status and access to health care'.

HEALTH IN EUROPE

Although the World Health Organisation is an international body, it is divided into regions. The European region of the WHO covers many member states from the Pacific shores of Russia, to the Mediterranean and Greenland in the North and has a population of 850 million people (WHO 1993). After Health for All was started in 1977, the European region decided in 1984 to implement a strategy comprising 38 targets for health based around four interrelated themes (Box 1.3).

Box 1.3 Health for All – interrelated themes (WHO 1993)

- Ensuring equity in health by reducing gaps in health status between countries and between groups within countries.
- Adding life to years by helping people achieve, and use, their full physical, mental and social potential.
- Adding health to life by reducing disease and disability.
- Adding years to life by increasing life expectancy.

Europe is made up of many states, some of which have great industrial wealth, but nevertheless the region still has great potential to improve health, particularly in terms of inequalities within the European region but also within the individual countries themselves.

Since 1984, there has been progress with the targets in terms of reduced infant and maternal mortality, as well as reduced mortality from ischaemic heart disease and increased life expectancy across the European region. Also advances have been made in terms of environmental pollution and quality of drinking water and the availability of primary health care provi-

sion in most countries has increased.

Areas that still need to be addressed include mortality from cancer, inequalities in health status between countries and within countries, high rates of suicide, drug and alcohol abuse and tobacco use (WHO 1993).

Since 1984, the targets have been updated, the latest version being adopted by the WHO Regional Committee for Europe at its 48th session in September 1998 (WHO 1998a) (Box 1.4). These new targets can be broken down into various categories. The new targets are part of a Health for All policy framework for the WHO European Union called Health 21

Box 1.4 WHO targets for health – categories (reproduced from World Health Organisation 1998a, with permission)

Goals	Equity in health	Target 1–2
	Quality of life	Target 3–5
	Better health status	Target 6–10
Strategies	Lifestyles conducive to health	Target 11–13
	Health environment	Target 14
	Appropriate care	Target 15–17
Support	Health for All development strategies	Target 18–21

Target 1   Solidarity for health in the European region. By the year 2020, the present gap in health status between member states of the European region should be reduced by at least one-third.

Target 2   Equity in health. By the year 2020, the health gap between socioeconomic groups within countries should be reduced by at least one-fourth in all member states, by substantially improving the level of health of disadvantaged groups.

Target 3   Healthy start in life. By the year 2020, all newborn babies, infants and preschool children in the region should have better health, ensuring a healthy start in life.

Target 4   Health of young people. By the year 2020, young people in the region should be healthier and better able to fulfil their roles in society.

Target 5   Healthy ageing. By the year 2020, people over 65 years should have the opportunity of enjoying their full health potential and playing an active social role.

Target 6   Improving mental health. By the year 2020, people's psychosocial well-being should be improved and better comprehensive services should be available to and accessible by people with mental health problems.

Target 7   Reducing communicable diseases. By the year 2020, the adverse health effects of communicable diseases should be substantially diminished

through systematically applied programmes to eradicate, eliminate or control infectious diseases of public health importance.

Target 8   Reducing non-communicable diseases. By the year 2020, morbidity, disability and premature mortality due to major chronic diseases should be reduced to the lowest feasible levels throughout the region.

Target 9   Reducing injury from violence and accidents. By the year 2020, there should be significant and sustainable decrease in injuries, disability and death arising from accidents and violence in the region.

Target 10   A healthy and safe physical environment. By the year 2015, people in the region should live in a safer physical environment, with exposure to contaminants hazardous to health at levels not exceeding internationally agreed standards.

Target 11   Healthier living. By the year 2015, people across society should have adopted healthier patterns of living.

Target 12   Reducing harm from alcohol, drugs and tobacco. By the year 2015, the adverse health effects from the consumption of addictive substances such as tobacco, alcohol and psychoactive drugs should have been significantly reduced in all member states.

Target 13   Settings for health. By the year 2015, people in the region should have greater opportunities to live in

---

Box 1.4 Cont'd

healthy physical and social environments at home, school and in the local community.

Target 14   Multisectoral responsibility for health. By the year 2020, all sectors should have recognised and accepted their responsibility for health.

Target 15   An integrated health sector. By the year 2010, people in the region should have better access to family- and community-orientated primary health care, supported by a flexible and responsive hospital system.

Target 16   Managing for quality of care. By the year 2010, member states should ensure that the management of the health sector, from population-based health programmes to individual patient care at the clinical level, is orientated towards health outcomes.

Target 17   Funding health services and allocating resources. By the year 2010, member states should have sustainable financing and resource allocation mechanisms for health-care systems based on the principle of equal access, cost-effectiveness, solidarity and optimum quality.

Target 18   Developing human resources for health. By the year 2010, all member states should have ensured that health professionals in other sectors have acquired appropriate knowledge, attitudes and skills to promote and protect health.

Target 19   Research and knowledge for health. By the year 2005, all member states should have health research, information and communication systems that better support the acquisition, effective utilisation and dissemination of knowledge to support Health for All.

Target 20   Mobilising partners for health. By the year 2005, implementation of policies for Health for All should engage individuals, groups and organisations throughout the public and private sectors and civil society, in alliances and partnerships for health.

Target 21   Policies and strategies for Health for All. By the year 2010, all member states should have and be implementing policies for Health for All at country, regional and local levels, supported by appropriate institutional infrastructures, managerial processes and innovative leadership.

Box 1.5   Health 21: four main strategies for action (WHO 1998b)

- Multisectoral strategies to tackle the determinants of health, taking into account physical, economic, social, cultural and gender perspectives and ensuring the use of health impact assessment.
- Health outcome-driven programmes and investments for health development and clinical care.
- Integrated family/community-orientated primary health care, supported by a flexible and responsive hospital system.
- A participatory health development process that involves relevant partners for health at home, school and work and at local community and country levels and that promotes joint decision making, implementation and accountability.

(Box 1.5), the main aims being 'to promote and protect people's health throughout their lives and to reduce the incidence of the main diseases and injuries, and alleviate suffering they cause' (WHO 1998b).

Various strategies have been adopted to propel the framework forward (Box 1.5). The WHO Regional Office for Europe urges member states to 'incorporate' this policy framework for the 21st century in their own individual health

policy. This appears to have happened with the Labour government's White Papers on health (see below), particularly with regard to issues surrounding inequalities in health, improving mental health, reducing non-communicable diseases such as cancer and cardiovascular disease and in terms of collaboration and partnerships for health.

Alongside the above WHO European strategy for health are the initiatives put forward by the European Community. Indeed, the community works in partnership with many international organisations including the WHO. Although many of the policies of the community relate to economic and financial systems, some policies that relate to health are now emerging. A good example of this is the public health policy that was developed in 1993 and is being revised at the present time due to changes and challenges within the field of public health.

The aims of the 1993 public health policy, which were included in the Maastrict Treaty, are as shown in Box 1.6 and 'mirror' the aims of the WHO European health strategy.

To facilitate the policy, the European Commission proposed the development of eight

---

Box 1.6 Aims of the public health policy – European Community (European Commission 1998)

- The community shall contribute towards ensuring a high level of human health protection by encouraging cooperation between member states and, if necessary, lending support to their action.
- Community action on health protection should be focused on the prevention of disease.
- Community activities in the field of public health should concentrate particularly on the major health 'scourges', including drug dependence.
- In these areas, the community is to cooperate with other organisations active in the field.

Box 1.7 Five key areas for England (Department of Health 1992)

- Coronary heart disease and stroke
- Cancers
- Mental illness
- HIV/AIDS and sexual health
- Accidents

Box 1.8 Five key areas for Scotland (Scottish Office 1992)

- Coronary heart disease
- Cancers
- HIV/AIDS
- Accidents
- Dental and oral health

---

public health programmes. These included: action on AIDs and other communicable diseases; cancer; drug dependence; health promotion; health monitoring; pollution-related diseases; injury prevention and rare diseases (European Commission 1998). There appears to be no rationale for the choice of these particular projects.

THE UK GOVERNMENT

The main way that governments who are signatories to the Alma-Ata Declaration put Health for All into operation is through the use of targets for health. After consultation documents were produced in the late 1980s and early 1990s the Conservative government in the United Kingdom finally produced health targets for England, Scotland, Wales and Northern Ireland.

The English White Paper, entitled *The health of the nation*, was published in 1992 after due consultation throughout 1991 with various groups, individuals and organisations who expressed interest after the publication of a Green Paper with the same name.

The health of the nation document was seen by the Conservative government as a unique initiative although, as the UK government was a signatory to the Alma-Ata Declaration, it had taken 14 years to produce a response to the Health for All strategy. The White Paper acknowledged the reliance on the Health for All concepts to inform the strategy for England. These concepts were about 'adding years to life' and 'adding life to years' as well as discussing the contribution of 'public policies' that relate to health, 'healthy sur-

roundings', 'healthy lifestyles' and 'high-quality health services'.

Five key areas (Box 1.7) were chosen because they were seen as areas where, although they may be major causes of illness and premature death, improvements could be made, measurable targets and objectives could be set and good/efficient interventions were available. Within each of the five key areas, specific targets were set with a time limit, e.g. 'to reduce death rates for both CHD and stroke in people under 65 by at least 40% by the year 2000' (DoH 1992).

McCallum (1997) argues that the areas chosen for action were those where targets could be set, monitored and measured and therefore were limited, thereby making *The health of the nation* a top-down agenda, with the government setting the priorities. A White Paper, *'Scotland's health – a challenge to us all'*, was published in Scotland in 1992 (Scottish Office 1992). This also concentrated on five areas of priority (Box 1.8). Within each of these priority areas there were specific targets. The document went on to discuss areas of personal behaviour and lifestyle where improvements in health could be made, along with environmental issues and initiatives related to schools and the workplace. A very brief discussion of how different organisations can work together to achieve the strategy and related research and monitoring conclude this White Paper.

Vignette 1.1 Health promotion in primary care

I am a district nurse and member of a primary health-care team which does not include a practice nurse. Health promotion activities offered by the practice are jointly carried out by the district nurses and health visitors.

Historically health promotion and health education performed by the district nurse was on a one-to-one basis in the patient's home. Working in this practice, however, allows the practitioners a wealth of scope in developing their own health promotion roles. My special interest is in a cardiovascular screening clinic offered to every patient between the ages of 16 and 60 years. The protocol for the clinic was jointly drawn up by myself and the health visitor involved and approved by the GPs.

This clinic is now well established, offering appointments in the evening principally to enable clients in full-time employment to attend. The documentation used has been evaluated and amended to suit the needs of the staff and clients involved. The clients are requested to complete a lifestyle questionnaire disclosing their smoking, drinking, eating and exercise habits. Also requested is a family history of cardiovascular disease. From the information collected and the results of the tests (blood pressure, urine analysis, weight, etc.) carried out by the nurse, an overall picture emerges which becomes the basis for discussion.

If the client should request assistance to give up smoking, reduce weight or alcohol consumption, there are support groups within the health centre which meet regularly. Should the test results give cause for concern, the client is advised to return within normal surgery time to have them repeated before the GP becomes involved.

As a district nurse, I recognise the importance of good health to the individual and the intangible benefits to the community. Playing a major role empowers me to give clients comprehensive information enabling informed choice concerning their own health.

These targets became key areas where primary care initiated health promotion. A good example of this is seen in vignette 1.1.

A similar strategy for health was developed in Wales (Welsh Health Planning Forum 1989) where they identified 10 areas for health gain, which included broad areas related to not only physical health but also social, emotional and psychological health (Box 1.9).

The Northern Ireland Strategy (Northern Ireland DHSS 1992) includes four broad themes and eight key areas (Box 1.10).

New strategies for public health

In February 1998, two new Green Papers were launched for consultation, on public health strategies for England and Scotland (DoH 1998, Scottish Office 1998). Both Green Papers were very similar in content and set out to address some of the issues that were neglected in the previous White Papers published in 1992. Wales also published a Green Paper entitled *Better health, better Wales* (Welsh Office 1998). The Green Papers were followed up in 1999 by new White Papers for England and Scotland. The White Paper *Towards a healthier Scotland* (Scottish Office 1999) gives a framework for public health in

Box 1.9 Ten key areas for Wales (Welsh planning forum 1989)

- Maternal and early childhood health
- Mental handicap
- Injuries
- Emotional health and relationships
- Mental distress and illness
- Respiratory illness
- Cardiovascular disease
- Cancers
- Physical disability and discomfort
- Healthy environments

Box 1.10 Four main themes and eight key areas for Northern Ireland (Northern Ireland Department of Health & Social Service 1992)

Four main themes:
- a greater emphasis on health promotion and disease prevention
- the continued improvement of acute hospital services
- a shift from institutional care to care in the community
- targeting health and social need

Eight key areas:
- maternal and child health
- child care
- accidents and trauma
- physical and sensory disability
- mental health
- circulatory diseases
- cancers
- respiratory diseases

Box 1.11 Health headline targets for the period 1995–2010 (Scotland) (Scottish Office 1999)

Coronary heart disease
• Reduce premature mortality by 50%

Cancer
• Reduce premature mortality by 20%

Smoking
• Reduce smoking among 12–15 year olds from 14% to 11%
• Reduce the proportion of women smoking during pregnancy from 29% to 20%

Alcohol misuse
• Reduce incidence of men and women exceeding weekly limits from 33% to 29% and 13% to 11% respectively

Teenage pregnancy
• Reduce rate among 13–15 year olds by 20%

Dental health
• 60% of 5-year-old children with no experience of dental disease

---

Box 1.12 *Saving lives: our healthier nation* – targets (Department of Health 1999)

By the year 2010:
• cancer: to reduce the death rate in people under 75 by at least a fifth
• coronary heart disease and stroke: to reduce the death rate in people under 75 by at least two-fifths
• accidents: to reduce the death rate by at least a fifth and serious injury by at least a tenth
• mental illness: to reduce the death rate from suicide and undetermined injury by at least a fifth.

Box 1.13 Public health responsibilities for primary care trusts and primary care groups (Department of Health 1999)

• To improve the health of, and address health inequality in, the local community.
• To develop primary and community health services by improving the quality of those services and dealing with poor performance in primary care service providers.
• To commission services for their patients from NHS hospital trusts.

Scotland by considering action for better health on three levels:
1. *life circumstances* – to target and improve unemployment, poverty, poor housing, limited educational achievement and all other forms of social exclusion
2. *lifestyles* – to reduce smoking, drug and alcohol misuse, to encourage a healthier diet and improve physical activity
3. *health topics* – to target certain health topics: child health, dental and oral health, sexual health, including teenage pregnancies and sexually transmitted diseases, coronary heart disease (and stroke), cancer, mental health, accidents and safety.

The health headline targets for Scotland 1995–2010 are highlighted in Box 1.11.

The English White Paper *Saving lives: our healthier nation* (DoH 1999) has two aims: 'to improve the health of everyone and the health of the worst off in particular'. Specific targets in priority areas have also been set (Box 1.12).

The emphasis within the public health strategy is to tackle inequalities, although no specific targets have been set, and for 'people, communities and government to work together in partnership to improve health'. Various ways to tackle health problems have been initiated and include health skills programmes, NHS Direct, health action zones and healthy living centres and promoting research into public health through a new health development agency.

The new strategy also highlights the need for primary care trusts and groups 'to play a leading role in improving health and cutting inequality, working closely with their local communities'. Their key responsibilities are set out in Box 1.13. District nurses will play a key role in implementing particularly the first two responsibilities.

A strength of the new public health strategies is the acknowledgement that social and economic issues affect health and that prevention is an investment rather than a cost. Also, each of these papers relates back to the NHS White Papers published at the end of 1997. This is an improvement on previous public health strategies that appear to have been in direct competition with NHS health-care reforms (McCallum 1997).

The Welsh Green Paper *Better health, better Wales* (Welsh Office 1998) supports the moves away from the lifestyle approach to health and uses the following areas as the main focus for tackling the underlying causes of ill health:

• healthy workplaces
• community safety
• personal and family support
• social exclusion.

Critique of health targets

The World Health Organisation, along with many governments within Europe, has a health strategy based upon targets. Many of these targets are illness focused and quantitative in nature, thereby making them easy to evaluate but giving any strategy a reductionist, medicalised conception of health.

Baum & Sanders (1995) contend that the philosophies of Health for All do not translate easily into strategies based around targets. This is because goals and targets are seen as reductionist and measurable but, as is well documented (Seedhouse 1986), health is a difficult concept to define and means different things to different people, therefore setting health targets as a strategy to improve a nation's health is absurd. It is an improvement to see that some recognition has been given to the social, political and economic contexts of health and illness in the new White Papers.

In terms of the new public health strategies, the emphasis on inequalities has been welcomed. However, the targets are still seen as very disease focused and no specific targets have been set in relation to reducing the inequalities (Reid 1999, Whitehead 1999).

HEALTH AUTHORITIES AND HEALTH BOARDS

In 1988 the Acheson Report (HMSO 1988) was published in England and suggested that an increased emphasis should be placed upon public health. This would include a public health function for health authorities, including appointment of directors of public health to monitor the population that the health authority served and to produce an annual report on the health of this population. These recommendations were also adopted by the rest of the United Kingdom.

These reports have now been produced for a decade and can be a source of useful local data for district nurses to utilise. Unfortunately, it has been noted by Robinson & Eklan (1996) that community nurses generally do not make use of these data and that directors of public health do not make use of local data collected within primary care teams to assist health authority/board planning. This seems to lead to a considerable duplication of effort on both sides.

The White Papers related to the NHS reforms published in 1997 reiterate the role that health authorities and health boards have in terms of their public health function. *The new NHS: modern, dependable* (DoH 1997) and *Designed to care* (Scottish Office 1997) list health needs assessment and health improvement amongst the key functions, with 'health improvement programmes' being the way in which health authorities and boards can fulfil these functions, the director of public health's annual report being the starting point.

The new NHS goes on to state that the 'family doctor or community nurse is often the first port of call for patients when they need health advice'. Therefore in England, primary care groups have been established 'in each area to work together to improve the health of local people'. In Scotland similar groups called local health-care cooperatives have been developed which will be required to 'support the development of population-wide approaches to health improvement and disease prevention which required lifestyle and behavioural change'. This later statement relates to the traditional approach to health promotion whereas the English version talks about 'community development and improving health in its widest sense'. It is commendable that both White Papers continue to consider the impact that primary care teams can have on their local population and to encourage this trend.

HEALTH PROMOTION IN PRIMARY CARE

Primary care is increasingly being seen as a setting for health promotion. This idea of the reorientation of health services is one of the elements of the Ottawa Charter that the British government appears to have endorsed (DoH 1997, Scottish Office 1997). The increased emphasis on health promotion in primary care has been implemented primarily via the GP Contract which was introduced in 1990, when it was made a contractual requirement for GPs to run health promotion clinics within general practice.

The government of the time felt that the general practice setting was where health promotion should take place (DHSS 1986), the aim of the White Paper *Promoting better health* being to 'shift the emphasis in primary care from the treatment of illness to the promotion of health and prevention of disease'. This decision was made despite a lack of research evidence to support this premise. It is true to say that 'general practice offers numerous and at times effective opportunities for health promotion' (Kemm & Close 1995) and research evidence states that over 70% of registered patients consult their general practitioner at least once a year (Office of Health Economics 1994).

Naidoo & Wills (1994) suggest several other reasons why primary care is the key setting for health promotion (Box 1.14).

There has been much criticism of health promotion within primary care since the introduction of the GP Contract. Doyle & Thomas (1996)

Box 1.14 Reasons why primary care is a key setting for health promotion (Naidoo & Wills 1994)

- Primary care teams provide better access for people in the community.
- Users and providers tend to be on 'equal terms', therefore health messages are communicated more effectively.
- Support of patients with chronic conditions may prevent the need for hospitalisation.
- Prevention and primary care are cheaper options than hospitalisation.

---

suggest that this may be because of the way that health promotion was originally introduced into practice by the contract, where initially health promotion clinics were unfocused and non-targeted. In 1993, a 'banding' system was introduced in which health checks concentrated on risk factors for cardiovascular disease, this being followed by the present system in 1996 where GPs submit annual proposals on health promotion to health promotion committees for ratification. It must be argued that the constant changes over the last eight years have led to primary care staff being dissatisfied and health promotion becoming 'discredited'.

Another issue has been the evaluation of the effectiveness of health promotion within primary care. Two large national studies, the British Family Heart Study (Family Heart Study Group 1994) and the OXCHECK Study (ICRF 1994), have evaluated approaches to health promotion within primary care. Both studies were quantitative in nature and used 'hard' indicators to measure outcome and a pre/post-test study design. Results indicated that the impact of the health promotion interventions on the population being studied was negligible. These studies, although useful, have both been criticised for their narrow focus in terms of exploring individual risk factors for heart disease and not considering in depth the broader social factors such as social class, income and poverty (Cowley 1995). Cowley goes on to suggest that if health promotion is to succeed within primary care, a broader view of issues affecting the health of the population should be adopted rather than a framework based on a medical model of health. Similar opinions are expressed by Daykin & Naidoo (1997) who consider that organisational constraints within primary care itself 'may limit the scope and effectiveness of health promotion'.

Doyle & Thomas (1996) also suggest that collaboration between departments of public health in health authorities, health boards and primary care teams needs to be addressed. This would mean that locally based health promotion projects would articulate with work being done in

---

Vignette 1.2   Locally based health promotion projects

Nurses have been identified as the key providers in health promotion and screening activities in the community setting. Health promotion is an integral part of the district nurses' role in promoting individual assessment and care for sick patients and their relatives in the home, but this role has been extended to provide a new well woman clinic session for females within the practice population of 11 500 patients.

It has been identified that government targets for a reduction in the percentage of cervical cancer deaths by cervical screening would not be reached owing to the number of women failing to attend the clinic. This was due, in part, to a change of working patterns by GPs to exclude evening sessions.

A district nurse and health visitor undertook a recognised course in breast and cervical screening, supervised by two interested GPs. This enabled them to initiate a new clinic session for cervical smears and

teaching breast self-examination. The nurses carried out a survey of female patients which identified a preference for a female smear taker at an evening clinic.

A local protocol, including procedure for audit, was written by the nurses and agreed by the GPs. Information on women's health issues was researched and a stock of relevant informative literature was provided for the clinic.

Audit of the clinic sessions, which were initiated 1 year ago, demonstrates a significant increase in women attending, including previous defaulters, satisfaction and an increase in the number of referrals to colposcopy.

The professional skills and knowledge gained by the district nurse have enhanced personal development and status, with further training in women's issues projected.

Menopause workshop sessions have been initiated for interested clients.

---

primary care (Vignette 1.2). They go on to suggest that there should be a strategic approach to health promotion within primary care, the advantage of which would be prioritising specific health promotion needs for the population that the practice serves but that the strategy should also link with national strategies. An important tool of this process would be the community profile, discussed later. Cook (1995) suggests some key points that need to be considered when examining health promotion within the primary care setting (Box 1.15).

It is hoped that the philosophies of the White Papers will assist with identifying health promotion needs within primary care through the community health profiles that will be undertaken by the primary care groups and local cooperatives. The development of self-managed integrated nursing teams should also allow for a more focused approach and permit district nurses an increased involvement with group health promotion (Vignette 1.3).

Health promotion and nursing within primary care

Literature from the late 1980s onwards emphasises the importance of the role of the nurse in health promotion. A staunch advocate in this area

Box 1.15   Key points for consideration when examining health promotion in a primary care setting (Cook 1995)

- People who are at risk and are willing and ready to change should be targeted.
- Trying to change too many risk factors at once is counterproductive.
- An essential element of health promotion within primary care is teamwork.

Vignette 1.3   Group health promotion

As a district nurse, I am currently involved in collecting data for a community health profile for a local health-care cooperative (these groups are replacing individual fundholding practices in Scotland). In the past I have been involved in doing neighbourhood studies and practice profiles and although myself and colleagues have used the information to inform our own community practice, it is refreshing to know that information that I am collecting at present for the LHCC will also be 'fed back' through the primary care trust to the health board to inform their decisions.

---

was Malher (cited by Rundle 1992) who, in his role as the Director General of The WHO, stated: 'Nurses will become resources to people rather than resources to physicians: they will become more active in educating people on health matters'. In recent years there have been government documents supporting the health promotion role of the nurse. The Department of Health (1989) recommended in *Strategy for nursing* that 'Health education and health promotion should be a recognised part of health care: all practitioners should develop skills in and use every opportunity for health promotion'. Although not so explicit, the Scottish *Strategy for nursing, midwifery and health visiting* (Scottish Home and Health Department 1990) also talks about the role encompassing 'the promotion of health and the prevention of illness, disease and disability'.

The Department of Health (1992), in *The health of the nation*, suggested that all nurses should develop their roles as health educators and, in terms of nurses working in the community and their influence on health, stated that 'Together with GPs, they are in the front-line of NHS care and have direct influence over the general health of the population'. Although implicit within *Scotland's health – a challenge to us all* (Scottish Office 1992), the message for nurses is not so obvious.

The NHS Executive (1993) also suggests that primary health care nurses are developing skills in public health and that these skills will allow them to 'identify groups most in need of health support, treatment and guidance'.

Cook (1995) asserts that one of the main ways in which community nurses will deliver effective and efficient health promotion will be through teamwork. Self-managed integrated nursing teams are very much the way forward for nursing in primary care and, indeed, the NHS Executive (1993) made teamwork a key to progress for community nursing. Cook goes on to suggest that teamwork allows community nurses to identify, through community profiling, priority groups in their locality to whom health promotion initiatives can be targeted. The individual skills of each of the team members can be utilised effectively to promote health through different opportunities in different settings. In the case of district nurses, they are uniquely placed to be involved in health promotion initiatives with the elderly and their carers in the home. This is a very traditionalist view and in the new climate of integrated nursing teams, there is no reason why district nurses could not be

involved in health promotion in a clinic setting with people of all ages (Vignette 1.1).

There is some research related to community nursing and health promotion in the United Kingdom. One study by Littlewood & Parker (1992) explored community nurses' attitudes to health promotion using a survey approach amongst district nurses and health visitors in one regional health authority. Results indicated that the majority of the community nurses questioned felt that they did not have enough time to 'carry out health promotion'. The results also indicated that, generally, community nurses agreed that they had a central role in health promotion and most of them held similar views on health promotion whether they were health visitors or district nurses.

District nursing and health promotion

Another study (Sourtzi et al 1996) examined the health promotion activities that community nurses carry out in the course of their work. The methods used were a questionnaire, observation and interviewing and the sample included 100 district nurses over four district health authorities. Findings indicated that district nurses 'had little involvement in organised health promotion activities at individual and group level' and that much of what they perceived to be health promotion was carried out in patients' homes but that a minority of them were involved in community health promotion projects, along with their health-visiting colleagues. This agreed with the findings of an early study by Cant & Killoran (1993) who found that district nurses had a comprehensive role in health promotion during home visits. They assert that teamwork is fundamental to the success of health promotion within the setting of primary care.

Thomas & Wainwright (1996) considered a small study where district nurses and health visitors were interviewed about 'their health-promoting role and the ethical concerns they experience within it'. Findings indicated that district nurses tended to be more 'judgemental about their clients' behaviours', used scare tactics and negative role modelling. They also tended to value 'results and outcomes' and would use 'active persuasion' to achieve this.

Many definitions of health promotion suggest that health education is part of health promotion (Tones & Tilford 1994). One example of a small qualitative study carried out to explore district nurses' perceptions of health education (Cantrell 1998) indicated that district nurses perceived health education to be a significant part of their role, this role being facilitated by the uniform and the one-to-one relationship built up with patients in their own homes. Constraints were time, resources and organisational factors. District nurses suggest that perhaps GPs and managers should be made more aware of their health education role.

Although traditionally health promotion has been seen as more of a remit for other community nurses, particularly the health visitor and practice nurse, health promotion and health education should be on the agenda of all district nurses. First, because it should be on the agenda of all nurses (rules 1 and 2 of The Nurses, Midwives and Health Visitors Rules; UKCC 1983), second, district nurses can build up effective relationships with patients and their families and third, because district nurses work within the primary care setting and can help to facilitate community health needs through community profiling and the assessment of health needs using a team approach.

The Standing Nursing, Midwifery and Health Visiting Advisory Committee (1995), in a report on the contribution of nurses, health visitors and midwives to public health, suggests that the public health function of all nurses and midwives is 'fundamental to delivering health improvement to local people' and that district nurses are effectively using clinical audit to reassess practice in terms of the health needs of local populations (SNMAC 1995).

COMMUNITY PROFILING AND HEALTH NEEDS ASSESSMENT

District nurses have an important role in assessing and facilitating the health needs of the populations that they serve. One aspect of this process involves community profiling or health needs assessment.

The terms community profiling, health needs assessment, caseload profiling and community assessment seem to be used interchangeably although they have slightly different definitions and philosophies.

Health needs assessment

Robinson & Elkan (1996) suggest that one definition of health needs assessment 'is as a process of measuring ill health in a population'. They go on to suggest that there are problems with this definition because there are people within any population who need to be protected from ill health and these people are not included. Also, there is no mention of what should happen once these health problems have been detected. Some authors also have concerns over the use of the phrase 'health needs' (Hawtin et al 1994, Neve 1996). The debate surrounds the issues of how to define a health need, who defines health needs, how to choose between competing needs and how to evaluate whether needs have been met.

Health needs assessment can be applied to whole populations, as is the case with directors of public health who, under the NHS and Community Care Act (DoH 1990), are required to assess the health needs of the population served by their health authority or health board. Health needs assessments tend to be carried out by an organisation or statutory body for planning proposes and to be based on quantitative data with little or no consultation with the community that is being assessed, i.e. this approach is usually 'top down'.

Community profiling

The term that seems to be the broadest and the one that is used commonly is community profiling (Hawtin et al 1994). Community profiling can be defined as:

A comprehensive description of the needs of a population that is defined, or defines itself, as a community, and the resources that exist within the community, carried out with the active involvement of the community itself, for the purpose of developing an action plan or other means of improving the quality of life in the community. (Hawtin et al 1994)

Some form of community profiling (sometimes called the neighbourhood study) has been part of the district nurse role description since the mid 1980s, when the training of district nurses moved into higher education and was aligned with that of health visitors. Indeed, one of the key district nursing responsibilities in the 1980s was 'promoting new developments to meet changing health care needs' (Turton & Orr 1993). It could be argued that this could only be achieved if district nurses were aware of the health needs of the community that they served. A small Scottish study (Worth 1996) found that district nurses played little part in the identification of community health needs. The Audit Commission (1999) also reported that more than half the district nurses surveyed said 'that their teams were not involved in profiling the health needs of their local community'. Therefore it appears that there may still be some way to go to achieving a public health role for district nurses.

Goodwin (1992) has contended that community nurses have an important role to play in community profiling but as Robinson & Elkan (1996) point out, information gathered by community nurses is not normally utilised by health authorities and health boards and there appears to be much duplication of effort to gather similar information. Neve (1996) suggests that the primary health-care team is ideally placed to identify health needs (Box 1.16).

One of the differences between a health needs assessment and a community profile is the involvement of the community within the process (Burton 1996, Hawtin et al 1994). Also, whereas a health needs assessment may rely heavily on quantitative data that has already been collected such as mortality/morbidity statistics, information from the census and the General Household Survey, the community profile should also collect qualitative data from individuals in the community. The process of undertaking a community profile is as important as the outcomes (Burton 1996) and the profiles should not only consider the health needs of a community but should also look at the strengths and resources that the community has to offer. These philosophies are also integral to the community development approach. Burton (1993, 1996), suggests the 10 steps shown in Box 1.17 when producing a community health profile.

A number of issues have been identified in the literature that need to be addressed if a comprehensive community profile is to be achieved. These include the time involved in undertaking a community profile (Twinn et al 1990), the ad hoc way in which data are collected (Billings & Cowley 1995) and the lack of a standardised approach (Cowley 1995). Neve (1996), in a small study, also found that for primary health-care teams, lack of financial incentives and appropriate skills, lack of support from team members, distrust of qualitative methods and defining a community from practice boundaries were barriers to community profiling.

Box 1.16 Why the primary health-care team is ideally placed to identify health needs (Neve 1996)

- They have frequent contact with patients.
- They have access to quantitative data on their practice population and health.
- They are a small unit and should be flexible enough to respond to identified needs.

Box 1.17 Ten steps to producing a community profile (reproduced from Burton P, Hanson L 1996 with permission)

Step 1 Assembling a group: size, who should be involved, how the group should be organised
Step 2 Identifying your initial priorities: what are the aims and what do you hope to achieve?
Step 3 Planning the time scale
Step 4 Identifying your resources
Step 5 Gathering data: existing data sources, need to consider whether data is qualitative or quantitative
Step 6 Analysing need
Step 7 Presenting results
Step 8 Working with others
Step 9 Monitoring, evaluation and review
Step 10 Celebrating achievements

Caseload profiling

This approach can be part of the community profiling exercise and tends to be a quantitative examination of a caseload, perhaps in terms of age/sex, dependence, services used, length of time on caseload, numbers of admissions and discharges.

Community assessment

This is the same as community profiling but is suggested by Neve (1996) as a less judgemental term than health needs assessment.

Planning and implementation

Once a community health profile has been achieved, it is important that needs are prioritised and that the planning process begins. This like the profiling, should be undertaken jointly between all members of the primary care team (Vignette 1.4). Naidoo & Wills (1994) indicate that 'planning is important because it helps direct resources to where they have most impact'.

After priorities have been set, it is important to consider what the aims and objectives of each particular health promotion project might be. For example, the aim for the priority chosen in vignette 1.4 might be: within 6 months to facilitate a network of at least 20 carers who will be encouraged to exchange ideas/solutions to problems, thereby reducing stress levels. Objectives might be to:

- informally speak to all carers of dementia patients who are being visited regularly by district nurses
- produce a leaflet about the network
- ascertain who in particular would be involved with the network and how it would operate.

Ewles & Simnett (1995) argue that setting aims and objectives gives the initiative clear focus and 'you know what you are trying to achieve'.

Once aims and objectives have been set, decisions have to be made about how these can be achieved. In vignette 1.4, a written leaflet and information may be required about how carers become part of the network. Perhaps the network may need to meet at least once to decide how it will operate in terms of supporting each other. Perhaps the issue of confidentiality needs to be considered, if people are willing to give out their phone numbers so the network can be supportive.

Once the initiative is set up, what involvement will the primary care team have?

Resources are another issue that need to be considered in the planning stage. Again, in relation to vignette 1.4 and the aims and objectives, various resources such as time, preparation of a leaflet and room availability are just a few things that need to be considered. Have any other members of the primary care team been involved in a similar type of project?

Vignette 1.4   Community health profiling

As a district nurse, I have been involved recently, along with other members of the primary care team, in completing a community health profile. The experience, although time consuming, has been worthwhile with many lay members of the community involved with collecting data through questionnaires and focus groups. One member of the public stated that being involved with the profile had 'given her something to concentrate on over the last few months' and that she had noticed 'an increased community spirit within the area'.

My involvement with the project consisted of designing and sending out a questionnaire to voluntary groups serving the community and then following this up with telephone interviews. Once the profile was complete it became obvious that there were a number of areas that could be addressed by our team. One that I am particularly interested in is the support for carers who are looking after relatives with dementia. I think the nursing team could really have an impact on this group of clients and I would like to see a support network 'up and running'.

Evaluation

Evaluation is very important for any health initiative and must be considered during the planning stage. There are various reasons why we need to evaluate:

- *evidence-based practice* – being able to justify what you are doing
- *dissemination of practice* – giving evidence to other district nurses and members of the

primary care team about what is successful/not successful in terms of practice

- *resources* – being able to give an account of how resources have been used efficiently and effectively
- *reflective practice* – perhaps this has been a great success and you have the evidence to prove it or perhaps changes need to be made if the initiative is to continue or for future initiatives.

There has been much literature devoted to evaluation of health initiatives (Hawe et al 1990, Kemm & Close 1995, Naidoo & Wills 1994), so here we only raise some of the broad issues that need to be considered.

- *What to evaluate?* You will not be able to evaluate all aspects of each initiative, therefore you will need to decide what to look at. In terms of vignette 2.4, you might assess whether you have achieved a network of 20 carers in 6 months. You may also wish to send out a questionnaire to these carers to find out what they feel about the network.
- *When to evaluate?* Evaluate the initiative too early and the effects may not be evident. Evaluate too late and the initial success may now seem the norm.
- *How to evaluate?* What methods are you going to use? For this vignette it could be questionnaires, interviews, focus groups or just the numbers that may now be involved in the network.
- *Who is the evaluation for?* Obviously the evaluation is for the individuals involved and the primary care team. It may also be for trust managers who may have resourced the initiative, the carers who are contributing to the network and other district nurses/professionals who are interested in the project. Dissemination of the evaluation should also be considered. It could be by word of mouth, a written report, a conference presentation or a journal article.

Remember that the only way to measure the success of an initiative objectively is through evaluation.

CONCLUSION

District nurses have a key role to play in both health promotion and public health. As the Audit Commission report (1999) states, for district nurses 'in the future, there is likely to be greater emphasis on providing health education and advice to enable people to maintain their health and independence for as long as possible'. This is related to health at an individual level but district nurses are also expected to participate in community health needs assessment through integrated nursing teams, primary care groups, local health groups and local health-care cooperatives. The changing climate in primary care demands that district nurses should take a more community-centred/public health approach to their role, thereby providing supporting evidence for their work within the locality that they serve.

REFERENCES

Audit Commission 1999 First assessment – a review of district nursing services in England and Wales. Audit Commission, London

Baum F, Sanders D 1995 Can health promotion and primary health care achieve Health for All without a return to their more radical agenda? Health Promotion International 10(2): 149–159

Billings J, Cowley S 1995 Approaches to community needs assessment: a literature review. Journal of Advanced Nursing 22: 721–730

Brown P, Piper S 1997 Nursing and the health of the nation: schism or symbiosis? Journal of Advanced Nursing 25: 297–301

Burton P 1993 Community profiling – a guide to identifying local needs. School for Advanced Urban Studies, Bristol

Burton P 1996 Producing a community health profile:some pitfalls and how to avoid them. In: Burton P, Harrison L (eds) Identifying local health needs. Policy Press, Bristol

Cant S, Killoran A 1993 Team tactics: a study of nurse collaboration in general practice. Health Education Journal 52(4): 203–208

Cantrell J 1998 District nurses' perceptions of health education. Journal of Clinical Nursing 7: 89–96

Catford J 1996 Moving into the next decade – a new dimension? Health Promotion International 11(1): 1–3

Cook R 1995 Health promotion in the primary care setting. Health Visitor 68(6): 289–290

Cowley S 1995 Health promotion in the general pratice setting. Health Visitor 68(5): 199–201

Daykin N, Naidoo J 1997 Poverty and health promotion in primary care: professionals' perspectives. Health and Social Care in the Community 5(5): 309–317

Department of Health 1989 Strategy for nursing. HMSO, London

Department of Health 1990 The NHS and Community Care Act, HMSO, London

Department of Health 1992 The health of the nation. HMSO, London

Department of Health 1997 The new NHS: modern, dependable. HMSO, London

Department of Health 1998 Our healthier nation. HMSO, London

Department of Health 1999 Saving lives: our healthier nation. HMSO, London

Department of Health and Social Security 1986 Promoting better health HMSO, London

Doyle Y, Thomas P 1996 Promoting health through primary care: challenges in taking a strategic approach. Health Education Journal 55(1): 3–10

European Commission 1998 Communication on the development of the public health policy. Internet source: http://europa.eu.int/search97cgi/

Ewles L, Simnett I 1995 Promoting health – a practical guide. Scutari Press, London

Family Heart Study Group 1994 Randomised controlled trial evaluating cardiovascular screening and intervention in general practice: principal results of a British family heart study. British Medical Journal 308: 313–320

Goodwin S 1992 Community nursing and the new public health. Health Visitor 65(3): 78–80

Hawe H, Degeling D, Hall J 1990 Evaluating health promotion. Maclennan and Petty, Sydney

Hawtin M, Hughes G, Percy-Smith J 1994 Community profiling: auditing social needs. OUP, Buckingham

HEA 1998 OHN: developing the debate. Healthlines 53: 10

HMSO 1988 Public health in England. HMSO, London

Imperial Cancer Research Fund OXCHECK Study Group 1994 Effectiveness of health checks conducted by nurses in primary care: results of the OXCHECK study after one year. British Medical Journal 308: 308–312

Kemm J, Close A 1995 Health promotion – theory and practice. Macmillan, Basingstoke

Levin L, Ziglio E 1996 Health promotion as an investment strategy: considerations on theory and practice. Health Promotion International 11(1): 33–39

Littlewoood J, Parker I 1992 Community nurses' attitudes to health promotion in one regional health authority. Health Education Journal 51(2): 87–89

McCallum A 1997 Public health, health promotion and broader health strategy. In: Illitte S, Munro J (eds) Healthy choices. Lawerence and Wishart, London

Naidoo J, Wills J 1994 Health promotion – foundations for practice. Baillière Tindall, London

Neve H 1996 Community assessment in general practice. In: Burton P, Harrison L (eds) Identifying local health needs. Bristol, The Policy Press

NHS Executive 1993 Nursing in primary care – new world, new opportunities. Department of Health, London

Northern Ireland Department of Health and social services 1992 Regional strategy for health and personal social services in NI. DHSS, Belfast

Office of Health Economics 1994 Health information and the consumer. Office of Health Economics, York

Reid D 1999 OHN: the pros and cons. Headlines 65: 8

Robinson J, Elkan R 1996 Health needs assessment – theory and practice. Churchill Livingstone, New York

Rundle R 1992 Parsons revisited: a reappraisal of the community nurse role. In: Jolly M, Brykczynska G (eds) Nursing care – the challenge to change. J. M. a. B. G. Edward Arnold, London

Scottish Home and Health Department 1990 Strategy for nursing, midwifery and health visiting, HMSO, Edinburgh

Scottish Office 1992 Scotland's health: a challenge to us all. HMSO, Edinburgh

Scottish Office 1997 Designed to care. HMSO, Edinburgh

Scottish Office 1998 Working together for a healthier Scotland. HMSO, Edinburgh

Scottish Office 1999 Towards a healthier Scotland. HMSO, Edinburgh

Seedhouse D 1986 Health: foundations for achievement. John Wiley, Chichester

SNMAC 1995 Making it happen. Department of Health, London

Sourtzi P, Nolan P, Andrews R 1996 Evaluation of health promotion activities in community nursing practice. Journal of Advanced Nursing 24: 1214–1223

Thomas J, Wainwright P 1996 Community nurses and health promotion: ethical and political perspectives. Nursing Ethics 3(2): 97–107

Tones K, Tilford S 1994 Health education: effectiveness, efficiency and equity. Chapman and Hall, London

Turton P, Orr J 1993 Learning to care in the community. Edward Arnold, London

Twinn S, Dauncey J, Carnell J 1990 The process of health profiling. Health Visitors Association, London

United Kingdom Central Council for Nursing, Midwifery and Health Visiting 1983 Nurses, midwives and health visitors rules. UKCC, London

Welsh Health Planning Forum 1989 Strategic intent and direction for the NHS in Wales. Welsh Office, Cardiff

Welsh Office 1998 Better health, better Wales. Welsh Office, Cardiff

Whitehead M 1999 The saving lives White Paper: making it work. Health Education Journal 58: 209–210

WHO 1979 Formulating strategies For Health for All by the year 2000: guiding principles and essential issues. WHO, Geneva

WHO 1986 Ottawa charter for health promotion. International conference on health promotion, November 17–21. WHO Regional Office for Europe, Copenhagen

WHO 1993 Health for all targets – the health policy for Europe. WHO Regional Office for Europe, Copenhagen

WHO 1997 The Jakarta declaration on leading health promotion into the 21st century. Fourth International Conference on Health Promotion: New Players for a New Era, July 21–25. WHO, Geneva

WHO 1998a Health for all targets – the health policy for Europe. WHO, Copenhagen

WHO 1998b Health 21 – health for all in the 21st century. WHO, Copenhagen

Worth A 1996 Identifying need for district nursing: towards a more proactive approach by practitioners. NT Research 1(4): 260–269

FURTHER READING

Naidoo J, Wills J 1998 Practising Health
Promotion–Dilemmas a Challenges. Baillìere TindalL,
London
Naidoo J, Wills J 2000 Health Promotion: Foundations for
Practice. Baillìere Tindall, London

Ewles, Simnet 1999 Promoting Health: a practical guide.
Baillìere Tindall, London

2

Demography and social change

Lis Cook

Key points

- Caring for an ageing population
- Care provision in the community
- Partnership in service delivery
- A diverse and multicultural society
- A government-led initiative to reduce inequality in health care

The district nurse has traditionally been at the centre of health-care provision for those patients who remained at or were discharged to their own home. However, the environment of care is changing on several fronts. In response to the needs of a changing population and developments in health care, the focus on care provision has moved from a predominantly hospital-based service to a community-orientated service. Health-care services alone cannot meet the extended range of health and social care provision now required. The care arena that the district nurse now functions in requires new and varied applications of existing skills. Indeed, in many cir cumstances, additional skills are essential to meet the needs of the patient and of the public. The ultimate aim of maintaining and improving the health of the population within the 'district' has remained the same for district nursing, despite the change in terminology to 'community'.

CARING FOR AN AGEING POPULATION

The 20th century has seen the most rapid advance in technology and to none has it been more evident than to those who have lived through it. The present generation of older people has experienced a number of major changes in society. It has lived in an environment where there was initially no health service free at the point of delivery. Instead, there was the support of a family whose duty was to care and where women were at home to do so, with whatever resource they had available to them. Over the ensuing years they have witnessed a number of changes including those listed in Box 2.1.

Box 2.1 Health and social changes

- vast swings in employment
- the introduction of a National Health Service
- the Labour government's move to corporate responsibility for health, housing and education
- an increase in overall wealth
- a move to privately owned housing
- the Conservative government's promotion of personal responsibility.

They have lived in and adapted to a continually changing environment, where the extended family has been replaced by the nuclear family. Attitudes towards and views of the older person have changed, in the light of financial independence through pensions and physical independence through better health. However, it must be remembered that increasing age heralds a reduction in ability to adapt to change and to the speed of adaptation.

Health of an ageing population changes with the environmental and social factors that impinge upon it. However, health care is influenced primarily by need and the changing health-care needs of an ageing population are what we shall now focus upon.

During the latter half of the 20th century there have been five major influences on the environment of care facing the older person:

1. Employment patterns have changed.
   - High unemployment has created a desire for a younger workforce with consequent pressures on older employees to retire early (Ashton & Maguire 1986).
   - Women have become an established part of the workforce and are beginning to adapt family life around a full- or part-time career (OPCS 1991).
2. Family life has changed.
   - Adult sons and daughters are less likely to remain in their parents' home.
   - One-third of children are born into a one-parent family (OPCS 1993).
3. Community life has changed.
   - House planning is designed to accommodate sectors of need separately, i.e. blocks of flats, estates of family houses, sheltered housing complexes.
   - Commuter lifestyle is gradually closing small local businesses, in favour of large shopping complexes.
4. Health services have changed.
   - NHS residential nursing care in hospitals and homes is virtually extinct and the private sector has blossomed.
   - Nursing care in the community is delivered by nurses, with a range of skill mix, who no longer undertake many social care tasks.
   - Medical and pharmaceutical advances have revolutionised treatment for many diseases, removing the threat to life and reducing the need for hospital admission and length of stay in hospital.
5. Life expectancy has changed.
   - The percentage of people whose age at death exceeds 65 years has increased from 35% in 1919 to 82% in 1992 (Markowe 1994).
   - The population profile has altered from one with a high birth rate, relatively low perinatal mortality rate and high death rate in the older populace to a gradually decreasing birth rate and increasing number of elderly, surviving into their 80th year and beyond (Baly 1995).

The consequences of the changes are significant. Unemployment has shortened the active working life for many. Whilst for some this has been of great benefit, removing them from a tedious or strenuous occupation to free time for new interests and occupations, for others it has imposed financial constraints, social isolation and loss of self-esteem at an even earlier stage (Banerjee 1996). Middle-aged women, previously the main carers for the elderly, have become noticeably absent from the home, as employment opportunities for them have expanded.

The casual social and supervisory care of older relatives, often given unconsciously by young adults remaining in the family home, is now much less likely to happen, as the pattern of family life changes. Partnerships, single parenting and dispersal of family units are much less conducive to establishing a regular caring contact with an elderly person, especially if there is no link of relationship by marriage. Lone parenting demands a great deal and leaves little scope for attention to elderly relatives.

Social and caring support from neighbours has been a mainstay for many older people, who rely on neighbours for shopping, minor household help and alerting services in the event of illness. The continuing trends towards detached housing, door-to-door car travel and lack of 'street life' are discouraging neighbourliness. Added to this, the loss of local shopping facilities, libraries and other amenities hinders the establishment and maintenance of social contact.

For many years elderly people, from the frail to those with complex care requirements, had their needs met in the continuing care environment of hospitals, whose 'long-stay' beds were often occupied until the patients' eventual deaths. Many elderly people existed in a fragile balance between 'relative wellness' and acute hospitalisation (Allen 1994). Improving medical and pharmaceutical knowledge in chronic disease management has reduced the number of patients requiring admission to or long stays in hospital, but has increased the number of elderly patients within the community requiring specialist and short-term, often intensive support. The resulting burden of care falls not just upon the health-care system but also upon the families, friends and neighbours of the elderly chronically ill.

The implementation of the 1990 NHS & Community Care Act (DOH 1990) radically altered that care scenario. Now there are virtually no long-stay beds in the NHS and a full range of community care has necessitated the introduction of a wider nursing skill mix. The move to community has, however, introduced many much broader implications for care and these will now be considered in detail.

A CONTINUING MOVE TO CARE PROVISION IN THE COMMUNITY

The NHS & Community Care Act (DOH 1990) was the government response to a crisis in health and social care. National statistics had indicated that the number of 75–85 year olds would nearly double in the following two decades (OPCS 1992). Care demands began to outstrip the service's ability to meet the need, on a number of levels.

Resources

Insurance contributions, which fund the rising cost of health care, have remained at a fixed level, made by the increasingly small number of the population in significant employment. Although private health insurance has been promoted, which should theoretically reduce the public cost of health care, its limited use has never significantly reduced NHS costs.

Personnel

The bulk of nurse preparation and service delivery had traditionally been within the acute sector and in a mixed skill environment. This had been labour and cost intensive, due to the additional resources required for accommodation and domestic amenities.

Social support

The demands upon social services, as existing family and neighbourhood support diminished

---

Vignette 2.1 June's Story

June was well known to the community nursing services. She was 50 years old and was diagnosed as having motor neurone disease in 1990. Her problems included hemiplegia, obesity, poor vision and urinary and faecal incontinence. June's husband Tom had been her main carer but there was a gradual increase in support from the GP and DN services as Tom's health deteriorated.

Following an admission to hospital for surgery a case conference was held by the social services department. A case package was compiled which met June's requests to remain at home but failed to address the physical and emotional stressors on herself, Tom and indeed the professional and voluntary sectors involved. In addition, the enormous cost of the package exhausted the community care budget for the area within 6 months severely curtailing services for the rest of the community. The low priority given to the health professionals assessment had a two-fold effect.

Firstly, it failed to meet June's needs and those of her husband. Secondly, it had a negative effect on the relationship between health and social care professionals.

---

and expectations of the service from the public grew, became manifest in the number of older people utilising services. Home helps, meals on wheels and day care centres became victims of their own success, with ever-increasing waiting lists. Admissions to private nursing and residential homes, funded largely by Social Services, rose rapidly.

The escalating numbers of elderly will surely mean a continuous rise in service demand over the next decades, which should influence service provision (Easchus et al 1996).

To a lesser extent there was also a move to reestablish the rights of older people in society: the right to have an informed choice regarding care, the right to remain in their own homes wherever possible and the right to remain autonomous and self-caring wherever possible (Gordon 1993). In retrospect, it is easy to be cynical in realising that it took a financial crisis to highlight the more altruistic aims of care in the community. However, it is also only in retrospect that, several years on, the government have discovered that 'the community' is not a cheap option.

Whatever the main motivator of change, the concepts underlying the move to care in the community were entirely valid. The emphasis on personal involvement, greater choice and overall assessment and care delivery were in accordance with models of nursing care and the move to patient empowerment. Difficulties emerged because one agency was given the lead role for community care delivery, i.e. social services. Although the crucial role of GPs and district nurses was emphasised, the reality often fell far short of the rhetoric (Vignette 2.1).

In some areas as many as 35% of nursing home residents are considered to have been inappropriately placed (Bennet et al 1995). This may, in part, have been due to a failure to share the responsibility of purchasing care between Social Services and health authority or trust health professionals, such as district nurses.

AN INCREASING EMPHASIS ON PARTNERSHIP IN SERVICE DELIVERY

District nursing had until the 1990s enjoyed a period of considerable autonomy. Many enterprising nurses had established excellent working relationships with GPs, Social Service departments and voluntary services. It could be claimed quite legitimately that they enjoyed a position of considerable standing in the community (DHSS 1986) and therefore had influence. In many rural areas they were the linchpin around which needs were identified, services were coordinated and care was delivered and evaluated. Indeed, the nursing process was the forerunner of modern-day care management.

The shift of responsibility for community care away from district nursing called for a period of reflection to reestablish the district nurse's role and allow a reevaluation of skills. The rapid spread of GP fundholding concentrated the minds of nurse managers and a real opportunity for innovation began.

As a knowledgeable health-care professional, skilled in assessment, planning, delivery and evaluation of care, the district nurse is in a unique position to assist older people in the community to identify their care requirements.

However, district nurses are not the only stakeholders in health and social care provision. The burgeoning care industry that swiftly followed the 1990 legislation saw a host of new faces. The range of personnel that may now be involved in care provision for an older person with complex needs, e.g. following a stroke, could people a small army. The risk to the patient and the family is that their home can begin to feel as though it has been invaded (Cook 1997).

If we take into account the range of staff filling each role over a given period of time, the addition of students and observers at various intervals and the preponderance of auditors at all stages, the players become a substantial cast! In order for the cast to be fully effective they must work in partnership.

A variety of successful models of care are in progress around the country. In Aberdeen the skill and experience of district nurses in a holistic approach to patient care assessment and management were recognised in their appointment as full-time care managers, employed by the Social Service department. This model echoes that used in America, where case management by community nurses is evolving in complexity and effectiveness. The potential for improved self-management and the consequent alteration in amount and type of health resource utilised by the patient is seen as beneficial not only to the patient, but also to the primary care provider and the health-care organisation (Scott & Rantz 1997).

Other areas have utilised nursing expertise in the formulation of joint assessment and care documentation, notably West Lothian, where two enterprising nurses gained funding to work within the Social Services department one day a week, using the opportunity to demonstrate their skills and forge stronger links.

If all roles are potentially valid within any specific care context, how do we decide which role to pursue, as district nurses, if we are to offer maximum benefit to the patient? This can perhaps best be illustrated by considering a fairly typical care scenario.

There are a number of different roles that the DN could take as shown in Box 2.2.

Box 2.2 District nursing roles

- *Coordinator*. Organise further bath assessment and screening, review medication and continue initial assessment.
- *Key worker*. Do bath assessment and screening and admit to caseload for ongoing assessment. Arrange home visit by GP.
- *Referrer*. Refer to GP for review of medication; refer to practice nurse for screening of bloods and urine; refer to occupational therapist for assessment; refer to care manager for continued assessment.

In deciding on the DN's appropriate role in this instance, a number of factors must be considered, under three main headings.

1. *Patient*
   - What has the initial response been to the visit?
   - How receptive would they be to another face?
   - Would they significantly benefit by referral elsewhere at this point?
2. *Nurse*
   - How well have you been able to establish a rapport?
   - How much of the continuing assessment are you able to do?
   - Are you the most effective person to assess at this point?
3. *Setting*
   - Is speed of assessment an issue?
   - Will an assessment carried out by the nurse be valid elsewhere?
   - Will other professionals' expertise be available as a resource to aid assessment, without face-to-face contact?

There are, of course, side issues to muddy the waters. These include the current debate over the divisions between health and social care, illustrated by the apparently insoluble question 'Is a bath a health or social care function?' The introduction of GP fundholding and the consequent contracting issues which often ensued brought the health and social care issue to a head, diverting nursing from the holistic approach to care provision.

The emphasis on responsibility as ultimately lying with Social Services ensured that care provision could not be seen to have reduced following the implementation of Care in the Community (NHS & Community Care Act 1990) and the response in many areas was for bathing and 'tuck down' services to be created, as a social requirement. It would be easy for district nurses to abdicate all responsibility for social aspects of care in the face of resource restraints. However, there remains a crucial consideration for all potential referrals and that is – would a nursing assessment benefit them?

It is the author's opinion, based on many years experience of district nursing, that one bath visit, carried out by a DN, can be utilised as a comprehensive assessment opportunity, allowing appropriate referral to be made and care needs to be identified. Although initially time consuming, the insight into patient care needs far outweighs the resource implications of DN time and allows much more effective targeting of resources to benefit patients (Vignette 2.2).

Vignette 2.2 Miss Dove

A referral comes to the district nurse via the practice nurse from the GP. He has recently spoken to a patient who has concerns about her elderly aunt. The aunt is 82 years of age and lives alone in a semi-detached house, nearby. Although she has kept relatively good health throughout her life, she is growing frail and less mobile and the niece fears that her personal hygiene is suffering, as she is reluctant to have a bath. Despite discreet offers of help from the niece the aunt has refused to consider her assistance as 'it wouldn't be right'. However, she had given permission for the niece to speak to the doctor about any help she might get.

At this point there are various options to take, but the appropriate one would seem to be that of an initial assessment undertaken by the district nurse.

The district nurse (DN) telephones the aunt, Miss Dove, to make an appointment and assessment begins. She is pleased to note that Miss Dove's hearing and speech are unimpaired and that she has retained her memory of conversations with her niece about getting help.

The following day the DN visits Miss Dove. Miss Dove takes several minutes to answer the door and can be heard shuffling along the hallway in loose-fitting slippers. On opening the door she appears to be struggling for balance and in some pain raising her arm to the high doorknob. She recognises the uniform and responds to the nurse's greeting by inviting her in. The nurse observes that Miss Dove has obvious arthritic changes to her hands, which may be affecting her other joints and causing the impaired gait.

As a health professional the DN is usually in the privileged position of having inherited credibility. However, as a guest in a patient's home, it would be inappropriate to exploit this privilege by exhaustive or excessively intrusive questioning. The skill therefore is in eliciting information through general conversation and by encouraging the patient to volunteer information through a social chat. Where specific information is required, the framing and referencing of questions is crucial to the degree of comfort the patient feels in discussing personal health and social care matters.

Utilising the skills of therapeutic gossip, the following points are noted during the assessment process.

Single lady, 82 years old. Closest relative is niece, who pops in twice a week and usually stays for an hour or so to take tea. One elderly neighbour doesn't get out, the other neighbours are a new couple who both work and contact is really only on a nodding basis.

Large house, rather untidy and dusty, with a number of loose rugs. Miss Dove does her own cleaning, cooking and washing. Gas cooker and single tub washer in the kitchen. Gas fires in kitchen-diner and sitting room; usually at least one is on. Downstairs lavatory, no heating and one long flight of stairs to bathroom and bedrooms. Convector heater on landing and in main bedroom. Heated towel rail in bathroom, which has integral toilet, bath and basin. Miss Dove usually washes upstairs in the bathroom – fairly quickly because it is cold – and, once downstairs, remains so until bedtime as the stairs are difficult to negotiate. She last got into the bath 2 years ago, but nearly didn't get out again as she couldn't pull herself up easily.

The temptation is often to cover every aspect of daily living at the first visit. However, assessment is an ongoing process and dealing with presenting problems whilst completing the assessment is often a good way of establishing a trusting relationship with a new patient.

The DN notices that Miss Dove smells of urine and surmises that impaired mobility may be a cause, but there are several other possibilities, i.e. urinary tract infection, stress incontinence, etc. In a tactful approach to the topic she suggests to Miss Dove that the GP may be able to help joint pain and mobility problems which will enable her to get about more easily. She also offers to give Miss Dove an 'MOT', to check her blood pressure, urine and blood chemistry and offers information about bath aids which Miss Dove could access and which the occupational therapist would assess for.

The increasing number of elderly people in society, together with the decreasing amount of informal carer support, will result in rising demands on all caring agencies. District nurses can maximise their effectiveness by constantly reviewing the care scenario and moving from one role to another as patient care needs require. Where collaborative approaches to care provision between health and social care services exist, a degree of flexibility in all professional roles will ensure a patient-focused service. The demand upon individual professionals, however, is not just in terms of delivering care but in generously sharing their knowledge and expertise appropriately. The benefit to the patient is in reducing the number of different carers in and out of a home during assessment and provision of care, whilst accessing and utilising the broad knowledge base of a large number of individual professional carers.

Little research has been done to measure the effect on patients and their families of complex care packages being delivered in the home. An assumption seems to have been made that patients prefer to be at home and there appears to be no evidence to dispute this. However, the reality is that for some families, the home has become a 'venue for care' first and a home second. The responsibility of having an elderly relative living in the home is often great and as professional carers, we must be aware of the added imposition of having continual 'visitors' who demand time, take up private space and often ask repetitive questions!

Respecting and acknowledging the skill of others is as applicable to nurses as it is demanding of them. There is an increasing range of professionals currently offering care to older people in the community, in the home and in residential settings. The established Social Services departments will already have formal and informal networks for communication and joint working. These vary across the country but usually take the form of joint training initiatives (Cook 1998a), joint planning, joint assessment (Cotterill et al 1997), case conferencing and joint staff meetings. Where voluntary sector care provision is introduced then nurses must initiate communication and establish links where appropriate, to maximise quality and continuity of care.

In complex care scenarios, it is often the case that over time different tiers of care are added. District nursing services may be attending a patient for a health-care treatment, home help services may be attending to supervise personal care, voluntary services may be involved in supporting the patient and carer, who could also be in need of care. Avoiding repetition and duplication of efforts must be addressed as a collaborative exercise, by all agencies involved in care.

The peculiarities of service documentation systems and the smoke screen of confidentiality put up by many health-care professionals should not be insurmountable in achieving a streamlined information flow. There are now good working models of patient-held records, utilised by patient and health and social carers alike, which reduce the previously tedious round of basic information gathering done by each agency (Hayward 1998). Moreover, the use of shared records gives the DN a window into the daily life of the patient and a showcase to demonstrate her considerable skill in collaborative working and recording of care episodes. Where such practice is not common the DN has an opportunity to take the lead in joint documentation initiatives, utilising the considerable research literature available.

However, sharing documentation is only the first step in collaboration. Careful and reflective care management may highlight areas where care can be shared, particularly where overlaps in care are apparent. Whilst it is not efficient use of resource for a DN rather than a home help to go into a patient's home to give him lunch, if a DN will be in the home carrying out a nursing task during the middle of the day, it is not inappropriate for her to give the patient a pre-prepared meal and hot drink, whilst she is there. Colleagues who have argued against 'domestic tasks' being undertaken whilst in the home on a nursing visit seem to have had no problem offering drinks and assisting patients with meals when they are on the ward, in hospital. What is the difference?

Similarly, voluntary carers have taken on, with appropriate preparation, tasks such as medication giving, insulin injections, etc. due when they are present. This concept of 'trading places' makes best use of resources when employed effectively and, most importantly, it reduces the number of care personnel invading the home, whilst still utilising their knowledge and expertise (Cook 1998b).

As was stated earlier, the move to Care in the Community (NHS & Community Care Act 1990) has seen a swell in the number of voluntary sector nursing and residential homes. District nurses have an increasing role within the residential sector as health-care providers and as an expert resource to social carers. It has been calculated that one misplaced resident in an independent nursing home may result in a life cost waste of £42 000 (Bennet et al 1995). Initial difficulties around resourcing of nursing care to residential homes were due to the contract difficulties of practice-based DNs. It is anticipated that these will resolve with the dismantling of the internal market and the implementation of new legislation (DoH 1997, Scottish Office DoH 1997, Welsh Office 1998a). Primary care groups and local health-care cooperatives should be able to respond to the overall needs of patients in residential home settings. Many areas already have well-established patterns of contact, where visiting DNs hold regular 'clinics', as well as room calls. Indeed, treatment rooms designed specifically for the use of district nurses are now available in many residential homes.

The role of expert resource should be fully exploited and residents should have access to the full range of equipment and aids available to their contemporaries at home. Advice on moving and handling and appropriate use of lifting aids for residential care staff can only be of benefit to patients. Access to residential care and transfer to nursing care establishments is currently arranged only via an initial Social Service assessment. This should be in consultation with the district nursing service and is an opportunity for effective nursing assessment to ensure transfer to an appropriate care placement.

It is in this capacity that a DN can adopt another role, that of advocate. Advocacy is a concept often talked about as part and parcel of nursing, yet recent literature indicates the inability of a service provider to act as a fully independent representative of the patient's wishes (Mallik 1997). The advocacy role therefore can only really be effectively carried out when the nurse has an informed and ongoing relationship with the patient and when district nursing service provision is no longer required, i.e. when the care environment is changing.

Older people are individuals with the range of needs and personalities evident in society as a whole. It would be quite wrong, therefore, to assume that there is a uniform answer to care provision, which nurses have access to. The skill that a DN can offer is the ability to assess a person from a health and social care perspective, with an open mind as to how care needs can be met. This will be informed by the knowledge of existing service provision but open to consideration of other solutions. The problem-solving approach to nursing can equally be applied in generic care settings in the community.

Enabling older people to retain control in the face of decline, often with the added burden of what Dr Lisbeth Hockey labelled 'cumulative multiple trivia syndrome', a condition of disability brought about by no one single disease but by a series of minor problems, is a privilege accorded to few. The DN is one of the few. She has the education and experience to identify the health and social care requirements, she has the communicative skill and established professional credibility to advise and advocate on the appropriate service to meet the need and she has the expertise to devise, deliver and evaluate care. American research describes the relationship between the chronically ill patient and the nurse care manager as 'bonding'. Whether district nurses in the UK would use that description is questionable but their patients may well agree with the description, offered by one patient, of the relationship moving from the nurse 'knowing her stuff' to 'knowing me' (Lamb & Stempel 1994).

With increasing age there is often increasing vulnerability caused by illness, infirmity, poverty, powerlessness and dependence. The DN is a key member of the team of health and social care professionals who can minimise that vulnerability and improve the quality of an increased lifespan.

A DIVERSE AND MULTICULTURAL SOCIETY

The ability of the DN to care in any community setting has never been more relevant than in today's society. Not only do we have a population whose financial and social status varies vastly, we also have a culturally and racially diverse society within geographically small areas. Statistics show that approximately 6% of the total population in Britain is from ethnic minority groups. Added to this figure are the additional minority groups undetected by the present classification system, e.g. those of Irish descent would be classified as 'white' and although culturally and ethnically individual, would not be identified within the present system of recording (OPCS 1992). The delivery of an equitable and appropriate nursing service, responsive to diverse needs, calls for particular skills and flexibility, which may be called upon even when working within a single area or with attachment to a single GP practice. If the DN is to offer a patient-centred service then the individuality of the patient must be reflected in the approach to care.

As a person's culture influences his perception of and response to illness, the DN must provide care that is meaningful for and sensitive to the patient within that culture (Lynam 1992). This approach may be considered from a number of perspectives, one of which is patient comfort.

Whatever the reason for a district nursing visit, assessment, care management, care delivery, screening or support, patient comfort is a vital ingredient in realising maximum patient and carer well-being. Comfort is used here as an expression of the overall state of feeling in relation to the district nursing visit. Physical comfort is important, of course, and should be a goal to aim for in care provision, but total physical comfort is not always achievable despite the best endeavours of all concerned. Emotional comfort, although a much more nebulous concept, can be achieved even when physical discomfort is present. In order for the patient to feel comfortable during the nursing visit, a complex communication process is utilised, often without either party being conscious of its occurrence. Lynam (1992) argues that a practitioner cannot identify with the client's perspective or involve the client in discussions regarding care if she cannot communicate effectively.

A DN may communicate with people at different levels. This depends largely on the patient's knowledge and understanding of his condition and the treatment and care the nurse is providing. She may adjust the language used and the speed at which information is given, as well as the type of information and the level of reinforcement. Often there is a subtle change in the way she relates to people. A student on placement with a DN for 2 weeks observed at least five different initial approaches made to a patient's house.

1. *Formal*. Prearranged appointment. Ring bell, wait for answer. Introduce self on doorstep. Wait to be invited in.
2. *Semi-formal*. Prearranged appointment. Ring bell, wait for answer. Introduce self as entering.
3. *Less formal*. Prearranged day. Ring bell and enter, calling 'Hello, it's the nurse, can I come in?'.
4. *Informal*. Half-expected, pop in visit. Ring bell and enter, calling 'Hello, it's the nurse'.
5. *Friend*. Visit any time. Ring and enter, calling 'Hello'.

When these visits were analysed, there were a number of factors involved in the use of the different approaches. The most obvious factor was familiarity. The less well the patient knew the nurse, the more formal the initial approach. This conforms to established communication processes. However, there were also a number of patients who, although equally familiar with the nurse in terms of numbers of contacts, were approached in different ways. The approach varied as the DN engaged in tactics to increase patient comfort with and within the nursing visit.

Where a patient was visibly alone, socially or geographically isolated and starved of personal contact, their nursing visit was often perceived as a welcome break and a social interlude in addition to a treatment session. The approach as 'a friend' reinforced the patient's sense of well-being and self-esteem as part of the therapeutic intervention.

The 'informal' visit approach was used where patients or carers were anxious about their use of nursing or indeed any professional's time. They were often visibly worried about 'being a nuisance' and only felt comfortable receiving care if it caused a minimum of fuss or if they could give recompense in some way. This approach, usually accompanied by the patient or carer giving the nurse a cup of tea, enabled comfortable acceptance of the nurse's visit.

The 'less formal' visit was often adopted when carrying out supervisory or screening visits, to allow the patient and/or carer a degree of control over the character of the visit. It enabled a refusal of service from a diffident and often underassertive patient or carer, without that refusal being seen as impolite. Again, this allows maximum comfort with the initial visit, even if a future visit or screening opportunity is refused.

The 'semi-formal' and 'formal' visiting approaches, even with long-established patients and carers, was adopted to maximise their control over personal environment and care service. This approach enabled patients with little control of their disease or disability to exercise control over access to nursing care. It also enabled carers within a family home to retain the privacy and sanctity of personal space, so crucial to comfort and well-being.

The nuances of the initial approach to a district nursing visit offer an insight into the cognitive approach to caring required in a multicultural and multiracial society. As individuals, we all learn a complex set of rules which guide and inform our attempts to establish relationships and to communicate within those relationships. We are usually comfortable with the peculiarities of communication within our

---

Vignette 2.3 A misunderstanding

A district nurse born and raised in the North of England, where 'to doubt' someone is to question his or her correctness, spent several weeks of uncertainty on moving to Shetland to work. Many of her patients used the expression 'I doubt you're right, nurse'. It required eventual reassurance from a colleague that, in fact, this was an expression used in Shetland to concur with a statement, not the reverse!

---

own environment. As developing individuals, we quickly learn that there are different rules, in school, in college, at work and beyond, that we must learn to conform or adapt to. The DN is no exception.

To work effectively within a variety of cultures and races requires more than a passing familiarity with the language. If the concept of 'comfort' is fully explored, it requires a knowledge of custom and practice and a respect for the individual, which merits adaptation of nursing practice, wherever appropriate, to reflect the culture and tradition of the patient (Vignette 2.3).

This knowledge can often best be passed on to the nurse by the patient or by other informed members of the community. Local health councils, Citizens Advice Bureaux, translators, min-isters of religion, etc. are all valuable resources, as are relevant texts (Karseras & Hopkins 1987).

However, the DN must first be willing to recognise a knowledge deficit and then to invite input in a manner that values the contribution that another culture, and indeed the patient within that culture, has to offer. The emphasis on the client's perspective is common throughout nursing literature but is particularly relevant here (Benner 1984).

There are excellent examples of the resourcefulness of nurses across the UK in meeting the needs of our diverse society. Even accounting for issues of gender, age and social class, the ethnic population is more disadvantaged and as a result is more likely to become ill (Bassett 1994). In order to address this inequality, local initiatives should be supported by policy and by resource, if true effectiveness is to be achieved and measured (Vignette 2.4).

Vignette 2.4 Adaptability

In Glasgow, a nurse working with older people from an ethnic minority group was struggling to apply theories of health promotion designed to meet the needs of white, retired Glaswegians from social classes 3–5. Her client group met in a day-care centre, set up and run by younger members of the same ethnic group who were second- and third-generation Scots, by place of birth.

Attempts at promoting self-help were diminished by the popularly held belief that the young people should be doing everything, as had been the case in their country of origin, prior to their emigration. Neither the older people in this ethnic group nor their younger counterparts had experience of present-day practice within their country of origin, so a sense of loyalty to former custom and practice prevailed. This insight into the rationale behind their failure to respond to health promotion initiatives allowed the nurse to adapt her practice. Her response to the dilemma, however, went beyond the ordinary.

She successfully applied for funding to go to the country of origin of many of her patients, the Punjab. She took with her a translator, a nurse co-worker from the centre and a video camera. Having arranged site visits prior to her departure through a number of health and local ethnic group representatives, she filmed her trip. A number of older people were interviewed with the assistance of the interpreter, giving a unique insight into current lifestyles of the elderly within the Punjab and into their health and social care. The film was edited into video format.

It has been useful in terms of facilitating the patients in the day centre to come to terms with the changes in the society that they have left behind and therefore giving themselves permission to move on. Moreover, it has clearly demonstrated the respect that the nurse has for their culture and her willingness to adapt and maintain her care (White 1997).

Vignette 2.5 Rose

Rose was dying from cancer. As the last patient on the district nursing caseload that evening, she would continue to receive care until her death, expected in the next few hours. Her husband was visibly upset, but calm when the nurse gave him the news that Rose would soon die. He said he would inform the priest and asked if it would be all right if the family came round. The nurse readily agreed.

Over the next hour Rose's peaceful passing transformed into something of a spectacle. The priest was preceded by 11 of Rose's sons and daughters-in-law, several grandchildren, neighbours, friends and other relatives, who all packed the small sitting room where Rose lay. They joined the priest in fastening Rose's hands around a large candle and giving her the last rites. Whilst prayers were said in the sitting room, ever more

people arrived in the kitchen and the original sustenance of tea being offered soon gave way to that of whisky. When Rose died at 2 am, every person there came to say goodbye, in their own way. It was some time before the nurse could eventually remove the melted candle wax from her fingers, regain what little control she had had over her care and perform last offices.

It had not been the usual peaceful passing that the DN had experienced many times in the cold stillness of the night, not what she had expected when Rose's husband had asked if the family could come round, but it had been a death in keeping with the customs and tradition of this Irish Catholic family. Most important of all, in the final moments of her life, Rose would have been comforted by what she may have heard or felt of the love and esteem shown by all around her.

Although it is neither practicable nor desirable that all nurses undertake such an endeavour, it does highlight the need to communicate effectively with the patient.

Empathy and understanding are keys to promoting comfort, particularly where areas of acute sensitivity are exposed, in areas of taboo around sex and death, for example. Within even a small, relatively homogeneous community, there can be a large divide in religious persuasion, social mores and customs. Assumption is never a safe option when nursing, particularly in

the community, where the nurse has less control over the environment than in hospital (Yoshida & Davies 1982) (Vignette 2.5).

A GOVERNMENT-LED INITIATIVE TO REDUCE INEQUALITY IN HEALTH CARE

The National Health Service has a duty to respond to the needs of all the population, including culturally and ethnically diverse groups, through the work of planners, commissioners and providers of care. In recent years the trend to consider health in a medical model has been overtaken by the view of health adopted by the World Health Organisation, as a 'state of complete physical, mental and social well-being'. Evidence for the existence of inequalities in health was produced initially by the Black report on inequalities in Health (DHSS 1980) and confirmed 18 years later in the Acheson Report (DoH 1998). An apparent lack of interest in the subject by the previous government has been replaced by a committment by the current labour government to address health inequality and the social and environmental factors that contribute to ill health (DoH 1998, Scottish Office DoH 1998, Welsh Office 1998b). As knowledgeable community health professionals, district nurses have a role to play in involving the public in the decision-making process about health care and in informing planners and commissioners of the needs of their patient groups.

The community is an ever-changing population and health professionals must be alert to the effects of health policy on individuals and groups within it. For example, the most recent trend of health-care policy in the community has reflected the increasing numbers of older people, with a consequent de-emphasis on child and maternity care. This disadvantages ethnic minority families whose community patterns are still based on the extended family and higher birth rates (Bassett 1994).

Inequalities may exist not only in range and amount of provision but also in access. This dilemma is amply illustrated by the discrepancy evident in health services for men and women. Many women still function in two roles, those of unpaid domestic worker within the home and as a worker for money outwith the home (Oakley 1982). Access to health-care services that do not offer crèche facilities is therefore restricted. Although women attend GPs more than men do, they often attend on behalf of children and elderly and disabled relatives. Self-care, rest and leisure are of low priority (Macintyre et al 1996) which leads to the low uptake of regular physical activity by women (DoH 1996) and the increased risk of later ill health from, for example, osteoporosis. In addition, past history indicates that women's health and dietary needs took second place to men's for significant periods of time during the two world wars. Prolonged periods of poor nutrition in women are evident now in the elderly population, in bone deformation and circulatory deficiency. The habits of an earlier lifestyle are hard to break and in many households the men still receive the best cuts of meat. The DN is in an ideal position to influence dietary habits and to improve women's nutritional status, particularly during ill health and convalescence, by emphasising the improved healing rate that good nutrition will offer.

Women live longer than men do, but their experience of health differs. They are more likely to report psychological distress, requiring support and counselling time, an intervention that many GP appointment systems are not designed to facilitate. District nurses will spend a great deal of time in patients' homes where carers are predominantly women. Encouraging a proactive approach to health amongst carers by facilitating a separate assessment of their needs will begin to address inequality, by providing advice and help in a person-friendly environment, the home.

Inequalities are not due solely to gender. They may also exist because of social and financial pressures, influencing access to good-quality housing, food and work and leisure facilities. Primary care groups and local health-care cooperatives will direct the new public health agenda. Equitable provision of services in accessible areas, addressing locally directed needs and utilising a community development approach will begin to address current service discrepancies.

District nurses in South Lanarkshire actively canvassed their 'elderly forum' to establish the kind of integrated evening service that would meet the needs of the population. The service, launched in January 1999 and coordinated by a district nurse, combines health and social care under one management system, with direct access for the public.

Whilst the newly designed community care service will enable attention to be paid to local issues, it must be remembered that it may have adverse effects. Mobile populations, such as travelling people, may not be represented in the community profile and consequently the care they receive will be less likely to be tailored to their needs.

The DN can add value in her role with the new groups, as a conduit for local information. She can convey the details required to identify any local need and facilitate service requirements being addressed in future planning and provision.

In order to be served, however, a patient must first be recognised. Recognition will only occur when preconceived ideas of cultural norms do not obstruct vision. To be aware of one's own

limitations, in knowledge, in skill, in understanding and in empathising with a patient, is vital. Patients and relatives can be wonderful teachers as well as pupils, with a plethora of new experiences to share. The relationship between patient and nurse can be cemented in interdependence, each enabling the other to give culturally sensitive and appropriate care.

The nature of change within the community, the health service and nursing ensures that district nurses will continue to learn, from their patients, the public, their colleagues and themselves, as they care.

REFERENCES

Allen S A 1994 Medicare case management. Home Healthcare Nurse 12: 21–27

Ashton D, Maguire M 1986 Young adults in the labour market. University of Leicester, Leicester

Baly M 1995 Nursing and social change, 3rd edn. Routledge, London

Banerjee A K 1996 Caring for the elderly: problems and priorities. British Journal of Hospital Medicine 56(4): 159–161

Bassett C 1994 Not just a black and white issue. Journal of Community Nursing 8(6): 12 16

Benner P 1984 From novice to expert: excellence and power in clinical nursing practice. Addison-Wesley, Menlo Park, California

Bennet M, Smith E, Millard P H 1995 The right person? The right place? The right aims? An audit of the appropriateness of NHS placements post Community Care Act. Department of Geriatric Medicine, St George's Hospital Medical School, London

Cook L 1997 Operation overload. Nursing Times Exhibition, London

Cook L 1998a A multidisciplinary training video for use in primary care. Queen's Nursing Institute, Edinburgh

Cook L 1998b Clinical view. Nursing Times 94(22): 47

Cotterill G, Lawrence J, Reid J 1997 The formulation of an assessment tool to facilitate joint working. Queen's Nursing Institute, Edinburgh

Department of Health and Social Security 1980 Inequalities in health: the Black report. HMSO, London

Department of Health and Social Security 1986 Neighbourhood nursing: a focus for care (Cumberlege report). HMSO, London

Department of Health 1989 Caring for people: community care in the next decade and beyond. HMSO, London

Department of Health 1990 NHS and Community Care Act. DoH, London

Department of Health 1996 Health related behaviour: an epidemiological overview. HMSO, London

Department of Health 1997 The new NHS: modern, dependable. Stationery Office, London

Department of Health 1998 Our healthier nation. HMSO, London

Department of Health 1998 Inequalities in Health The Acheson Report, Stationery Office, London

Easchus J, Williams M, Chan P et al 1996 Deprivation and cause specific morbidity: evidence from the Somerset and Avon Survey of Health. British Medical Journal 312: 324–325

Gordon R 1993 Community care assessments: a practical legal framework. Longmans, Harlow

Hayward K 1998 Patient-held oncology records. Nursing Standard 12(35): 44–46

Karseras P, Hopkins E 1987 British Asians – Health in the Community. John Wiley, Chichester

Lamb G S, Stempel J E 1994 Nurse case management from the client's view: growing as insider-expert. Nursing Outlook 42(1): 7–13

Lynam J 1992 Towards the goal of providing culturally sensitive care: principles upon which to build nursing curricula. Journal of Advanced Nursing 17: 149–157

Macintyre S, et al 1996 Gender differences in health: are things really as simple as they seem? Social Science Medicine 4. 617–624

Mallik M 1997 Advocacy in nursing – a review of the literature. Journal of Advanced Nursing 25: 130–138

Markowe H 1994 Health trends in the past 75 years. Health Trends 26(4): 98–105

Oakley A 1982 Subject women. Fontana, Glasgow

Office of Population Censuses and Surveys 1991 General household survey. HMSO, London

Office of Population Censuses and Surveys 1992 1991 Census. HMSO, London

Office of Population Censuses and Surveys 1993 Mortality statistics: perinatal and infant: social and biological factors: review of the Registrar General on deaths in England and Wales, 1991. HMSO, London

Scott J, Rantz M 1997 Managing chronically ill older people in the midst of the health care revolution. Nurse Administration Quarterly 21(2): 55–64

Scottish Office Department of Health 1997 Designed to care. Stationery Office, Edinburgh

Scottish Office Department of Health 1998 Working together for a healthier Scotland. Stationery Office, Edinburgh

Welsh Office 1998a Putting patients first. Stationery Office, London

Welsh Office 1998b Better health – better Wales. Stationery Office, London

White I 1997 A study tour of the Panjab. An innovation award. Queen's Nursing Institute, Edinburgh

Yoshida M, Davies M E 1982 Parenting in a new culture: experiences of East Indian, Portuguese and Caribbean mothers. Multiculturalism 5(3): 3–5

3

Policy and political ideology

Sue Howard

Key points

- The provision of health care
- The British economy
- The nature of politics
- The function of political parties
- Political ideology
- Politics and health-care policy
- Patient/client empowerment
- Devolution
- Current policy development

INTRODUCTION

Before embarking on this chapter, it is necessary to set out its parameters. Whilst the main aim is to introduce the reader to some of the political thinking that has shaped the way that health care services and district nursing in particular is delivered, it will, by necessity, provide only a limited view of politics and policy development which, by nature of their complexity, are the bases for study in their own right. The reader is therefore directed to the end of this chapter for additional reading.

There is much to be gained by recognising the old adage that nothing takes place in a vacuum and this is particularly relevant to health-care provision. Whilst there are many local influences on the way that district nursing is carried out, for example local health care initiatives, the forces that drive decision making at local level are often influenced and shaped by a much wider arena. This is frequently referred to as the context in which care takes place. The main purpose of this chapter, therefore, is to explore the context in which district nursing takes place, particularly in relation to policy development and political ideology.

THE PROVISION OF HEALTH CARE

The provision of health care along with education is an area fraught with problems regardless of the political party in power, largely because it accounts for a massive part of government expenditure and there are many different views not only as to how the money should be spent but also the standard and type and amount of care to be made available. Since the NHS was founded by a Labour government in 1948, the government of the day has been viewed by many to be the sole provider of health care. It is therefore not surprising that in times of perceived shortage in the service, the public looks to the government not only to address the problem but also to pay for its resolution.

Daintith & Isaacs (1990) demonstrate this point neatly.

The twentieth century will be remembered chiefly, not as an age of political conflicts and technical inventions, but as an age in which human society dared to think of the health of the whole human race as a practical objective.

This quotation leads to the view that it is not only politics in themselves which ultimately shape health-care provision but raises the pertinent question as to whether a system of health care which is all embracing is in reality a viable option. Many of the opinions relevant to this are reflected in the individuals' beliefs and values or, put very loosely, their ideology, which will be identified later in this chapter.

THE BRITISH ECONOMY

Britain is a capitalist economy which by its nature is dependent on the market place to produce and distribute goods and services. Robertson (1993) defines capitalism as:

any economic system where there is a combination of private property, a relatively free and competitive market and a general assumption that the bulk of the workforce will be engaged in employment by private (non-governmental) employers engaged in producing whatever goods they can sell for profit.

The implications for health of a 'free-wheeling' capitalist system were, according to Marxists, inequality, exploitation and conflict. These, according to Baggott (1994), were clearly apparent during the 19th century when there was widespread material deprivation and poverty. The standard of care which different classes received was also unequal, largely because it was market based. Implicit in this is the fact that people received only the care and treatment that they could afford.

It could, however, be argued that since the Second World War a mixed economy has developed with certain key functions owned and managed by the state (the public sector). One of the key requirements of an economy dependent on its workforce is that the workforce is healthy. This is because the economy is dependent upon it in terms of the work it is able to undertake and, equally as importantly, the resources to pay for state welfare provision. In an economy such as Britain's there is a need for flexibility of the workforce as the evolution of different types of work requires different skills. In order to maintain this flexibility and the possible resulting swings in unemployment, state benefits need to be at a sufficient level to support people in times of need.

It was with these factors in mind that, following the Second World War, there was a recognition that it was not always possible for individuals to protect themselves from the many vagaries which impacted on their health and a support system was required to assist them in times of need. From this, a national welfare state system was created and the National Health Service was established as part of the development of the new welfare state on the principles shown in Box 3.1 (Fatchett 1994).

THE NATURE OF POLITICS

Historically, politics is an area in which district nurses have had very little involvement other than at the 'sharp end' of community care when the availability of resources may not have been what was required to implement the care. The increase in political issues in pre- and post registration curricula, however, has led to a much greater understanding of the politics of health care and how nurses can best influence them. The relevance of politics to nursing was also enhanced by the election of the first two nurse Members of Parliament, Laura Moffat and Anne Keen, on 1 May 1997. Indeed, if the future of the nursing profession is to be secured and an equitable standard of care provided for patients, nurses must become more aware at every level of politics (Masterson & Maslin-Prothero 1999).

It has been argued that politics have arisen out of conflict and that if everyone held the same beliefs and behaved in the same way, there would be no need for their existence (Gough et al 1994). This is a very appealing thought, not only for district nurses as one of the major providers of care in the community but all individuals involved in health-care provision. Certainly, conflict has a profound impact on the way that care is delivered.

The fact that there is such a multiplicity of individuals and groups within society, each wanting different things, makes the question of how the country is governed extremely complex. A clear example of this is the conflict in opinion which frequently exists when new hospitals (particularly those for patients suffering from mental health problems) are to be built. Clearly, if anarchy is not to prevail, then conflicts must be managed and resolved peaceably. Implicit within this is the need for a system which will enable decisions to be taken. In Britain, this system is political (Butler 1992).

THE FUNCTION OF POLITICAL PARTIES

Political parties are the core of the political system in Britain but other organisations also impact on political activity. In relation to health care, professions, professional organisations and trades unions will put forward their political views and demands and can potentially have a major impact on the development of health-care provision.

The nursing workforce remains very much a 'sleeping giant'. Its huge size (over 500 000 people in the UK have trained as nurses, most of whom are women) means that nurses have enormous potential as agents of social change and promoting health and wellbeing. It does not take too much to imagine what the impact might be if over half a million people become empowered, assertive and articulate agents of change for better health. (RCN 1999)

The primary function of the political parties is to ensure that there is competition of potential leaders in the House of Commons to give the electorate a choice at general elections. The chain of responsibility between the electorate, Cabinet of elected members and Parliament is fundamental to British parliamentary democracy. Implicit in the function of the British government is the need to gain and maintain public consent through the voting system in order for them to exercise power. Political parties also have additional functions (Box 3.2).

Political parties have one primary function and a number of subsidiary functions which assist in the running of the political system in Britain. The primary function is the acquisition

---

Box 3.1   The principles on which the NHS was established

- It aimed to cover the whole of the population.
- It aimed to provide equal access to people in need of health care.
- It was free at the point of use.
- It was comprehensive in cover.
- It was to provide services of a good standard for everyone.
- It was based on notions of public service.
- It aimed to be egalitarian in ethos.
- It aimed to treat individual patients with respect as persons in the collective interest.

Box 3.2   Political parties – additional functions (Forman & Baldwin 1996)

- The provision of a framework in which the public can participate in political processes.
- The reflection of a wide range of interests and views of the population.
- The provision of legitimate frameworks for the debate of political issues, largely through their annual conferences.
- The organisation of political campaigns at local, national and international level.
- The increase in membership and fundraising.

and retention of a mandate from the public that affords them the power to govern and the secondary functions are those relating to the development of local and national initiatives.

Britain has often been described as having a two-party system of government as only the Labour and Conservative parties have formed governments since 1945. As a result, more recent health-care policy has been developed on the ideologies of these two parties.

POLITICAL IDEOLOGY

Ideology is a concept frequently used but one that is very difficult to define. It is open to many interpretations in both academic and everyday circles. A workable definition is that of a 'world view' which includes an individual's perception of the social world and incorporates both its substance and how it works. Ideologies are often described as being highly relative and subjective in that they are in some way shaped by our life experiences and our social and class position (Robertson 1993). Ideology is also a word frequently used within the social sciences and as a result has the potential for many different interpretations. For the purpose of this chapter, ideology is defined as 'a complete and self-consistent set of attitudes, moral views, empirical beliefs and even rules of logical discourse and scientific testing' (Robertson 1993).

Kingdom (1991, p. 192) argues that, 'The most common basis for distinguishing parties ideologically is in terms of a left–right dichotomy'. This tends to parallel the distinction between collectivism (all members of society work together for the common good) and individualism (people only look after themselves). Put very simply, in relation to the Labour and Conservative parties, Labour would be on the left of the continuum and the Conservatives would be on the right.

Whilst the NHS was based on collectivist ideology, it is important to note that the notion of collectivism is not always easy to apply in relation to health-care provision. For example, some parents would probably pay to have developmental checks carried out on their children in order to safeguard their future health and others would

not. By the same token, if all sick and disabled people were required to meet the total cost of their own care a substantial number would be unable to raise the necessary funds. As a result it is incumbent on whoever is in power to ensure that resources are available by other means, for example the state, private or voluntary provision.

It is equally important to note that ideas and beliefs are not formulated in a vacuum and are dependent on many extraneous factors, in particular life experiences and social developments throughout history. As a result, whilst political ideologies are the 'starting block' for political action they will inevitably change over time and in recent years it could be argued that there has been much more 'meeting in the middle' of the major political parties in terms of their ideologies.

The political ideologies of the Conservative and Labour parties have dominated since the inception of the NHS. It is therefore necessary to discuss these two political perspectives here, as their particular ideologies form the basis for the developments in health-care provision and ultimately the ways in which district nurses are required to work.

The Conservative party

A fundamental belief of the Conservative party is that the state should not be the main vehicle in achieving improvements in society. Whilst recognising it has a part to play, it encourages the individual attributes of initiative, competition and choice. Implicit in this is:

- that individual ability should be rewarded. A natural progression from this is that the acquisition of wealth should not be discouraged
- the development of private health care is essential as it provides individuals with the choice to dispose of their individual wealth as they so wish.

The basic view of conservatism as defined by Thatcherism is that economic activity will be increased by minimum state interference. As a result, a free market will develop (Dowding 1996). This is achievable by three methods (Box 3.3).

> **Box 3.3** Three methods for developing a free market
>
> - Controlling NHS inflation by controlling the supply of money.
> - Controlling of the professions and unions. If these can be controlled then the demands they make in terms of pay awards and procedures are severely limited.
> - Faith in the free market and the ability of employers to operate it.

Heywood (1992) argues that 'Conservatism is neither simple pragmatism nor mere opportunism. It is based on a particular set of political beliefs about human beings, the societies they live in, and the importance of a distinctive set of political values'. It is certainly these values which led to the Conservatives' strong opposition to the Labour government's implementation of the National Health Service in 1948.

The Labour party

The Labour party was founded on the viewpoints of two different groups: first, those who were concerned with defensive matters, for example improving the pay and conditions of working people, and second, those who wanted a socialist society. The main argument of socialism is that it is opposed to an economy in private hands that runs purely for profit. It offers a different explanation of capitalism as identified by the Conservatives, which is based on self-interest and competition, viewing it as creating high inequalities in wealth and power. Socialism can be defined as 'a political and economic theory of social organisation which advocates that the community as a whole should own and control the means of production, distribution and exchange' (Robbins 1987).

According to Klein (1995), there were four key principles underpinning the inception of the NHS: comprehensiveness, equality, universality and collectivism. It is perhaps useful to consider the extent to which these principles are present in today's health-care provision, particularly when set against successive governments' well-publicised commitment to the principles of the NHS. There are many competing arguments which

> **Box 3.4** Arguments why the current ideology may be at an end
>
> - Demand will always outstrip supply. There will always be new technology and treatments. The recent publicity regarding the prescribing of Viagra is a good clear example of this.
> - The current system is selective in terms of accessibility of care and treatment. Treatment by 'postcode' prevails whereby individuals receive treatment dependent on whether their particular NHS trust deems it a priority.
> - Individuals providing health care are unable to meet need.
> - Politicians are being set up to fail. For example, they are agreeing to reduce waiting lists when in fact it is merely shifting resources from an area which is also in need of funding.

> **Box 3.5** Arguments why the current ideology will continue
>
> - Health-care provision is fundamental to our beliefs as a caring society.
> - As a member of a civilised society every individual has a right to health care.
> - There is a need to care for the most vulnerable

may be used to signal that the future of the current health-care system is uncertain (Boxes 3.4 and 3.5).

Other methods of funding have not been explored; for example, increasing taxation to be spent specifically on health care. However, political parties need to consider the impact that this would have on their successful election. It is perhaps not surprising that they are unwilling to 'raise their head above the parapet' by implying either overtly or covertly that if the public requires a comprehensive and dynamic health service then the public is going to have to pay for it by a substantial increase in taxes.

POLITICS AND HEALTH-CARE POLICY

The notion of social policy is closely linked to the existence of the welfare state which means that providing welfare services for the population is the responsibility of government. The foundation of the NHS in 1948, which established a system of largely free health care for everyone paid for mainly out of taxation, set up Britain as a pioneer in welfare. It is interesting to note, however, that the level of spending on welfare in the United Kingdom is now less than in comparable advanced industrial societies although 'the composition of the spending is close to the international average' (Klein 1995, p. 566).

Spending on welfare is, along with comparable countries, by far the largest part of public expenditure in the United Kingdom. It is unlikely that this will change essentially for two reasons. First, virtually the whole of the population has a stake in welfare services and it is on this basis that votes (and elections) can be lost and won. The public sector is also a major employer with an influential vote. Second, the political parties which have dominated British politics throughout the 20th century have all, albeit in different ways, viewed the state as a source of welfare.

Throughout the 20th century social policy has proved to be one of the greatest headaches for successive governments not only because of the factors already identified above but also because it potentially involves the whole of the population and their rights to access benefits. It is also difficult to deliver welfare services which are true to the ideology of equal access and provision as they are, by their nature, extremely complex and also potentially without limit.

The *Concise Oxford Dictionary* (1995) defines policy as 'a course of action or principle adopted or proposed by a government, party, individual, etc.'. In relation to health-care provision, Klein (1995) develops this further and provides a very comprehensive definition: 'Welfare policy making is about choices concerning the welfare services in a community, about their range, about how they should be paid for, about how they should be delivered and about who should benefit from the welfare state'. This supports the notion that regardless of the political party in power, policy development is closely entwined with the welfare state and also regardless of the party in power, the population looks to the government of the day to pay for and in most instances to actually provide the services which are required.

As previously identified, the political party which takes up government also governs the process of policy making, but the process is much more complex. The fact that political parties may share similar ideology does not necessarily mean that they share the same views. This is evident in instances where Members of Parliament vote against their own party on certain issues or may in extremes 'defect' to a different political party.

In addition to this, there are many groups who wish to influence the way policy is developed from a national perspective. For example, legislation regarding employment of the disabled could involve input from many different groups with a specific interest.

In recent years much of health-care policy development has centred around cost reduction or at the very least making better use of available resources. A clear example of this type of policy development is health-care NHS trust mergers. On face value, it would appear sensible to implement systems which effectively reduce management costs by combining roles or indeed bringing together duplicated services. It has been argued, however, that the evidence to support widespread mergers is in extremely short supply. Edwards & Passman (1997) claim that it is not always possible to identify the specific problems mergers are meant to address. Probably highest on the list is cost reduction but clearly this needs to be explored alongside other essential issues. For example, what are the likely costs of redundancy packages and, equally as important, what is the cost of the improved communications systems required in order for the merger to function effectively?

PATIENT/CLIENT EMPOWERMENT

At a macro level patient empowerment needs to consider the whole nature of power, government function and the ideas and beliefs which underpin decision making. Implicit in this is their contribution to the shaping of health-care policy.

The terms 'empowerment' and 'autonomy' in health care could be argued to be inextricably linked. For example, if individuals are enabled to

---

Box 3.6   Issues surrounding patient empowerment

- Patient empowerment assumes that individuals and communities wish to take control.
- It is something which is 'bestowed' on the patient. For example, the nurse is the enabler to the patient becoming empowered.
- There is no clarity in terms of what the patient is being empowered to do.
- It is incumbent on the professionals to decide who they will empower.
- Empowerment, by its nature, must be set within the existing health-care structures.

Box 3.7   Arguments for and against the value of devolution

Positive
- The result of devolution makes provision more sensitive to local need.
- Eradicates unnecessary decision-making machinery and bureaucracy.
- Enables local people to voice opinions on local issues.
- Enables local people to decide the amount of money they wish to pay for essential services.

Negative
- Administrative costs are multiplied for essential services.
- It may cause friction regarding resource allocation.
- It does not provide the populations of each of the countries with an equal say in each other's affairs.
- It may weaken the United Kingdom's position in Europe as each country may have different or opposing views.

---

make certain decisions regarding health care then it also means that they have the ultimate responsibility for the specific course of action they choose. However, the extent to which empowerment is attainable within a health-care system is open to debate (Fatchett 1998). The main reasons for this are shown in Box 3.6 (Masterson & Maslin-Prothero 1999).

It is also interesting to note that a dichotomy exists in the professional language used about patient involvement. Although our current health-care system seeks to 'empower patients and clients', at the same time they are berated for their lack of 'compliance'.

However, it could be argued that if the care we provide is to be fully effective then patients must be involved in that care. This view is supported by Johnstone (1993) who states that:

For community care to succeed and for vulnerable people and their carers to exercise real choice in where and how they live, depends not only on the commitment of professionals to new ways of working, but a power shift away from providers to service users.

The importance of patient, client and carer involvement continues to be a main focus of policy development in the government's strategic intentions for nursing, midwifery and health visiting. It is important to note, however, that the quest for a comprehensive health-care system, which attempts to make the most appropriate use of resources with patients at its heart, is not new to the current Labour government. In 1987, the then Conservative government had a difficult time in relation to allocation of money as doctors vied for funds for their own specialities. This is clearly identified in the government's Green Papers of the time, which all promoted the empowerment of individuals to make decisions regarding their own health as opposed to having decisions made for them by professionals.

DEVOLUTION

The word 'devolution', when applied politically, involves transferring power from central government to a lower or regional level. The purpose is to enable countries, regions or localities to decide on their own priorities and fund them according to their own choices. The process of devolution was first debated in the United Kingdom in the late 1970s when proposals were made to establish separate assemblies for Scotland and Wales with each country holding power over its own internal affairs.

Both positive and negative arguments have been put forward on the value of the devolution process as outlined in Box 3.7.

Devolution is of course crucial to the future development of health-care policy. For example, the government's White Paper on its proposals for a Welsh Assembly stated that 'a directly elected Assembly will assume responsibility for policies and public services currently exercised by the Secretary of State for Wales' (*Times Higher Education Supplement* 12 September 1997, p. 4). In terms of health-care policy, this could effectively provide a different agenda from that of England, Scotland or Northern Ireland. The situation regarding nurse education across the four countries is equally as interesting. Agreements with other European countries render it possible for nurses to take up posts across Europe (in theory at least); however, differences in policy in the four countries could effectively mean that a nurse could enter Europe to work but not necessarily England, Wales or Northern Ireland. The debate is just beginning but clearly close collaboration will be essential.

Scotland now has its own law-making Parliament. In relation to health-care provision, it has the power to pass laws on health, education, social work, housing and economic development and the environment. In relation to health specifically, it has responsibility for the NHS in Scotland which will include public and mental health. It includes the terms and conditions of NHS staff and GPs and also the education and training of health-care professionals. One of the key differences that devolution makes is that individual countries can tailor their resources to the specific health-care needs of their people.

CURRENT POLICY DEVELOPMENT

The changes in health-care policy identified by the Labour government in the last two years need to be set against profound economic changes, largely brought about as a result of the factors shown in Box 3.8.

Public expectations continue to rise. In their daily lives people are no longer ready to tolerate waiting for services. 24 hour shopping and direct line services mean instant access is the norm. People want accessible health care, delivered promptly and to a uniformly high standard. (DoH 1999)

To address these issues, the government has developed a variety of methods with which to make the services more responsive to individual need.

Box 3.8 Economic changes

- Much less job security. This is apparent within both the health-care system and society at large. In health care specifically there are many examples of restructuring and the subsequent removal of management posts.
- The increase in single parents and the concomitant increase in the number of women undertaking paid work.
- A huge increase in the numbers of people accessing the benefits system, due in part to the increase in households who have no one in employment.
- Increase in demand for pensions for the elderly as the number of people reaching pensionable age increases.
- Increase in people's expectations regarding the type and quality of services available.

CONCLUSION

It has been stated that politics is a 'legitimate part of nursing knowledge' (Masterson & Maslin-Prothero 1999). It could, however, be argued that politics is not only legitimate but essential if district nurses are to shape the future of their own profession and have an important place in the development of patient/client care. In order to do both of these things, an understanding of the different political agendas is crucial.

As identified in previous chapters, the government's nursing strategies for England, Wales and Northern Ireland pose major and interesting challenges for the future of nursing. In addition, the pace of change of health-care provision since the inception of the current Labour government makes it imperative that district nurses do not view issues that affect them or their patients and clients in isolation from the 'big picture'. The development of *A higher level of practice* by the UKCC (1999) is a clear example of this, as implicit in the need to recognise practitioners working at a higher level of practice is the need to assess the impact this development will ultimately have on pay and manpower planning. These are two issues that will always remain at the heart of any government's future plans.

Finally, and on a positive note, we live in a world where the powers of communication are increasing at an unprecedented rate. Most major national health and social care policy documents can be accessed and downloaded from the Internet, making it likely that district nurses in the future will have a much greater opportunity to gain information and ultimately influence the political agenda

REFERENCES

Baggott R 1994 Health and health care in Britain. Macmillan, London

Butler J 1992 Patients, policies and politics: before and after Working for Patients. Open University Press, Buckingham

Daintith J, Isaacs A 1990 Collins reference dictionary of medical quotations. Collins, Glasgow, p. 87

Department of Health 1999 Making a difference. Strengthening the nursing, midwifery and health visiting contribution to health and health care. Department of Health, London

Dowding K 1996 Power. Open University Press, Buckingham

Edwards N, Passman D 1997 All mixed up. Health Service Journal 12 June: 30–31

Fatchett A 1994 Politics, policy and nursing. Baillière Tindall, London

Fatchett A 1998 Nursing in the new NHS: modern, dependable? Baillière Tindall, Edinburgh

Forman F N, Baldwin N D J 1996 Mastering British politics. Macmillan, Basingstoke

Gough P, Maslin-Prothero S, Masterson A 1994 Nursing and social policy: care in context. Butterworth-Heinemann, Oxford

Heywood A 1992 Political ideologies: an introduction. Macmillan Education, Basingstoke

Johnstone C 1993 The reality for community nurses. Primary Health Care Journal 3(4): 10–12

Kingdom J 1991 Government and politics in Britain. An introduction. Polity Press Blackwell, Cambridge, Massachusetts

Klein R 1995 The new politics of the NHS, 3rd edn. Longman, Harlow

Masterson A, Maslin-Prothero S 1999 Nursing and politics: power through practice. Churchill Livingstone, London

Robbins L 1987 Politics and policy-making in Britain. Longman, New York

Robertson D 1993 A dictionary of modern politics, 2nd edn. Europa Publications, London

Royal College of Nursing 1999 Imagining the future: nursing in the new millennium. A summary report of the views of nurses involved in the RCN Futures Project. RCN, London

UKCC 1999 A higher level of practice. UKCC, London

FURTHER READING

Parliament Publishing Services, Central Office of Information 1996 Aspects of Britain. HMSO, London
This book is one of a series which, overall, explore the different facets of politics and policy development. This particular book provides a factual briefing and describes the functions and workings of the House of Commons and House of Lords. It also outlines the growth of parliamentary government over the centuries.

Fatchett A 1998 Nursing in the new NHS: modern, dependable? Baillière Tindall, London
This book provides a clear interpretation of the context in which nursing currently takes place. It traces the many changes in the health service in recent years and explores issues relevant to them.

Robertson D 1993 A dictionary of modern politics, 2nd edn. Europa Publications, London
A very useful guide to the complex terminology that surrounds the world of politics in an easy-to-read format.

Masterson A, Maslin-Prothero S 1999 Nursing and politics: power through practice. Churchill Livingstone, London
This is essential reading for anyone who wants anything more than a very superficial overview of politics as they apply to nursing. It provides a very practical approach to the role of political parties, political structures and power, supported by questions for discussion.

4

Multiprofessional working

Fiona Redworth Dianne Watkins

Key points

- Definitions
- Primary health-care team
- Teamworking
- Team development
- Team descriptions
- Interdisciplinary collaboration

INTRODUCTION

The importance of multiprofessional working has emerged as a recurring theme in district nursing. It is important that district nurses understand the principles of teamworking and how barriers to effective teamwork can be overcome. In this chapter, a model of collaboration will be advanced to demonstrate effective strategies for teamwork in primary care.

DEFINITIONS

There seems to be a great deal of literature available which seeks to answer the question 'What is multiprofessional working?'. Yet, the one thing that is clear from this abundance of accessible literature is that there is some confusion about the definition of terms used to describe teamwork in the community. These terms, which include *interprofessional*, *interdisciplinary* and *multiprofessional teamwork* and *collaboration*, are often used indiscriminately and interchangeably. It seems appropriate then to start the chapter by considering what is meant by the term 'multiprofessional working', how this varies from some of the other terminology outlined above and where the district nurse fits in to such definitions. From reviewing the literature the following definitions emerge.

Interprofessional suggests that there is some sharing of work and specialised knowledge amongst personnel from different professional groups. The key here is about relinquishing professional authority, breaking down boundaries and working together towards common goals. This, Øvretveit (1996) believes, requires a high level of integration, where the team members' 'work and clinical decisions are governed by multidisciplinary policies and by group decisions made at team meetings'.

There are few examples which can be drawn from practice to illustrate this approach to primary health care. Some attempts to work as an interdisciplinary team are made in vignette 4.1.

Here is an example of staff in the team beginning to forego professional authority through the idea of a rotating chairperson. Whilst it might be argued that this is tokenistic in nature, the team see it as a positive move towards interprofessionalism. The team have established some common goals in terms of accessing professional education and are demonstrating some efforts to break down boundaries, by all working on the development of a community health profile, group protocols and clinical audit.

Interdisciplinary. Here again, the emphasis is on sharing common goals but the boundaries are further diminished to embrace staff who are not affiliated to a professional group, such as voluntary workers, but whose aim is improved care for the patient or client. Breaking down boundaries between professional groups is a contentious exercise. Opening this up to people who are traditionally perceived as 'outsiders' is even more difficult to achieve. Yet, this is obviously an approach which the government believes that PHCT members should be working towards.

Multiprofessional is a venture which is based on cooperation between professionals. In this case, however, the conventional models and demarcations of professional power and knowledge are preserved. Such an approach to work, in the area of palliative care, is represented in vignette 4.2.

Vignette 4.1   The interprofessional team

The staff of the Pwll Glas PHCT are all based in new, purpose-built premises which are owned by the NHS trust. The nursing team comprises two part-time practice nurses, one full-time health visitor and a district nursing team of three. Lisa, the district nursing sister, acts as a community practice teacher and therefore there is also a district nurse student attached to her team. There are three general practitioners (GPs) in the team and, as this is a training practice, one trainee GP. The team members believe that they are committed to the education of professionals. As well as training other staff, the practitioners take every opportunity to pursue further education openings. At present, one of the GPs, one of the practice nurses, the district nursing sister, the health visitor and a community staff nurse are all enrolled on professional education programmes which lead to academic qualifications.

The PHCT holds fortnightly meetings at which there is a rotating chairperson who formalises the agenda, to which all team members contribute, and ensures the smooth running of the meetings.

The PHCT members are in the process of completing a health needs profile of the community. From this they plan to set annual team objectives. The team has also developed a number of group protocols and all members take part in auditing clinical practice.

Vignette 4.2   Multiprofessional working in palliative care

During a visit to a 'terminal' patient, Tina, a district nursing sister, establishes that the pain relief the patient is prescribed is not adequately controlling her pain. Tina has recently completed a palliative care course and feels confident in her ability to recommend appropriate analgesia for the GP to prescribe. Tina contacts David, the GP, and makes some suggestions to him about a new pain relief regime. David, who acknowledges that he has little experience in this field, consults his BNF and finds that Tina's recommendations are appropriate. David, however, feels reluctant to take the advice of a nurse about the prescription of controlled drugs and therefore elects to contact the medical consultant at the local hospital for guidance. The consultant confirms that Tina's recommendations are appropriate and David therefore goes ahead and makes the alterations to the patient's analgesia. Both David and Tina are satisfied with the new arrangements made for the patient.

In this vignette the traditional roles of GP and district nurse are maintained whilst ensuring that the patient receives the best care. This model of multidisciplinary working suggests restrictive patterns of operation and this is clearly the case for Tina. Nevertheless, it is apparent, from both experience and the literature, that this is the most prominent model in the primary health-care setting (Pearson & Spencer 1995, Wiles & Robison 1994).

Multidisciplinary also involves cooperation between staff but suggests that staff may be associated with groups which do not have a professional remit. This term will be examined in more detail later in the chapter.

Two commonly used suffixes are attached to the above terms and again both require definition.

Teamwork as the term suggests, involves a group of people who work together, towards common goals and objectives which, in the case of primary health care, focus on the patient. Wiles & Robison (1994) view teamwork as a contentious issue and assert that nurses do not appear to be perceived or treated as equals within primary health care. The scenario outlined in vignette 4.2 conforms to this definition.

Collaboration involves the sharing of more than common goals. It requires shared knowledge, shared values, shared responsibility, shared decision making, shared outcomes and shared visions. In a truly collaborative relationship, Henneman et al (1995) assert that power is shared and is based on knowledge and expertise rather than on role or title. This is nicely illustrated by the situation outlined in vignette 4.3.

Whilst this might seem like a simple exchange, it is important and, indeed, according to authors such as Field & West (1995), unusual in that the main attributes of collaboration are present. The district nurse and GP are working together to make a decision about patient treatment. Each professional recognises her responsibility in the process and both are able to contribute their knowledge and expertise in order to arrive at a decision.

As West & Poulton (1997) demonstrate, the reality in primary health care is that we have yet to achieve true collaboration and continue to function within a model of teamwork.

The term most frequently used within the community setting to describe teamwork in relation to health is the primary health-care team.

PRIMARY HEALTH-CARE TEAM (PHCT)

Structure

The PHCT comprises the professionals who offer first-tier health provision within a defined local community setting. Øvretveit (1996) believes that establishing the membership of the PHCT is a crucial means of drawing boundaries around the team. He suggests that the most common membership distinction is between 'core' and 'associate' members. Core members are likely to be full time in the team, governed by team policy, managed by a team leader and have formal voting rights. District nurses normally form part of the core team together with general practitioners, health visitors (HVs) and practice nurses (PNs). Other professionals, such as the social

---

Vignette 4.3 Collaborative working

DN   Hi Delyth, I have just been visiting Mrs Jones and her venous ulcer is not improving with the current treatment. I would like to start her on compression bandaging. Could you give me a prescription for her, please?

GP   Have you done a Doppler assessment on her, Enid?

DN   Yes, I have fully assessed her and she is suitable for compression treatment.

GP   Fine, I'll write that for you now. Who is going to collect it?

DN   Can one of the receptionists drop it off at the chemists so that Mr Jones can pick it up later?

GP   No problem, Caroline will be going over soon anyway.

DN   Thanks Delyth, see you later.

GP   Yeah, see you, Enid.

worker and community psychiatric nurse, are associate team members and are likely to be associated with more than one team and thus are part-time members of the team.

Function

James (1995) believes that the principal function of the PHCT is to act as the gatekeepers of health care by assessing the need for referral and access to NHS resources. Within this province, the team takes on four key functions (Box 4.1).

Box 4.1 Four key functions of the PHCT (James 1995)

1. *Clinical functions*, which relate to the professional backgrounds of the individual team members.
2. *Pastoral functions*, through responding to the wider implications of the context of care and approaching each care event holistically by supporting the family as a unit.
3. *Health promotion*, through the judicious use of health promotion models and strategies to enhance the health of the communities that they serve.
4. *Research and data collection*, in order to contribute towards the production of the data required to provide a complete service to the community.

Historical development

The term 'primary health-care team' was first mooted as early as the 1920s in the Dawson Report (Ministry of Health 1920), where using health centres to deliver care was commended. There was no real potential for primary health care to develop, however, until the rationalisation of the NHS in 1948, through the NHS Act (Ministry of Health 1946). James (1995) points out that even after this Act there was no genuine opportunity for teamworking to become a reality, and that the creation of a tripartite structure of health care did little to integrate health services in the community. The status of GPs was regarded to be inferior and their financial rewards were meagre compared to hospital doctors in the early years of the NHS.

The Gillie Report (1963) recommended the development of group practices and the affiliation of community nursing services to such practices. Yet, despite these recommendations and the introduction of the GP Charter in 1966, which allowed for reimbursement costs of ancillary staff, little progress was made in the development of PHCTs.

It was not until 1973, which saw major reforms to the NHS, that attempts were made to align community health services and general practice. Care was now organised to serve distinct geographical areas but community services and general practice continued to work independently of each other and this resulted in duplication and, indeed, omission in care.

In the early 1980s comprehensive reviews of the organisation of community nursing services in England (Cumberlege Report, DHSS 1986) and in Wales (Edwards Report, Welsh Office 1988) were undertaken and some significant recommendations relating to the delivery of the services were made.

The recommendations stemming from these reports, that the delivery of community health care and primary health care needed to be realigned, resulted in patterns of work whereby community nurses were attached to general practices. This, however, did not necessarily mean that sharing the same premises became the norm and indeed, today many community nurses are not physically based with their GP colleagues. What the changes did mean, according to Blackie (1998), was that the general practice became the basic organisational unit of primary health care.

Further legislative changes in the early 1990s, through the introduction of GP fundholding and the GP Contract, and the NHS and Community Care Act 1990 has shaped the face of primary health care. Today we see the formal attachment of community nurses to general practices, a phenomenal increase in the number of practice nurses, the development of the practice manager role and a shift in the focus of the work of the PHCT towards health needs assessment and health promotion. Although the individuals who have been swept along by the changes do not always welcome these, it is clear that PHCTs have now reached a situation where real collaborative work within the team becomes a possibility.

It is not pessimistic, though, to entitle this chapter 'Multiprofessional Working'. Rather, it seems that this reflects reality in terms of the patterns of working to which district nurses subscribe as a result of historical developments and team dynamics. Multiprofessional working thus forms a baseline from which we can all develop to form the type of PHCTs which documents such as *Primary care: the way forward in Wales* (Welsh Office 1996) and *Primary care: the way ahead* (Scottish Office 1996) encourage us to aspire to.

TEAMWORKING

The second part of this chapter reviews the principles of teamwork and identifies barriers to team members working effectively together. It will outline the key roles and skills required for teams to achieve success in working towards identified aims. In addition, it will also address the processes involved in building a team and will describe practical methods which will develop and facilitate teams towards working cohesively in the delivery of care to patients.

Principles of effective teamworking

Teams and how they function have become a popular area for research in both industry and the National Health Service. This has resulted in identification of 'principles of effective team working' which are outlined in Box 4.2.

Guzzo & Shea (1992) expand on these principles and, through a review of research-based evidence on team-working, make recommendations for the development of effective teams.

Box 4.2 Principles of effective teamworking (Pritchard 1995)

1. Team members share a common goal.
2. Each member has a clear understanding of the role and function of other team members and understands the contribution others can make.
3. The team pools knowledge and takes responsibility for outcomes.
4. The effectiveness of the team relates to its capacity to self-manage and become interdependent.

Principle 1

In relation to principle 1, Guzzo & Shea discuss the importance of not only sharing a common goal but also receiving feedback on one's individual performance when working towards achievement of the team goals. This motivates individuals within the team to work towards common objectives and thus the overall performance of the team is enhanced. Lack of common goals, aims or objectives was found to be a major stumbling block in PHCT members working together (West & Poulton 1997).

Principle 2

The second principle refers to knowing the role and skills of others within the team and respecting that all members have an equal contribution to make. Guzzo & Shea (1992) explain that all members must feel they are important to the success of the team and that their personal role is indispensable and essential to the team. People are then more likely to give their best knowing their input is appreciated by other team members. West & Poulton (1997) state, 'In primary health-care teams it is rare for individual contributions to be measured and feedback on performance given'. This obviously represents an area for development in relation to helping teams to function more effectively.

Principle 3

Expansion on the third principle, the pooling of knowledge and taking responsibility for outcomes, is discussed by Guzzo & Shea (1992) as the need for information sharing and built-in performance feedback. Team members need to illustrate the work they are involved with so it becomes visible to other team members.

Principle 4

Principle 4, the capacity to self-manage and become interdependent, relates to the ability to problem solve as a team. The more interesting and challenging the tasks, the more committed and motivated team members generally become

---

Vignette 4.4 Sue's story

Sue is a district nurse who works on a geographical basis. Her case load covers part of an inner-city area in South Wales. This area spans three PHCTs (general practices A, B and C) and whenever possible Sue tries to attend primary care meetings in the three different practices.

Sue finds great difficulty in identifying the goals each of the practices work towards. Practice A believes coronary heart disease (CHD) is a major problem and would like district nursing involvement, practice B is asking her to become more involved in the management of diabetes and practice C has no agenda and usually discusses case management of individual patients.

There is some discussion regarding how Sue could become involved with coronary heart disease but the team seem to be unclear as to what aspect they wish Sue to become involved with. Sue makes the point that CHD is a huge area and asks whether it is primary, secondary or tertiary prevention they would like her to take on. The team begin to disagree on what they believe to be the most important areas. Sue outlines her current practice in relation to CHD. No one seems to listen and Sue does not receive any feedback on what she is currently doing. It

seems the practice are concerned only with her undertaking more work as the practice nurse has recently resigned. Sue feels undervalued and demoralised.

Practice B asks Sue to become more involved with diabetes care. Sue outlines her current home visiting role with this group of patients but the general practitioner is keen for her to run a 'nurse-led' diabetic clinic in the surgery. Sue explains she does not feel adequately prepared to take on this role and expresses the need for further training. The GP advises her to go to the community trust to gain funding for a diabetic course. However, study leave is currently 'on hold' in the trust due to financial constraints. The GP continues to apply pressure on Sue to undertake this role and refuses to discuss the issue further.

Practice C continues to discuss individual patients as and when the need arises and Sue feels her work with practice C is reactive and not proactive.

The scenario outlined above highlights the problems district nurses face when trying to implement the principles of effective teamworking as a member of several PHCTs.

Box 4.3 Basic requirements for effective teamworking (West 1994)

- *Task effectiveness* – the extent to which a team is successful in achieving its task-related objectives
- *Mental health* – the well-being, growth and development of team members
- *Team viability* – the probability that a team will continue to work together and function effectively

---

(Guzzo & Shea 1992). The levels of participation which takes place between team members relate to how effectively the team is able to function. This has been examined by West & Poulton (1997) through observation of team members' participation in decision making and the frequency of team members' interaction. Observation of PHCTs revealed that conflict was often present between team members and other studies demonstrate that health visitors and midwives are commonly the least integrated members of the team (Wiles & Robison 1994). This is demonstrated in vignette 4.4.

The issues raised in vignette 4.4 clearly illustrate how the basic requirements for effective teamworking are not in place. There is no clarity of goals or tasks, there is little thought for the

well-being and personal development of the district nurse and the level of communication and participation between team members is limited. Basic requirements for effective team working are described by West (1994) and illustrated in Box 4.3.

Barriers to effective teamworking

Some of the barriers to effective teamworking have been raised earlier in the chapter when outlining the principles of effective teamworking. Barriers which can prevent team members from working together in the arena of primary care will now be expanded upon and summarised under the following headings:

- team composition
- managerial and professional accountability
- communication patterns
- roles and responsibilities
- team aim and purpose.

Team composition

Lack of clarity as to who forms part of the 'team' is one of the most fundamental barriers to teams functioning well (Øvretveit 1993, West 1994). This is a common problem in primary care as a variety of people may work directly from a general practice setting and consider themselves important members of the team, whilst other workers may contribute to the delivery of primary care but not use the general practice as a work base, and may or may not think they should be part of the team.

Box 4.4 would be an example of a 'core' PHCT. However, other professionals who would be involved in primary care provision but may not be practice based would include the midwife, the community psychiatric nurse, the social worker, the community learning disability nurse, etc. These individuals may or may not be regarded as core members of the team. Vignette 4.5 is a practical illustration of this.

Another factor which would influence decisions regarding team composition would be consideration of team size, as this has been identified as an important variable in determining team functioning (Stott 1993, West 1994). Belbin (1981) believes that in terms of team size, 10 should be a maximum number and three a minimum number. He states that somewhere in between these two numbers may represent the ideal.

Some authors comment on the impossible situation PHCTs may find themselves in as often the general practice and its attached staff will comprise many more than 10 members. This can make meetings difficult to handle (West 1994) and the principles of effective teamworking outlined previously difficult to achieve. The team may become less flexible as it grows larger and individual members may become more protective of their roles (Øvretveit 1993, Stott 1993).

A major problem for team composition in primary care relates to the inability for team members to choose new members according to personal characteristics which may 'fit' with the personalities of existing members. Many teams inherit individuals with whom they may have a personality clash or who have very different philosophies of working. Obviously the quality of teamworking is enhanced by the ingredients it is made up of. Rarely do PHCTs have the luxury of starting from scratch and choosing each member of their team according to the professional and personal contribution they would offer. Incompatibility between team members can be problematic.

Managerial and professional accountability

Different lines of management accountability can lead to conflict in teams, as each team member strives to meet the objectives set by the organisation for which they work. This, combined with meeting personal objectives in relation to individual performance review or personal development plans, can lead to confusion in also trying

---

Box 4.4 Examples of practice-based staff who could form a team

- Receptionists
- Practice manager
- General practitioners
- Practice nurses
- Health visitors
- District nurses

Vignette 4.5 Team composition

The district nurse has recently had reason to contact the community psychiatric nurse regarding a lady who has suffered from depression and hypertension for many years. The district nurse has been monitoring her blood pressure but feels that the lady has mental health needs which she is not able to meet.

The health visitor also contacts the CPN regarding a lady who she believes has postnatal depression.

The general practitioner also approaches the CPN in relation to a client with long-standing schizophrenia whose carers are not coping well with his recent relapse.

The CPN is not currently considered part of the 'core' PHCT although, as illustrated above, much of his work is carried out in the primary care setting.

For teams to work effectively a choice needs to be made regarding team composition. This decision in itself can lead to professional rivalry and immediate difficulties in communicating and collaborating across multiprofessional boundaries.

to meet team objectives. These structural barriers associated with diverse lines of management and different lines of accountability impact on team functioning (Jones-Elwyn & Stott 1994).

Lines of accountability for district nurses may be:

- NHS community trust
- primary health-care team
- district nursing team.

District nurses are usually employed by the local NHS community health trust and staff are often allocated to teams without any involvement from other members of the PHCT. This situation is probably changing and general practice staff are becoming more involved in recruitment of community trust staff. However, a reciprocal arrangement in relation to recruitment of general practice employed staff and involvement of community trust employees is usually absent. There is a distinct lack of control over those professionals who make up the wider membership of the team, such as social workers, and methods of working with individuals which overcomes these barriers is important to achieve.

Working to different 'protocols of care' devised by the various organisations involved in primary care can lead to conflict (Jones-Elwyn & Stott 1994, Øvretveit 1993, Pearson 1994). An example of these difficulties can be illustrated through wound care management, outlined in vignette 4.6.

Jones-Elwyn et al (1998) discuss whether individual team members are accountable to their line manager or to the team. This issue requires clarification for teams to be able to function effectively.

Communication patterns

District nurses and health visitors report the problems of teamworking as being associated with poor communication. A study by McClure (1984) found the main communication which occurred between members of the PHCT related to specific immediate patient problems and team objectives or strategies for teamworking were not discussed. This is confirmed in a study by Armstrong et al (1994) which identified that practice nurses were more concerned with task substitution than with working as a team.

Poor communication is one of the most frequently quoted reasons contributing to team ineffectiveness (Chaudry-Lawton et al 1992). As the team becomes larger, so these problems are likely to increase. An example of this is given in vignette 4.7.

District nurses communicate with a variety of professionals and non-professionals in planning packages of care. It is essential that all forms of communication, including written, verbal and telephone methods, are clear and concise at all times. Working as a member of a team involves observing the non-verbal behaviour of other

---

Vignette 4.6 Helen's story

Helen is a district nurse working to the trust protocol on wound care management. However, the team at the practice have decided to work with a community pharmacist to devise a 'practice protocol' on the best products to use in the treatment of wounds. The general practitioner is keen to reduce the financial burden associated with the numerous wound care products used in the surgery and this is a major factor affecting the decisions made.

Helen is confused regarding which protocol she should follow and feels the practice is dictated by finance rather than the most effective wound care products. She has reviewed the research evidence associated with the different products available and is sure of what products she would wish to use. This is reflected in the trust protocols. Helen ensures her own practice adheres to trust protocol and is research based.

However, when patients visit the practice nurse the products are frequently changed. Helen tries to discuss this issue with the general practitioner and with the practice nurse, to little avail. Both practitioners feel they are following a protocol of care and neither wishes to back down.

This illustrates an example of poor teamworking and confusion between managerial and professional accountability.

Ideally, a joint protocol developed by both parties would facilitate teamworking and improve continuity of patient care.

team members, active listening and meaningful dialogue. The full meaning of dialogue is not always understood. It should not be seen as something which 'naturally' takes place as a process of problem solving. True dialogue should fulfil the definition offered by Buber (1914) as 'a mode of exchange between human beings in which there is a true turning to one another, and a full appreciation of another not as an object in a social function, but as a genuine being' (cited in Senge et al 1994).

The above definition of dialogue includes a 'mutual respect' which accompanies good communication patterns. Research suggests this element is often missing from teams in primary care (Poulton 1995). Some authors suggest gender differences may exacerbate this situation. This difficulty, accompanied by deep-rooted professional divisions, is counterproductive to achieving mutual respect between team members (West 1994).

Vignette 4.7 Communication issues

The district nurse has received a discharge referral from the hospital for a 60 year old man who has suffered an acute myocardial infarction. He is said to be feeling anxious and is also hypertensive. The district nurse is asked to check his blood pressure.

On visiting the gentleman, the district nurse finds the practice nurse in the home. The patient has been referred to her through the hospital cardiac rehabilitation service which has been linking with general practice.

The patient is surprised to find two nurses visiting him and states that the general practitioner called earlier that morning to enquire after his health.

This demonstrates poor communication between members of the PHCT. The district nurse was not aware of the links with the practice on cardiac rehabilitation and feels it was an overlap of nursing activity for both herself and the practice nurse to visit.

Roles and responsibilities

Midwives and health visitors have been identified as team members who are the least integrated. A study by Wiles & Robison (1994) reports the problems of teamworking being associated with misunderstandings about individual roles and responsibilities. Other research outlines the problems associated with understanding and respecting the roles of other members of the team. Historically, general practitioners appear to understand the role of the district nurse better than that of the health visitor (Bond et al 1985) and the status of team members has been identified as a major stumbling block in effective teamworking. It is often assumed that general practitioners become the team leader, although they may have had little preparation for such a role (West & Pillinger 1996). Jones-Elwyn et al (1998) write, 'The team is in danger of becoming an unmanageable arena of professional conflicts, struggling to provide an ever more fragmented service'. There are a limited number of teams working in primary care who have received training to carry out such a role. This problem is exacerbated by professionals who undertake separate pre- and post-registration training and education. It therefore becomes difficult for team members to understand the role and function of other team members and to work together in a mutual respectful manner. Working in a multiprofessional manner is not part of traditional training programmes (Gregson et al 1991) and so expecting individuals in primary care to come together and understand each other's professional capabilities is somewhat unrealistic.

Team aim and purpose

There is frequently lack of clarity about team tasks in primary care (Øvretveit 1993, Pearson 1994, West 1994). Although teams meet and discuss pertinent issues, the majority of the dialogue focuses on reactive issues, rather than consideration of proactive team tasks which aim to meet the health needs of the practice population. A study by Poulton (1995) identified a positive relationship between a needs-based approach to primary care delivery and team effectiveness.

A common objective, accepted and understand by all team members, is fundamental to teamworking (DHSS 1981).

There are often conflicting goals and strategies between PHCTs and NHS community trusts. This leads to confusion for practitioners and difficulties in trying to identify professional and

---

Vignette 4.8 Conflicting goals and strategies

Sue has been issued with a 'strategy for primary care' by the community trust and has been asked to complete a 'personal development plan' which outlines her future educational needs.

Sue feels she would like to undertake a course in palliative care as she has a special interest in this area and much of her caseload involves the care of patients with a terminal illness. However, she covers three practices and they do not all see this as a priority.

Sue discusses her educational needs with her manager in the community trust who advises her to ask the practice teams whether they would support her in undertaking the palliative care course.

Practice A states this does not fit with their present needs, Practice B would prefer Sue to undertake a course in diabetes and Practice C are happy to support her.

This illustrates a classic example of an individual team member who is pulled in three different directions when trying to decide her personal development plan. Practice A and B will be unhappy with Sue if she undertakes the palliative care course.

---

personal educational needs. This situation in illustrated in vignette 4.8.

The barriers to effective teamworking have been highlighted above. Some of the problems may appear insurmountable and beyond the scope of this chapter to address, but research studies have demonstrated the effectiveness of team-building workshops (Spratley 1990). Other literature also suggests methods of working with teams to assist in their development. The next part of this chapter will discuss such methods.

TEAM DEVELOPMENT

When a team first comes together people tend to remain in their professional role and it is only when a task is initiated that other qualities begin to emerge. The most effective teams are those where members are valued not only for their specialist input but also for the personal qualities they possess. Team analysis allows for these qualities to be identified, which then assists the team in their decisions as to who may be best to take forward different elements of working towards team objectives.

It is possible to create the 'best team' to do the job, and although not all teams may contain individuals who naturally fall into specific roles, analysing team members and identifying areas of expertise allows teams to identify gaps and fill these accordingly by working together. In this way people perform jobs they enjoy and excel at, individuals are not forced into roles they find tedious and the team becomes motivated to achieve its task. In primary care, it is almost never possible to choose team members, so analysis of existing team members and identification of what they have to offer is an imperative first step.

The following framework has been used as a basis on which to analyse teams and initiate the process of team building. It has been developed by Chaudry-Lawton et al (1992) and is based around four Cs:

- clarity
- commitment
- communication
- celebration.

Clarity

Clarity of team roles, skills and responsibilities

It is important to begin by profiling the team and deciding who will become the team leader. There are several techniques which can be used to carry out this analysis. Belbin (1981) has identified eight major team roles (Box 4.5), and has produced a questionnaire which allows people to identify their personal attributes and the role they perform best.

Most people prefer to operate from one or two of the roles outlined in Box 4.5. Each role is briefly discussed enabling team members to distinguish for themselves which role their personal and functional expertise fits into.

There have been some changes to Belbin's original team roles: 'chairman' has been changed to 'coordinator' as this tends to move away from the hierarchical nature associated with the word

---

Box 4.5 Belbin's team roles (Belbin 1981)

Role characteristics

1. Company worker	Practical, well organised, turns ideas into action
2. Teamworker	Sociable and popular, counteracts friction, fosters a team spirit
3. Chairman	Clarifies, calm, able to get the team to work together, not always creative
4. Plant	Serious, creative thinker, does not always respond well to criticism
5. Completer, finisher	Conscientious, pays attention to detail, meets deadlines, anxious
6. Monitor, evaluator	Analytical and objective, good judgment, can lack tact
7. Resource investigator	Extrovert, will search for information and make outside contacts, elusive
8. Shaper	Dynamic, tries to direct the team, dominant, can be impatient

---

'chairman'. The second change is to replace 'company worker' with 'implementer', for similar reasons.

When profiling the team, it is important to value differences, to look for absent roles and roles which are under-or overrepresented.

Clarity of team leadership

A natural leader may emerge when compiling a profile of the team or teams may choose not to elect a team leader but nominate someone to take on a 'facilitator' role. Other teams may wish to opt for a revolving team leader or decide not to have a leader at all. The latter decision needs to be considered carefully, as teams without a leader/facilitator may achieve their task but may fail in terms of personal satisfaction (Chaudry-Lawton et al 1992). From personal experience teams without leaders can behave in an unruly fashion. Lack of ground rules, ambiguity and no 'one person' pulling ideas together and negotiating the allocation of tasks can lead to confusion and poor teamworking. However, some teams are now moving towards self-management where all of the team take responsibility for meeting the team aims and objectives.

Whatever the decision regarding leadership/facilitation or self-management, two important behaviours associated with a leadership role have been identified in some early work by Hersey & Blanchard (1977).

1. *Relationship behaviour* – this is about supporting others, respecting team members, recognising potential and rewarding good work.
2. *Task behaviour* – relates to the ability to identify clearly the focus of the task and providing direction as to how the task will be achieved.

Leadership in the 1990s has moved towards an empowerment, encouraging and coaching style (Chaudry-Lawton et al 1992). The coaching style of leadership requires the ability to listen, to allow all team members to participate, to give frequent constructive feedback and to recognise and reward progress. The emphasis here is on team development as well as on task performance. Characteristics of this are shown in Box 4.6.

The encouraging style of leadership is based on increasing the confidence of team members to achieve the task and calls for similar skills to those already mentioned under the coaching style. Skills of communication, recognising and rewarding potential are essential in getting the team to work effectively together.

The empowerment model of leadership allows team members to proceed alone and set their own goals for achievement of the task. This is the least interactive of the leadership styles mentioned. It recognises the expertise of team members and although the leader communicates warmly with the team, members are encouraged to achieve through using their own expertise.

Box 4.6 The skills of good leaders (Chaudry-Lawton et al 1992)

- To facilitate
- To coach
- To build relationships with others
- To manage boundaries
- To create a positive climate
- To focus on the broader vision

Clarity of people skills

The way in which people interact with one another is a key component in successful teamworking and it is imperative this is identified and discussed at the beginning of the team-building process.

Primary health-care teams can rarely choose their team members and, as already mentioned, they may well inherit personality traits which inhibit effective teamworking. Teams will need to be encouraged to work with all types of personalities and to mutually respect the views of others. Members must feel they are able to disagree and to be assertive without being intimidated by other members of the team.

Building relationships with others is a major element of the team-building process. This can be achieved through active listening and encouraging and supporting members to make their points heard. Team members need to be sensitive to one another and maintain a sense of humour to help relieve tension and anxiety. Positive people skills are highlighted in Box 4.7.

Box 4.7 Positive people skills

Able to:
- build relationships
- actively listen
- negotiate assertively
- be non-confrontational
- encourage and support
- show mutual respect and tolerance
- manage conflict
- maintain a sense of humour

Clarity of context

It is important to be able to recognise the political, social and intellectual issues relating to the environment in which teams work. In primary care the context is constantly changing and teams need to ensure they are aware of how their work fits with primary care groups and the wider arena of primary care.

All decisions made will need to reflect current health and social policy. Without reference to these contextual influences, teams can become insular and miss opportunities for joint collaborative ventures with other agencies involved in the provision of care.

Strategies for development within the team should take into consideration major external forces and use these forces to drive forward innovative tasks.

Clarity of task

The team requires clarity of the task to be achieved. This should be relatively easy to define but teams may require a formula to assist with this process. It may be useful to ask each team member how they see the task in hand and ask team members to clarify:

- the task to be achieved
- the existing knowledge team members have in relation to the task
- existing experience team members have in relation to the task
- existing expertise present in team members.

Adair (1986) suggests that targets should be set relating to the task and these should be:

- measurable
- time bounded
- realistic
- challenging
- agreed.

It is helpful if the team negotiates the targets, as this allows for ownership and motivation in achieving goals.

Commitment

Teams will not function effectively unless team members are committed to the task, the team, the organisation and to other team members.

Energies can be wasted if some members are enthusiastic but other members lethargic, thus leading the focus away from the task and onto relationships within the team. However, it is not always easy for all team members to feel immediate enthusiasm for working together to achieve a particular task. Some means of helping people to experience this excitement may be necessary. Chaudry-Lawton et al (1992) suggest three ingredients which help create enthusiasm and strengthen people's commitment to a team:

- ownership
- active role
- recognition for individual contribution.

Involvement of all team members in decisions and in agreeing the task and how it will be achieved will increase people's sense of ownership. The task becomes a vision for all and not the pipedream of one individual member. This collaborative approach must be seen as a mechanism for distributing responsibility fairly, ensuring all team members are accountable for their particular tasks.

Creating a team identity can also help with commitment and a team logo or name may help with this process. When the team meet it is important each person is allowed to 'have their say' and each member is made to feel their contribution is worthwhile.

Leaders are an essential part of building the commitment within the team. The leader should be seen as an integral part of the team, someone who listens to team members, who offers encouragement and support and who is available to discuss issues. The team should be able to talk about its progress and pitfalls and the promotion of ideas should be seen as a constant journey, rather than the end of the road.

Communication

This chapter has previously touched on many issues which relate to communication within teams, as this fundamental principle underpins all aspects of effective team working. Communication not only relates to exchange of information within the team, but also how the team communicates to the outside world, to patients/clients, within and outside the organisation. Box 4.8 illustrates a communication philosophy.

Box 4.8 Communication philosophy

- Communicate with respect for others.
- Value the contribution others make.
- Communicate clearly.
- Communicate to people that they are important.
- Don't make assumptions regarding the ability of others to understand your communication.
- Be patient.
- Actively listen to the responses of others.
- Don't jump to conclusions.
- Avoid unhelpful competition.

There needs to be communication regarding achieving the task and the elements which have to be considered to obtain results and communication about team members, their views, feelings and ideas. These issues have a positive pay-off in getting things done (Chaudry-Lawton et al 1992).

It may be advantageous to consider a range of factors when thinking about communication channels within and outside the team (Box 4.9).

Although the importance of communication in enhancing team working cannot be overestimated, it is worth remembering that 'overcommunication' can have a detrimental effect. Team members may tire of endless memos which contain trivial information. Ensure the transfer of information is necessary before passing it on to other members of the team.

Box 4.9 Communicating within/outside the team

Consider the following
- Why does the information need to be communicated?
- Who needs to know the information?
- Who should be responsible for communicating the information?
- What would be the most appropriate manner to communicate the information?
- When should the information be communicated?

Celebration

The celebration phase is about 'congratulating the team' on successes and acknowledging team

---

Box 4.10   Stages in team development (adapted from Handy (1990) and Chaudry-Lawton et al (1992))

Forming
Team is creating its own identity, finding out who everyone is and the part they play – **clarifying** roles and responsibilities, choosing a name, **clarifying** the task, the goals and objectives, **clarifying** the context.

Storming
Individuals begin to assert themselves and challenge the team identity, the task and the team purpose. People begin to question what others have to offer. They look for **commitment** from team members and begin to set ground rules. The purpose of the team is discussed and people begin to **commit** themselves to various roles and responsibilities.

Norming
The team begins to settle down and roles emerge which people feel they have an affinity with. Team requires

support and encouragement – may continue to challenge team purpose at times and requires **clarity**. There needs to be constant **communication** between team members to retain and redefine the focus and to **communicate** individual roles.

Performing
The team begins to perform. Team members balance the tasks to be undertaken and allocate workloads. There remains the need for reviewing progress and for sharing information. Team members must feel supported in the performing stage and this is achieved through constant **communication** which fosters respect and builds the self-esteem of those involved. The team should ensure there is time set aside for **celebration**. This may involve reaffirming the team's progress and discussion of both positive and negative issues.

---

progress. Chaudry-Lawton et al (1992) discuss the release of emotion as an important element of teamworking which helps reaffirm the team. The opportunity to get together and celebrate meeting targets increases motivation and ensures issues do not pass unnoticed.

Teams may not always be in a position to celebrate success but regular reviews also assist people in coming together to discuss obstacles and failures. This in itself can have positive advantages in that team members feel supported by the team and this in turn can enhance motivation. Celebration meetings also allow for all those involved to share their contributions and efforts. This allows for a release of tension and the opportunity to gain help and advice from others.

It is worth sharing any successes of the team publicly. This could take the form of a publication/and or posters in the workplace. Team achievement charts can also illustrate levels of performance and newsletters are useful to publicise to others the progress of the team.
The four Cs – clarity, commitment, communication and celebration – will now be applied to the phases of team development.

Phases of team development

It is well known that a team will go through several phases of development when it first comes

together. Although authors may name these phases differently, in essence the processes are the same. Handy (1990) discusses the infamous forming, storming, norming and performing as the stages in development. His explanation of these stages, coupled with the four Cs defined by Chaudry-Lawton, is constructed in Box 4.10 above to illustrate how they can be interlinked.

An awareness of the phases of team development helps with the process of team building. This, coupled with the four Cs, demonstrates some practical issues which can easily be addressed on an individual basis. All practitioners have the opportunity to facilitate the process of teamworking and should strive to apply the principles to their everyday work, thus enhancing cohesive effective teams in primary and community care.

TEAM DESCRIPTIONS

Having considered the principles of teamworking and how these can be achieved, the third part of this chapter seeks to develop a model of teamworking to which district nurses may be able to conform. Using Øvretveit's (1996) descriptions of a multidisciplinary team as a source, we consider the positions in which DNs currently find themselves within a team and how these can be modified to achieve best teamwork practice within everyday constraints.

Vignette 4.10   Jane's story

Jane is a district nursing sister employed by a NHS trust who heads a district nursing team of eight staff (three full time and five part time). Jane and her team are based in a health clinic which is located approximately half a mile from the GP surgery to which they are attached. The team's locality manager is based at the same health clinic. The health visitor also has her office at the same clinic although they rarely have time to meet.

Jane and her team have developed a number of innovative approaches to their work. For example, they have completed a health needs profile for the local community; they have developed a number of standards of care for practice; they have a team philosophy. Jane has not shared these innovations with other professionals as, in the past, any attempts at collaboration have 'fallen on stony ground'. There are no formal primary health-care team meetings. Staff from various disciplines make appointments with each other if they need to meet up.

Jane and her manager are currently in discussion with the general practitioners over the number of inappropriate referrals which they make to her team. This she attributes to their lack of understanding of her role.

Box 4.11   Five ways to describe a multidisciplinary team (Øvretveit 1996)

1. Degree of integration
2. Extent of collective responsibility
3. Membership
4. Client pathway and decision making
5. Management structures

Øvretveit (1996) outlines five ways to describe a multidisciplinary team (Box 4.11). These help to give clear definition to the approaches that district nurses are likely to meet in the primary health-care setting. The framework adds further weight to the argument that multiprofessional working is a realistic approach to teamwork in primary care which is worthy of discussion.

Degree of integration

This, Øvretveit (1996) asserts, addresses both subjective feelings about the degree of integration perceived by individual team members and objective measures of team integration. At one end of the scale is a loosely knit community of professionals where workers are organised within their professional services and managed by their service managers. Such an approach is illustrated in vignette 4.10

Vignette 4.10 describes a situation that many district nurses will identify with. It is evident here that links to a PHCT are tenuous. As previously mentioned, this is a phenomenon recognised by a number of authors who have studied the dynamics of PHCTs. For example, West & Poulton (1997) found that the separate lines of management in PHCTs prevented the development of shared objectives and could give rise to professional conflict. This is clearly evident in vignette 4.10.

Øvretveit (1996) identifies the other extreme of integration as the closely integrated team (Fig 4.1), where multidisciplinary policy and team decision making govern workloads and clinical judgement. The identification of a continuum suggests that there is room for manoeuvre from one element to the other. District nurses who find themselves in Jane's position thus may be able to take measures such as considering the clarity of the roles and leadership of the team, identified by Chaudry-Lawton et al (1992), to alter the configuration of the PHCT.

Extent of collective responsibility

The second description is where teams are accountable for pooling and using their collective resources to best meet the needs of the population that they serve. To achieve this, Øvretveit (1996) asserts that the team must be financed as a single entity. At present, because of the way that primary health care is organised, there are few examples of collectively responsible teams in Britain. However, at present, with the advent of primary care groups in England (DoH 1997), local health groups in Wales (Welsh Office 1998) and local health care co-operatives in Scotland (Scottish Office 1997), district nurses are ideally situated to

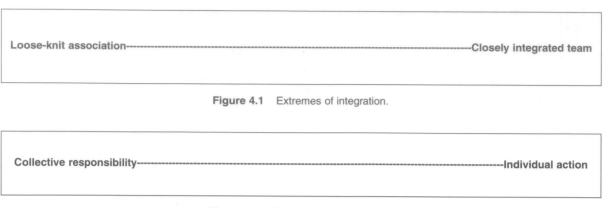

Figure 4.1 Extremes of integration.

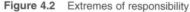

Figure 4.2 Extremes of responsibility

reassess the 'clarity of context' and 'clarity of task' of the team, identified above. These new initiatives offer more opportunity for PHCTs to act collectively to meet local health needs. The government is also allowing the chance to pilot new approaches to the delivery of primary health care, outlined in *Choice and opportunity* (DoH 1996) so there will be more scope for collective responsibility to become a reality. For example, Catherine Baraniak is a practice nurse project leader in Derby who is working on a pilot nurse-led PHCT which encourages collective responsibility.

What Øvretveit (1996) does not really address in any detail is the compromise that needs to be achieved between professional autonomy and collective responsibility. According to Henneman et al (1995) an antecedent of collaboration is that systems must be in place to allow participants to act autonomously and for this to occur, individuals must have a clear understanding and acceptance of their own role and expertise. If these conditions are realised, then there need not be a conflict between autonomy and collective responsibility.

Again, a continuum can be used to define collective responsibility (Fig 4.2). District nurses can take measures to move towards the optimum level of collective responsibility wherever their position is identified in a team analysis. Team analysis allows for these qualities to be identified. This then assists the team in their decisions as to who may best undertake different elements of working towards team objectives.

Membership

Øvretveit (1996) proposes that this defines the group's boundaries. It is likely that a mix of different professionals with different skills will be taken on as team members. Øvretveit (1996) recognises that a team is likely to consist of core members, which usually means full time in a team, and associate members, which means part time. The literature suggests that district nurses usually find themselves as core members of PHCTs. For example, Wiles & Robison (1994) found that over three-quarters of the district nurses who they interviewed considered themselves to be part of a PHCT.

However, this still means that there are many district nurses who do not currently fit into the core structure of a PHCT. There is a dearth of literature which gives indications of how the transition from associate to core member could be achieved. With the support of district nursing colleagues and managers, however, district nurses could facilitate their passage. Highlighting the district nurse's ability to contribute towards PHCT functions might be one strategy to adopt. By taking this approach, sufficient inroads may be made to enable a full team analysis to be undertaken.

Client pathway and decision making

This describes the team in terms of the passage of a client through that team. This

Table 4.1 Øvretveit's (1996) client pathways

Type	Pathway	Description
One	Parallel	Each profession has its own pathway. Team meetings are for cross-referrals.
Two	Allocation or postbox	Each profession has its own pathway. Members pick up referrals from team meetings and take these back to their separate professional pathways. Referrals are brought to the team meeting either by the team secretary or leader or by a team member.
Three	Reception and allocation	The team has a short-term response, with each member taking turns to fulfil. The team then acts as type two.
Four	Reception-assessment-allocation	The team has an assessment stage which occurs prior to deciding when or how to intervene. Clients are first allocated to a team member for an assessment and then for longer term work if this is judged to be necessary.
Five	Reception-assessment-allocation-review	Here a review stage is added after the intervention. The case worker presents a report to the team and, based on this, recommendations relating to further work are made by the team.
Six	Hybrid-parallel	A mixture of team pathways for some professionals and individual pathways for others who might work in a service which is separate from the team.

refers to both the time which is taken on the 'journey' and the process that the client is required to go through. In all, Øvretveit (1996) describes six different pathways to which a client might be exposed. These are illustrated in Table 4.1.

Whilst type five allows for the most effective collaboration, type one is likely to be the approach to teamwork which most district nurses will encounter. Rapport & Maggs's (1997) study confirms this. They found that district nurses feel that they are moving away from teamworking practice and that they have a strictly defined role where responsibility for care is not shared. This is the case in the team portrayed in vignette 4.11.

This vignette illustrates that the parallel pathway approach can result in duplication of care, lack of continuity for the patient and professional dissatisfaction and disharmony. Again, as suggested earlier in the chapter, a team analysis,

Vignette 4.11 Parallel pathway approach

Eira, a district nurse, is attached to one general practice in which there are four GPs and two practice nurses. Eira has been visiting Thomas Jones for about 3 weeks to dress his wound following the excision of a pilonidal sinus. As the wound is taking some time to heal, Eira asks the GP to see Thomas and Thomas attends an appointment at the surgery. The next day, Eira visits Thomas' home to find that he is not in. On making further inquiries, Eira discovers that Thomas has attended the surgery where the practice nurse has changed his dressing. Eira feels annoyed because nobody had consulted her about this change in arrangements despite the fact that she has been managing Thomas' care for some time.

particularly of roles, skills and responsibilities, might help to move the place of client pathways along the continuum for the district nurse. In which case the scenario outlined in vignette 4.12 may become the norm rather than the exception.

Vignette 4.12 Mr Williams's story

Mr Williams is due for discharge home from the elderly care unit of the local district general hospital tomorrow (Tuesday). He has Parkinson's disease and is likely to require support at home from a number of PHCT professionals. The hospital liaison sister makes the referral to Justin who is the team leader for the PHCT. Justin reviews the referral notes and asks Eleri, a member of the district nursing team, to make the first assessment. Eleri makes the assessment and decides that because of the interventions that Mr Williams requires, she should be the key worker for the patient. She reports this to the rest of the PHCT at the next weekly meeting. The team agrees that this seems an appropriate way forward and that Mr Williams' case is reviewed at the meeting in 1 month's time unless any changes occur.

Management structures

This is the fifth approach which Øvretveit (1996) uses to describe a multidisciplinary team. This he examines in terms of how the team is led and how the members of the different professions are managed. Again, Øvretveit outlines five different management structures. These range from a profession-managed structure, where each professional is accountable to a different line manager, to a single manager structure, where all professionals are accountable to the same manager.

Whilst the former approach is most commonly found in PHCTs (West & Poulton 1997), the approach which Øvretveit describes as 'team manager with contracts structure' is becoming more prominent within primary health care. This is especially the case since the introduction of GP fundholding. Within this management framework, a team manager, with a budget, contracts the services of the team members who are normally profession managed and thus has control over the members through the contracts which have been negotiated. Whilst Øvretviet envisages that there are benefits to the team of using this management structure, many district nurses relate that they have encountered difficulties when working within this structure. In vignette 4.13, Sion is often asked by his fundholding GP colleagues to undertake tasks which he feels are inappropriate. The GPs, on the other hand, are

paying for a service and believe that they should be able to direct the form of that service. Lack of cohesive managerial structure in this situation inevitably leads to conflict

Sion's situation is one that many district nurses can identify with. However, it need not be the only management structure for district nursing. Whilst district nurses might feel powerless to effect an organisational change, they may be able to raise the issue of management through a team analysis exercise. For example, while the employment issue may be impossible to overcome, the identification of an appropriate team leader could help to ensure that clear communication networks between all stakeholders of the team are established.

Vignette 4.13 Sion's story

Sion heads a team of six district nurses who are attached to a large fundholding general practice and who are employed by the local community health-care trust. Sion was not consulted by his community service manager when the practice recently renegotiated the community nursing contract with the trust. Indeed, Sion is unsure of what work he is committed to through the new contract.

Recently Sion and his team have received a number of what they consider to be inappropriate referrals from the GPs to take 'urgent bloods'. Sion is unsure of who he should approach about this problem. He sees that there are a number of alternatives:

1. the GPs
2. the practice manager
3. the trust community services manager.

Sion also feels some reluctance about approaching any of these people as he is concerned that he may appear ignorant if taking 'urgent bloods' has been included in the new contract.

INTERDISCIPLINARY COLLABORATION

Øvretveit's (1996) framework is a useful tool for district nurses which allows evaluation of the multidisciplinary team's structure and functions. This evaluation enables district nurses to establish their team's baseline from which they may be able to negotiate some change in approaches. Chaudry-Lawton et al's (1992) framework provides one method which can be used to review the position of the team. It would also guide district nurses to adopt strategies which will enable the team to make the transition from multiprofessional along a continuum to interprofessional collaborators. The use of an algorithm (Fig. 4.3) should aid district nurses in the analysis of their position in the PHCT and in the progress of their location along the continuum.

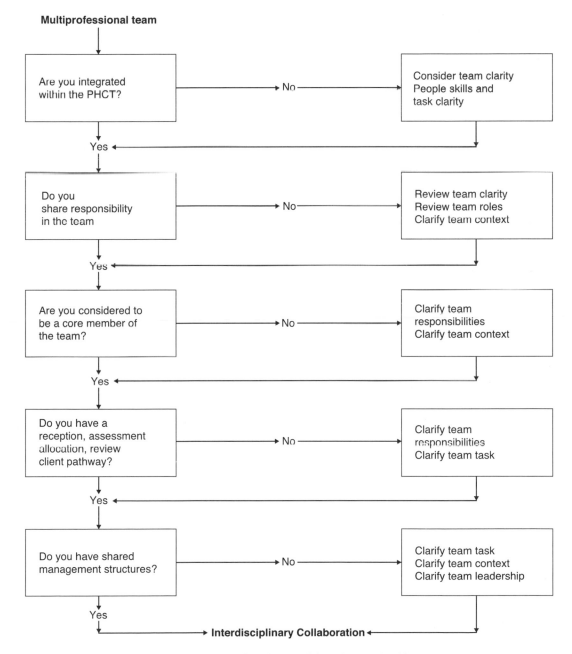

Multiprofessional team

Are you integrated within the PHCT? →No→ Consider team clarity / People skills and task clarity

Yes←

Do you share responsibility in the team →No→ Review team clarity / Review team roles / Clarify team context

Yes←

Are you considered to be a core member of the team? →No→ Clarify team responsibilities / Clarify team context

Yes←

Do you have a reception, assessment allocation, review client pathway? →No→ Clarify team responsibilities / Clarify team task

Yes←

Do you have shared management structures? →No→ Clarify team task / Clarify team context / Clarify team leadership

Yes←

Interdisciplinary Collaboration

Figure 4.3   From multidisciplinary teamwork to interdisciplinary collaboration: an algorithm.

CONCLUSION

This chapter has examined the issue of multiprofessional working for the district nurse and a number of different definitions associated with it. Through the examination of these definitions and an outline of the historical development of the PHCT, the chapter has demonstrated how district nurses have arrived at their position in the PHCT today. The chapter advances a description of an ideal team and gives some strategies which district nurses might adopt in order to engage in team building.

Finally, it is recognised that district nurses might find themselves in a number of different positions on a continuum as they strive towards interprofessional collaboration. With this in mind, an algorithm is developed which draws on the work of Chaudry-Lawton et al (1992) and of Øvretveit (1996), to indicate how district nurses might move from multidisciplinary teamwork to interprofessional collaboration.

It is evident from the discussions in this chapter that the district nurse is likely to face many barriers during the transition from teamworker to collaborator. What emerges through the deliberations, however, is that these barriers can be overcome. With careful analysis of the PHCT and the district nurse's position within that team, it is possible to adopt strategies which aid the transition from the current to the ideal arrangement. The use of the algorithm should aid this progression.

REFERENCES

Adair J 1986 Effective team building. Pan Books, London

Armstrong D, Tavabie A, Johnston S 1994 Job satisfaction among practice nurses in a health district. Health and Social care in the Community 2(5): 279–282

Belbin M 1981 Management teams: why they succeed or fail. Heinemann, Oxford

Blackie D 1998 The NHS: organisational history, reforms and influence on practice. In: Blackie C (ed) Community health care nursing. Churchill Livingstone, Edinburgh.

Bond J, Cartlidge A, Gregson B, Philips P, Bolom K, Gill K 1985 A study of interprofessional collaboration in primary care. Report No. 27. University of Newcastle upon Tyne, Newcastle upon Tyne

British Medical Association 1965 A charter for the family doctor service. BMA, London

Chaudry-Lawton, R, Lawton R, Murphy K, Terry A 1992 Quality: change through teamwork. Century Business, London

Department of Health and Social Security 1981 Care in the community. HMSO, London

Department of Health and Social Security 1986 Neighbourhood nursing, a focus for care. HMSO, London

Department of Health 1989 Terms of service for doctors in general practice, London, DoH

Department of Health 1990 NHS and Community Care Act, London, DoH

Department of Health 1996 Choice and opportunity – primary care: the future. HMSO, London

Field R, West M 1995 Teamwork in primary health care. Perspectives from practices. Journal of Interprofessional Care 9(2): 123–130

Gillie Report on the future scope of General Practice 1963 HMSO, London

Gregson B, Cartlidge A, Bond J 1991 Interprofessional collaboration in primary care organisations. Occasional Paper 52. RCGP, London

Guzzo R, Shea G 1992 Group performance and interrelations in organisations. In: Dunnette M, Hough L (eds) Handbook of industrial and organisational psychology. Consulting Psychologists Press, Palo Alto, California

Handy C 1990 Inside organisations. BBC Books, London

Henneman E, Lee J, Cohen J 1995 Collaboration: a concept analysis. Journal of Advanced Nursing 21: 103–109

Hersey P, Blanchard K 1977 Management of organisational behaviour: utilizing human resources. Prentice Hall, New Jersey.

James E 1995 Primary health care in the community. In: Sines D (ed) Community health care nursing. Blackwell Science, Oxford

Jones-Elwyn G, Stott N 1994 Avoidable referrals? Analysis of 170 consecutive referrals to secondary care. British Medical Journal 309: 576–579

Jones-Elwyn G, Rapport K, Kinnersley P 1998 Primary health care teams re-engineered. Journal of Interprofessional Care 12(2): 189–198

McClure L 1984 Teamwork, myth or reality? Community nurses' experience with general practice attachment. Journal of Epidemiology and Community Health 31: 68–74

Ministry of Health 1920 Report on the future provision of medical and allied services. HMSO, London

Ministry of Health 1946 A national health service. HMSO, London

Øvretveit J 1993 Coordinating community care. Open University Press, Buckingham

Øvretveit J 1996 Five ways to describe a multidisciplinary team. Journal of Interprofessional Care 10(2): 163–171

Pearson P 1994 The primary health care non team. British Medical Journal 309: 1387–1388

Pearson P, Spencer J 1995 Pointers to effective teamwork: exploring primary care. Journal of Interprofessional Care 9(2): 131–138

Poulton B 1995 Effective multidiscplinary teamwork in primary health care. Unpublished PhD thesis, University of Sheffield, Sheffield

Pritchard P 1995 Learning to work effectively in teams. In: Owens P, Carrier J, Horder J (eds) Interprofessional issues in community and primary health care. Macmillan, London

Rapport F, Maggs C 1997 Measuring care: the case of district nursing. Journal of Advanced Nursing 25: 673–680

Scottish Office 1996 Primary care: the way ahead. HMSO, Edinburgh

Scottish Office 1997 Designed to care. HMSO, Edinburgh

Senge P, Roberts C, Ross R, Smith B, Kleiner A 1994 The fifth discipline fieldbook: strategies and tools for building a learning organisation. Nicholas Breabey Publishing, London

Spratley J 1990 Joint planning for the development and management of disease prevention and health promotion strategies in primary health care. HEA, London

Stott N 1993 When something is good, more of the same is not always better. British Journal of Medical Practice 43: 254–257

Welsh Office 1988 Nursing in the community: a team approach for Wales. Welsh Office, Cardiff

Welsh Office 1996 Primary care: the way forward in Wales. Welsh Office, Cardiff

Welsh Office 1998 Putting patients first. Welsh Office, Cardiff

West M 1994 Effective teamwork. British Psychological Society, Leicester

West M, Pillinger T 1996 An evaluation of team building in primary health care. Oxford Health Education Authority, Oxford

West M, Poulton B 1997 A failure of function: teamwork in primary health care. Journal of Interprofessional care 11(2): 205–216

Wiles R, Robison J 1994 Teamwork in primary care: the views and experiences of nurses, midwives and health visitors. Journal of Advanced Nursing 20: 324–330

FURTHER READING

Øvretviet J 1993 Coordinating community care. Open University Press, Buckingham

Tovey P 2000 Contemporary primary care: the challenge of change. Open University Press, Buckingham

District nursing history

Helen Sweet   Rona Ferguson

Key points

- The origins of the district nurse
- The founding of the Queen's Institute
- Attitudes to home visiting
- The NHS and the role and professional image of the district nurse
- Transport, technology, organisation and their effects on the daily work of the district nurse
- Inter-and intraprofessional relationships
- Training and professionalisation
- The primary health-care team

INTRODUCTION

This chapter will concentrate on the development of district nursing from the 19th century, with particular reference to the growing professional role and the perception of that role both by the public and within the health professions. Information is based on documentary sources and oral histories. The latter have been gathered from district nurses from Scotland, England and Wales training and working from the late 1930s onwards, up to and including the present decade, and are presented as vignettes. As well as a wide range of secondary sources, the documentary evidence also includes some new material, notably the records of the Queen's Nursing Institute, newly catalogued by and held at the Contemporary Medical Archives Centre (henceforth referred to as CMAC) of the London Wellcome Institute, and information relating to district nursing associations from 1915 to 1935 provided by Burdett's Directories (throughout this period these contained an annual summary of public nursing institutions including district nursing associations, frequently providing a detailed 'breakdown' of their income and expenditure, area served, organisation, numbers of nurses employed and their conditions of service.

THE ORIGINS OF THE DISTRICT NURSE

Although Dickens' gin-swilling caricature of the district nurse (Sarah Gamp and Betsy Prig, two outdoor relief district nurses in *Martin Chuzzlewit*) is powerfully evocative and, as will be seen, not without some foundation in reality, it presents a monochrome image of the state of mid-19th century district nursing. It is probable that this contributed to its marginalisation within nursing as a profession (Sweet 1997). In fact, the predecessors of today's district nurse have a much more heterogeneous background, ranging from 'bible nurses' to 'corpse washers' and many shades in between, and although it is not within the mandate of this chapter to do so, their history can be traced to well before the 19th century (Hawker 1995, Loudon 1986).

Until the 18th century outside London there was a general reluctance to provide institutional nursing care (Abel-Smith (1960) claims from census data that 'as late as 1851 there were only 7619 patients [...] resident in hospitals, in the whole of England and Wales') and the (lay) nurse might be a formal or informal carer, also called a 'handy-woman', 'corpse-washer' or 'village nurse' private nurse or a member of the household, a midwife or 'monthly nurse', herbalist or bonesetter. She might apply leeches, dressings and poultices or practise blistering or bleeding. Any one or a combination of these might be carried out by a 'nurse' in the community either as a self-employed (often casually employed) independent practitioner, as member of a husband and wife 'team' or under contract to the voluntary hospitals and Poor Law relief committee. Dingwall et al (1988) describe this wide range of duties collectively as the 'techniques of preindustrial nursing'. It has been suggested that numbers of male nurses working as man-midwives,

attendants, asylum nurses and dressers may have been comparatively high until the mid-19th century.

During the mid-19th century first Elizabeth Fry's protestant Sisters of Charity (founded 1840) followed by other religious orders such as St John's (1848) and, from 1857, the bible nurses of the Ranyard Sisterhood supplied trainee and trained nurses to the provincial hospitals. In the community they provided nursing care to the sick poor in their own homes following the successes of French and German religious nursing organisations (Jones 1989). These recruited women from the 'handywoman' class to be trained as nurses and they later returned to the community to nurse the sick poor under supervision of the lady superintendent, whilst in many cases earning their keep by caring for private patients, as was also the case in later secular schemes. It should be noted that the nurse/superintendent arrangement represented a two-tiered, extremely hierarchical, class-based system (Williamson 1996). This 'did make an important contribution to the reconceptualisation of nursing' by combining the 'secular spirit of medical modernisation' with the 'spiritual concerns of the order' (Dingwall et al 1988), i.e. a relationship between nurse and patient based on spiritual salvation (religious reform) gradually incorporating social and sanitary reform.

At this stage there was 'vigorous competition in what historically was an unusually open market' with the changes in the Victorian economy both in costs and standards of living meaning that 'only a restricted section of the population could afford to pay for the cost of their medical treatment' (Digby 1994). Without detailing the complexities of and variations in Poor Law provision of 'indoor' and 'outdoor' relief during the mid-19th century, suffice it to say that pauper nurses were often recruited from within the workhouse to care for the sick in the workhouse infirmary and sometimes outside under the 'outdoor relief' system (Crowther 1986). Abel-Smith (1960) describes the workhouses as 'dumps' for the patients the voluntary hospitals had failed to cure or with types of illness they would not accept and that it was found 'that out of a total of 157,740 indoor paupers in 1869 about a third were sick', i.e. over 50 000 patients compared with less than 20 000 in general and special hospitals recorded in the 1871 census figures.

The result was a wide range of standards and duties carried out often just for token cash payments or special privileges such as improved rations and different dress, by nurses with minimal or no training under an equally variable range of supervision and management. They were frequently illiterate and often old and infirm; thus there was little to distinguish them from their fellow pauper patients. These working-class nurses were generally hired by the Board of Guardians and supervised by a lady inspector (Baly 1986).

At the other end of the spectrum it is worth noting an observation quoted by Summers (1997) that during the 1849 cholera outbreak one physician wrote, 'The nurse was then of more use to the patient than the doctor', i.e. where surgical intervention was inappropriate or, alternatively, where introduction of sanitarian principles (of hygiene rather than antisepsis) was paramount, the trained nurse was arguably of greater significance to outcome and to disease prevention than the doctor.

Similarly, the experience of terminal care provided by a trained nurse, Mrs Mary Robinson, in the home of William Rathbone when his wife died of consumption in 1859 provided the inspiration for his philanthropic establishment of district nurse training and provision for the sick poor of Liverpool from 1862 by establishing a training school attached to the Liverpool Royal Infirmary and founding the Liverpool Queen Victoria District Nursing Association (Hardy 1981). These provided district and private nurses and were supervised by a 'lady superintendent' who was a member of a 'committee of ladies' who ran the 'district nursing association'.

Subsequently a similar association was set up in Manchester and Salford in 1864. Dingwall et al (1988) describe the development of the Manchester and Salford Ladies' Sanitary Association and early 'Health Visitors' as having evolved from the district nurse/mission woman, utilising 'ordinary working-class women'.

Similar associations were formed in Leicester in 1867, Birmingham in 1870 and Glasgow in 1875, with the London Metropolitan and National Nursing Association being founded in 1874.

It can therefore be seen that by the 1870s there was a perceived need for an increase in skill, competence and status of the district nurse through better training and qualification. This also implied a need for organisation, regulation and improved professional image and public status. It is significant that at this time women were beginning to enter the medical profession and Abel-Smith quotes the following observation relating to the employment of skilled nurses in the homes of the wealthy as well as the poor:

There is no reason why the rich should not obtain for money services which are freely bestowed upon the poor. Ladies will now take fees as doctors, but they will nurse only for charity [...] Invalids of the upper classes would soon feel the advantage of being tended by a lady of refinement and scientific training, and would be willing to remunerate her services at such a rate as would in time repay the expenses of her preparatory study ... (Haddon, cited by Abel-Smith 1960)

FOUNDING OF THE QUEEN'S INSTITUTE

The Queen Victoria Jubilee Institute for Nurses (hereinafter referred to as the Queen's Institute) was set up and granted a Royal Charter in 1889 supported by the Queen's Jubilee Fund for 'the promotion and provision of improved means for nursing the sick poor in their own homes', receiving further financial support at the Queen's Diamond Jubilee in 1897 and following her death in 1901.

In response, many of the local nursing associations already in existence became affiliated to the Institute, with Scotland having its own separate branch and council. The Rural Nursing Association, which was founded in the West of England in 1888, established county nursing associations starting with Hampshire in 1891 and Lincolnshire in 1894. By the end of the 19th century there were over 900 Queen's Nurses on the Roll with the stipulated training changed to 1 year's hospital training, 3 months' midwifery and 3–6 months' 'training in district work'. The idea also spread throughout the Empire with the Canadian Victorian Order of Nurses being founded in 1897 and subsequently a 'Bush Nursing Service' being inaugurated in Australia and the King Edward VII District Nursing Service founded in South Africa in 1912 (Searle 1965).

Interestingly, during the battle for nurses' registration it was drawn to the attention of Queen's Nurses in 1904 that 'they are the one body of nurses whose system of work includes a "register", the Roll of Queen's Nurses, in which their names, training and reports are entered, and from which they are liable to be removed if they forfeit the privilege of remaining Queen's Nurses' (A. H. (1904): probably Amy Hughes, pro-registrationist). This system had therefore been running efficiently on a national basis for more than 20 years by the time state registration was finally achieved in 1919.

By 1892 the Local Government Board had authorised the appointment of district nurses by all boards of guardians stipulating a minimum of 1 year's training, a good 'moral character' and conditions of appointment similar to infirmary nurses (White 1978). This barred them from midwifery and placed them under the direction of the doctors who were to be instructed about the nurse's duties by the Guardians. The alternative was to use nurses supplied by nursing associations or the Queen's Institute. In addition, particularly in more rural areas, 'cottage' or 'village' untrained nurses or 'handywomen' were employed by voluntary agencies as domiciliary nurses within the community, working under the supervision of the trained nurses. The 1909 Royal Commission on the Poor Laws reported inadequacy in the provision of nursing for the 'outdoor' sick and set this as a high priority.

The more advanced state of professionalisation within medicine gave doctors a dominant and paternalistic position both in hospitals and the community, with authority over nurses (and patients) regarding patient management such as admissions and discharges, expenditure, treatment and even nursing care decisions such as requiring medical orders prior to bathing a patient (Walby & Greenwell 1994).

This inevitably placed nursing in a subordinate position to medicine despite its Royal Charter and patronage. However, the emergence of the better qualified and professionally supported Queen's Nurse must have presented the less financially secure general medical practitioners with a perceived threat to their livelihood, particularly in the decade before the introduction of the National Health Insurance (NHI) Act in 1911. This was fiercely defended by the local medical associations as illustrated by a case in 1908 in which a problem arose between Penwith Medical Union, Cornwall, and the local district nursing association in which nurses were accused of attending patients without referring them to a medical practitioner. The British Medical Association (BMA) took this up with the Queen's Institute, proposing a joint conference to discuss drawing up draft rules governing the work of district nurse-midwives in local district nursing associations, suggesting:

- representation of the medical profession on local district nursing associations
- confirmation of the position of district nurses working as auxiliaries to, and acting under instructions of, medical practitioners
- clarification of the situation where district nurse-midwives act as midwives without a doctor in attendance and/or attend private persons who could pay fees
- clarification of the situation where district nurses might leave the employment of the district nursing association and set up in private practice within the area in competition with the GP.

Replying to this and other suggestions, a Queen's Institute committee member commented that:

to set up a formal or semi-formal tribunal (even if there were the power to do it) and accord the [BMA] Association a locus standing for intervention would be more likely to encourage than allay friction [...] it is no part of the Institute's functions to help bring it about. It should not be forgotten that the two bodies are not on the same plane in this matter. The sole object of the Institute is the welfare of the sick poor, whereas the aggrieved doctors are fighting for their own hand. (Wellcome CMAC: The Queen's Institute Archives)

Whilst it is significant that this and other examples of interprofessional rivalries took place just before the 1911 NHI Act, other instances arose later in the 1930s. Although the 1911 NHI Act made considerable changes to the provision of medical care and was supported in principle by the Queen's Institute, comparatively few of the district nurse's patients fell directly under its provision.

Looking at the entries in Burdett's Directories and the records of the Queen's Institute from 1915 onwards, there were 2100 Queen's Nurses in 1914 although the number had fallen, possibly due to World War I, to 1989 by 1918. Listings of over 150 district nursing associations in England and Wales by 1920 suggest that an average starting salary of £40 per annum plus uniform was the norm, whilst the Royal College of Nursing recommended salaries were set at £85–120 pa for resident district nurses and recruitment was considered a high priority.

A pamphlet produced by the Queen's Institute around 1925 noted:

There are over 5800 nurses and midwives at work visiting over half-a-million patients annually and paying over 10 000 000 visits each year, but about 25% of the population of England and Wales live in an area where there are no district nurses and for the other 75% the existing service is not yet adequate. (Wellcome CMAC: The Queen's Institute Archive)

By the late 1930s it was estimated that there were 8000 district nurses working in Great Britain and these were more than 40% financially supported directly by the population they served, administered by voluntarily run local associations in almost every area. Just over half of these were Queen's Nurses (4566 in 1939). The Nurses' Registration Act of 1919 and subsequent formation of the General Nursing Council for England and Wales, plus the transfer of Poor Law administration to local authorities in 1929 and the growth of voluntarily organised district nursing associations affiliated to the Queen's Institute, imply some adoption of national standards.

ATTITUDES TO HOME VISITING

From these late 19th and early 20th-century origins, the notion of the 'home visitor' expanded to include the health visitor and the social worker. This was within the context of a religious philanthropic attitude towards welfare which was related to a wider concept of sanitarian health. However, critical attitudes to the home visitor were expressed both by the public and from within the professions themselves. Although the nurse coming into the home has been subject to accusations of condescension, the level of criticism, at least in popular belief, appears to have been considerably less than that shown to the health visitor and the social worker.

By the 1920s the district nurse viewed her role as that of carer of the sick at home; to help restore a person to health until he could continue with an independent life or to provide comfort and care to the dying. It was in essence responding to a need both immediately, in terms of the patient requiring treatment, and more generally, in being a service, which fulfilled a social need for healthcare provision for the poor. By definition, this role included an obligation to teach the patient and family appropriate basic nursing skills necessary to the maintenance of care when the nurse's visit was over. This instructive interaction with the family grew from a medical/health perspective and was directly related to the district nurse's approach to the care of the sick.

The health visitor, on the other hand, although a qualified nurse, was concerned not just about the sick patient's care but the well-being of the whole family and indeed the wider community. Leaving the hands-on nursing to the district nurse, the health visitor was given responsibility for instructing patients in preventive health procedures to deter the spread of disease and promote good health. Much of her time was spent advising mothers with young children in relation to hygiene and nutrition in the home. The object of the health visitor therefore was not an individual's medical health but rather society's health practices. Often regarded as a criticism of family management, and thereby implicitly of the woman and mother, health visiting (like social work) has been described sceptically as a form of 'social policing' and has suffered a less easy acceptance than district nursing in the public perception.

As home visitors, district nurses, health visitors and social workers have traditionally shared similar functions in being concerned for the welfare of individuals assigned to them for care and consideration. For example, the nurse provided health care to someone in poverty and poor housing (e.g. a woman in confinement with no money or provisions for the baby), the social worker was called in to tackle the issue of welfare rights and the health visitor advised on how to manage health and welfare in such conditions. All three were thus concerned with the needs of a person in a particular situation but in different ways. However, the public response to these roles has not been even-handed, the nurse being favoured over the health visitor and the social worker being regarded with a certain degree of disdain (Vignettes 5.1 and 5.2).

It is the golden rule of district nursing that the nurse must remember always that, unlike the hospital situation, she is the guest of the patient in his home. By all standards of etiquette, then, judgement and criticism are not acceptable and so her role as 'health-care worker' must be clear. By going to the doctor or approaching the nurse directly, the patient's condition is self-reported and the nurse is someone with a specific knowledge and skill, which the patient both lacks and needs. When engaged in dressing a wound, bathing an elderly patient, giving an insulin injection or delivering a baby, the nurse's function is not ambiguous. However, in many cases, particularly in triple-duty areas, the district nurse traditionally took on the health visitor's role. Having established a nurse–patient relationship, the wider concept of health care, including matters of health and hygiene, was more readily absorbed within it. This had the advantage that what might otherwise have been regarded as criticism could now be accepted as sound health advice.

Following from this relationship was a commonly practised role of confidante and counsellor so often taken on by the district nurse. Concerns over housing, money, family relationships and education would be discussed willingly with the district nurse by her patients in an unofficial manner without the threat of unsolicited intervention. In triple-duty district nursing more than any other, the merging of nurse, health visitor and social worker was evident. This produced a valuable set of strategic interventions. It was the 'tea and sympathy' advice and 'I'll see what I can do' approach from someone with a *medical* skill and useful connections rather than the *problem*-centered approach of the social worker with the dubious responsibility to both client and state. District nurses of the more recent past remember being respected by all and although they may obliquely refer to the 'odd one' who did not let them in the house, the reputation of the trusted and welcomed nurse prevails in both the individual and collective memory.

Vignette 5.1 Guest in the home

I said 'Well, who came yesterday?'; apparently it was the health visitor and the health visitor had told her she must clean her step and her stairs. 'She told me my stairs were filthy but you don't think they're filthy, do you?' I said 'Well, I suppose they could do with a bit of a clean or brush or something like that.' 'Well' she said, 'she looked at them down her nose and said how filthy they were!' That sort of put her off, you see, whereas I would go in to a house and gradually I might get round to that sort of thing but you were a guest in people's houses and whatever the house – whether it is filthy dirty or full of antiques or what ever – you were still a guest in the house.

Vignette 5.2 The public response

The great distinction for me was the welcome I received as a district nurse as opposed to the suspicion and the reluctance I met with as a health visitor … I think people just looked on you as someone who was interfering when you were a health visitor. Not all – there were some lovely mums who were glad of you to come in and chat and advise them about their babies but as a district nurse you only went because you were asked, you were only there at their request really because either someone was ill or they were having a baby and they needed you. As a health visitor, in a sense you were imposing yourself on them, you wanted them to see you as a friend … I don't think I was never allowed in … I was always welcome as a district nurse.

THE NHS AND THE ROLE AND PROFESSIONAL IMAGE OF THE DISTRICT NURSE

Prior to the introduction of the NHS in 1948, medical treatment was costly and many people called the district nurse before calling the doctor simply because it was cheaper to do so. Contrary to expectation, however, the new health service did not appear to make a great impact on the daily life of the district nurse except that it imposed the burden of fee collecting. This is largely because the district nurse had worked within the subscription schemes operated by the local district nursing associations where the collection of fees had not been an issue of importance for her. Members were not due to pay at the time of treatment and, more often than not, the nurse exercised discretionary powers regarding payment for non-members. Nurses relate that, if necessary, they put in the money themselves rather than ask for it of those who evidently could not afford it and the local association not uncommonly waived fees for the 'sick poor'. The most popular feature of the NHS, its being free to the patient at the point of use, merely legitimised an approach to health care which already prevailed in the district nurse's work.

At the inception of the NHS, the district nurse occupied what has been stereotypically represented as a vocational, maternal or semidomestic and dominantly female role as a generalist, located outside the hospital institution, concerned more with the 'caring' than the 'curing' role. Until the Public Health Act of 1936 this was largely supported through the voluntary sector rather than by local authorities. Even following NHS reorganisation in 1974, interprofessionally, many district nurse sectors came under hospital nurse management, whilst others were under the community-based control of health visitor directors of nursing. Either scenario continued to bar district nurses from direct participation in their own management, policy making and implementation (McIntosh 1985), referred to as 'separation from the political community'. Policy was largely decided through 'policy drift', 'extra-parliamentary' non-district nursing professional

elites and the medical establishment, and 'symbolic policy making'. Pay was modest.

The Rushcliffe Committee in 1943 gave the district nurse on average '£260 rising by annual increments of £10 to £340 inclusive of emoluments' compared to a situation in 1937 when 'the minimum salary of a Queen's Nurse had advanced almost imperceptibly to £70 a year rising to £100 with £10 extra for those practising midwifery' (Stocks 1960). An interdepartmental Committee on Nursing Services Interim Report in 1939 also pointed out this was a serious undervaluation. This led eventually to the introduction of Burnham salary scales.

Emoluments continued to vary at local levels, causing considerable variations in real pay at a time when most hospital nurses still 'lived in' with few living expenses. Also, since 1928 many hospitals had contributed to the Federated Superannuation Scheme for Nurses negotiated by the Royal College of Nursing, or a similar one of their own, but this was seldom an option for the district nurse as the district nursing associations rarely felt financially able to participate. However, the NHS proposals had highlighted the function of the district nurse within the context of the growing professionalisation of nursing and initiated protracted debates over salary and training.

With the NHS, the Queen's Institute tried to establish its position as adviser to the local health authorities, listing among the advantages it offered, the maintaining of high standards and status of the Queen's Nurse and consultation benefits through the experience of Queen's Institute Visitors (Wellcome CMAC: The Queen's Institute Archives).

In emphasising the benefits of its referencing system for the provision of suitable candidates for posts (in the form of detailed reports on nurses' particulars, appointments held, performance and details of employment) to be made available to subscribing medical officers of health and local health authorities, the Queen's Institute inadvertently increased the professional differential which placed the district nurse in a more marginalised relationship, subservient to medical colleagues. This contrasted with the hospital nurse who was becoming increasingly autonomous through specialisation and 'technicalisation'.

TRANSPORT, TECHNOLOGY, ORGANISATION AND THEIR EFFECTS ON THE DAILY WORK OF THE DISTRICT NURSE

Whilst World War II and the institution of the NHS were highly significant in affecting health and welfare, it is possible to overestimate just how much these impacted on the daily work of the district nurse. Given the pragmatic approach to home nursing practice with adaptability at its core, the wartime need to 'make do' only reflected the prevailing practice of nursing in the home (Vignette 5.3). The 'Queen's methods', learned at Queen's Institute training homes, exemplified adaptability by demonstrating how to utilise household items in the service of nursing care, for the maintenance of hygiene and reduction of the risks of cross-infection in the patient's home.

The nurse was even instructed to fold her coat inside out and place it on a clean newspaper to prevent the transmission of germs from one house to another. While the 'Queen's poke' is usually remembered with some fond-

ness, for some it epitomised the tradition-bound attitude of the Queen's Institute (Vignettes 5.4 and 5.5).

In practice, Queen's methods of this kind were often discarded for a more common sense and less cumbersome way of doing things. However, in the event of a supervisor's visit, they were dutifully practised to the letter. Suffice it to say that, the supervisor was rarely there when a baby had to be delivered in a tent in winter with only a candle in a jam jar for light.

The changes brought about by medical, materials and transport technologies are the key to many changes in image: a Queen's Nurse in the 1940s (Keywood 1985) wrote of the difficulties of nursing patients at a time when the outside lavatory, no running hot water, central heating nor electricity were the norm, interior sprung beds and lifting aids were rare and when equipment had to be sterilised by the patient on a very hit-or-miss basis by boiling or oven baking. Before the availability of sterile packs in the 1960s, the homely sterilising procedures taught by the Queen's Institute were accepted as necessary.

World War II brought an acute shortage of district nurses and so, prompted by their experience as nursing officers in the services, men returning to civilian life applied for training and were welcomed into the service.

James Orr was drafted into the Royal Army Medical Corps in 1940 and posted to various locations abroad throughout the war. After his demobilisation he decided to capitalise on his experience and applied for nursing training.

Vignette 5.3   Queen's method

Well, if you were going to do a dressing you had to spread papers on the floor and you had to make little, they were like little paper hats to put dirty dressing in. You see, there was nothing pre-packed.

Vignette 5.4   Queen's method

You consider the patient's house and you consider the furniture, you see. So you don't just plonk things down on a good sideboard or table, you put paper down. And you put, if you're doing a dressing, you put paper down. And there's the Queen's poke, it's like a wee hat that you could put on. But the swabs that you used went into the Queen's poke and then that could be discarded, you see. So, we used to make fun about making the Queen's poke...

Vignette 5.5   Queen's method

And we had to make our own dressings, and ... we would ask the patient for a biscuit tin, if they had a biscuit tin. And we lined it with a piece of white sheeting, and we made the swabs up in the patient's house. And sometimes some of the family helped you, sitting making the swabs up, and put them in the tin. And they put it in the oven and that was sterilised. And the same with your syringes. You asked them for a milk pan, something like that, and you would say to them, do you mind if you kept that aside from the household things? And they'd get a box, next time you went there'd be a box with all the equipment in it. Oh they were very cooperative.

Nurses were needed at this time and Mr Orr found no difficulty in being accepted into Ballochmyle Hospital which had acted as an emergency military hospital during the war. As in the army, he mixed well with the nursing sisters in hospital but, used to the 'unconfined air' of army nursing, opted for district training. Again, he was accepted easily and finally took up a post in Greenock where a male nurse for the district was specifically requested. 'Had I not been in the army I would certainly never have thought of it … it did certainly sow the seeds of my future.' Mr Orr married, raised a family and remained on the district until his retirement in 1984.

Men in the district nursing service were often used to deal with cases requiring heavy lifting or the more 'difficult' male patients. Membership of the Queen's Institute was not open to men until 1947 but by 1949 there were estimated to be nearly 100 male nurses working on the district. Exclusion from the practice of midwifery, which was required for higher posts, presented male nurses with a stumbling block to promotion for some time.

Developments in drugs such as penicillin and streptomycin in the 1940s and 1950s and oral hypoglycaemics in the 1960s and the introduction of sterile disposables such as syringes and dressing packs in the 1960s to some extent created a different patient profile and workload and simultaneously changed the nurse's image as shown in vignettes 5.6 and 5.7. As medical techniques and surgical skills improved, more medical conditions could be treated successfully in hospital, reducing the numbers of patients requiring long-term care in the home. This made an impact on the district nurse's caseload, with some chronic conditions being removed from the home to hospital for treatment or cure to be replaced with the need for more short-term after-care. The giving of regular antibiotic injections replaced four-hourly sponging and poulticing in many instances but this too was superseded by the use of drugs in tablet form which could be self-administered. No longer did the nurse have to make several visits to one patient but the patient could look after himself and the time required to carry out nursing duties on many visits decreased.

Vignette 5.6 New treatment

Discoveries of new drugs have done more than anything to change the aspect of nursing and in many cases injection therapy has replaced bedside care. This has also brought problems. Many nurses have suffered from dermatitis. The adequate sterilisation of syringes has been difficult to cope with and there have been many breakages … In some areas arrangements are made whereby all syringes issued to district nurses are autoclaved…

Vignette 5.7 Changing times

The fact that we had all the disposables and everything that, you know, as opposed to having to make up all the, the swabs and everything. That was all very time consuming. To go into a house and do a dressing with just a, with a pack, as opposed to going in and having to make up dressings, etc., and see that there was always plenty of these sort of things, was a big timesaver. And the fact that you had disposable syringes and everything … you had a sharp needle all the time. As opposed to the, the other ones that we used to have, because they didn't last forever and you always felt, well, I hope it's going to be sharp enough.

The nature of home nursing was changing and has continued to do so into the present decade. While the initial impact of new therapies and technical procedures was to reduce nursing required at home, improved design coupled with specific training has seen the nurse bring equipment and skills, hitherto confined to the hospital, into the home.

One of the most striking and beneficial practical changes to affect the district nurse during this period was the introduction of sterile packs, which represented a dramatic time- and energy-saving measure.

Although the benefits of prepacked sterile equipment were great, nurses were also struck by the wastefulness they involved (Vignette 5.8).

Transport and communications technology were very significant factors of change. For example, the increase in nurses' mobility as their mode of transport changed from pedal power to motor car resulted in a move from smaller geographically based practices to wider GP attachments and their being able to carry and use more

---

Vignette 5.8   Dressing packs

Well, we got disposable syringes, and then dressing packs came in. Well, when you think, if you open a dressing pack and all you require is a swab or something ... But, I must say, I was never called to question with what I ordered. I really got what was required. And we tried to economise as much as we could ... you had a towel in the pack of swabs and woolies, instruments, but you could, if you weren't requiring that, you see, a towel with your wee swabs out, if it was just a small sore or something that was requiring. And you got probes, you got all sorts of things, and while, I suppose, you had to look at the economy of it all, but I was never questioned.

Vignette 5.9   Transport

One night last winter Nurse received an urgent call to Grimisay. It was blowing a gale then, but the boat, the boatman and the Nurse braved it to the other side, and a message was sent to Hector to meet Nurse with the trap at low tide. Nurse was delayed, and when she got to the appointed place Hector had gone. (His horse had grown too restive.) So Nurse had to fight her way home in the dark on foot, struggling along in her oilskin and rubber boots, shining a torch and trying to avoid the rocks and the quicksands. It took her four hours, but she made it! (Gordon 1948)

---

sophisticated equipment. Stocks (1960) refers to this happening gradually from the 1920s, but notes that 'On Exmoor a Queen's Nurse still visited her patients on horseback in the late thirties'.

Many local authorities provided cars to replace bicycles. In the cities, nurses tended to use public transport or walked but in the extreme weather conditions in the more remote areas transport became problematic. Even if a car was available, and many district nursing associations had provided them in country areas, the weather and terrain were not always hospitable. In Scotland, island work could necessitate the most unusual methods with some nurses being carried on the backs of ferrymen across rivers, enduring gruelling boat journeys on stormy seas (Vignette 5.9), pulling women in labour on sledges to reach boats to the mainland and doing their rounds on horseback. In more clement weather, they simply walked for miles.

The telephone combined with the practice receptionist also became a more reliable and efficient method of communication than the slate outside the nurse's front door, yet symbolises a dramatic change in the pace of life and in community lifestyle. As early as 1935, a nurse wrote to the Queen's Institute in response to an enquiry into the perceived value of the telephone that 'she would be able to work much more usefully with the doctors, since she attended cases sometimes not seeing the doctors for days, not knowing when they will call, nor they when she will visit the patient'. Indeed, a report based on surveys of district nurses in 1934–35 was issued on behalf of the Queen's Institute aiming to reduce the telephone charges. This stated that: 'It was possible for the utility of the nurses to be greatly increased by taking advantage of modern inventions. The best way of organising district nursing associations was to provide a nurse with a motor-car or motor-cycle and to install the telephone in her house'. It added that: 'There was not enough work in some places to keep a nurse fully occupied, but she could not be moved as she must be at hand for midwifery cases. The provision of cars and telephones would enable the nurses to be centralised and would reduce the number required'. It claimed this would represent an economy of approximately £12 000 pa for rates of county councils and substantial savings for nursing associations.

This change in the balance between being a team member and an individual practitioner created an 'autonomy dilemma' for many nurses who saw their public, professional and self images change in just a few years. Baly (1977) remarked:

Nowhere have changes been more marked than in the community [...] High hospital costs have promoted research into how hospital equipment can be converted into 'do-it-yourself' home kits, and machines that were once the wonder of hospitals are now found as standard portable equipment in the back of the district nurse's car.

Throughout the 1950s and 1960s, women were increasingly encouraged to have their babies in hospital maternity units rather than at home.

In the cities, where a local authority midwifery service had been established for some time, this had less of an impact on the district nurse but in rural areas her workload was significantly reduced. However, in her combined role as health visitor, she retained responsibility for antenatal and postnatal care along with care of the newborn.

This gradual transfer of midwifery from the close community work of district nurses during the 1960s and 1970s has been recalled with mixed feelings by district nurses and midwives who recognised the benefits of maternity hospital care but traditionally defined their work as being intimately involved with 'their' patients from the moment of birth to the moment of death.

As unscheduled hours of work for the district nurse attending confinements decreased, making working patterns more predictable, increasing numbers of married nurses entered the service (as shown in Vignette 5.10). While it is taken for granted today that married women are no more or less able to perform their duties, this is an issue of distinct significance to many district nurses who worked through this period. The opinion that district nursing is unsuitable for married women, commonly adhered to by many elderly nurses, rests on a notion of the work which may challenge modern definitions. Some may see it as a romantic idea from a Golden Age that did not exist in reality but it is expressed through recalled experiences and it remains powerful. It is that of

the district nurse as dedicated to her community of patients, unbound by personal family obligations, fulfilling a role which is defined entirely by the needs of her patients, untiring in her efforts to console and care and always available. According to testimonies, this was indeed the way of life for many nurses, particularly those in rural or isolated districts, who literally trudged miles in the snow on a call, delivered babies in tents in the middle of the night, made meals or lit fires for people and went back to the elderly patient on his own at the end of a long day just to sit with him for a while. These were women – and they were almost exclusively women – whose lives were bound by the community they lived amongst and looked after. How, they ask, can a woman with a husband and family of their own give the same time and dedication? The question which remains unasked by them is whether or not they ought to. Has district nursing changed to accommodate modern attitudes or have attitudes adapted in the development of a new role for the nurse?

INTER- AND INTRAPROFESSIONAL RELATIONSHIPS

Throughout the interviews, we have found there are rarely any negative comments about the GPs with whom the district nurses worked. Of course, there are indications that occasionally things were not so perfect and that features of teamwork, such as regular communication and consultation, were inadequate. This suggests some lack of understanding of the nurse's professional ability and potential role on the GP's behalf, but it is in itself significant that this is rarely openly expressed (either by district nurses or by GPs interviewed for a separate study).

However, there is a noticeable change in relationships between the GPs and district nurses reflected in correspondence to the professional journals before and after the NHS. In 1932, when the economic recession was hitting the GP in less lucrative rural and poorer urban panel practices, there was a run of letters to the *British Medical Journal*, of which the following from a

---

Vignette 5.10 'A flea in a fit'

The day was different altogether then because one went up to the hospital first if you had a patient up there, as you know, and you scooted round then like a flea in a fit sometimes to get all the work and you know, because we covered so much more ground then. We didn't cover an awful lot of ground on the district before...

(Prompt) And did you approve of the change?
Yes I think I did, I think I do really ... because you see there were so many rules and regulations in the midwifery books, you know our rules, that really if you were doing general it was difficult to keep up to them. You were infectious, you might have been – dirty wounds, people dying – so yes, that was a good thing.

Vignette 5.11 GP correspondence

...the general practitioner has a hard job in these days to pay rents, rates and taxes, and school fees, if he can afford children. The district nurse now takes most of his midwifery, does antenatal and postnatal work, and, during these and other visits, is consulted on every ailment, which she diagnoses and treats. If she does not, she is told they will not in future contribute their pence to the association. She is then up before her committee, who are themselves often her most exacting and troublesome patients: all use her to save a doctor's bill. She does minor surgery and sends patients to hospital for advice and treatment ... She has been known to diagnose and treat a pneumonia case. In other words, she is one of the general practitioner's most dangerous opponents, and therefore he treats her as such and prefers the old 'Gamp', who is under his control.

Vignette 5.12 Less educated than the hospital nurse

At the same time they felt she [i.e. the district nurse] was less educated than the hospital nurse. I remember patients saying to me, you know, when are you going to qualify as a nurse, and that sort of thing ... People don't perceive hands-on nursing as being skilled nursing. The minute you gave them an injection or did anything ... and as you began to be more 'technical' I think your reputation as a skilled person rose.

Devonshire GP was fairly representative (Vignette 5.11).

It should be noted that several GPs wrote in defence of 'their' nurses who are described as 'valuable' in dealing 'with minor ailments, and above all relieving me of routine midwifery'. However, this contrasts with a complaint registered by nurses noted in a 1953 Ministry of Health Annual Report that doctors were 'taking advantage of the nurses by requiring them to attend at their own surgeries in order to do dressings and other treatments which they could otherwise have done themselves' (Boddy 1969, White 1985).

Similarly, there were moments of friction between district nurses and health visitors, not only on a personal level but as a professional group, such as the perceived anomaly in salary awards in 1957 (in December 1957 health visitors were awarded a 15% pay rise whilst district nurses, including those working in multiple roles as nurse, midwife and health visitor, received only 5%).

The following statement (Vignette 5.12) was reiterated in varying forms by several nurses when asked how they felt the general public saw them.

The public image was apparently also raised as a result of the change in employment agency from voluntarily run district nursing associations to a more free and autonomous mode of operation following the 1948 NHS Act, after which the district nurse was employed (directly or indirectly) by the local council. Before this, the nurse often had to request her 2/6d payment per visit from the patient or even to make the uncomfortable decision whether the patient could afford the standard charge and to later justify this assessment to the committee (Stocks 1960), although children, TB sufferers and patients with other infectious diseases were often paid for through local authority grants well before 1948 (Keywood 1985). Until this time she was at the beck and call of local committee members to whom she was accountable.

Nevertheless, in many areas the nursing association committee often continued to wield considerable power for some time, particularly where local government chose to subcontract this responsibility back to the nursing associations until reorganisation in 1969. The Ranyard nurses were still being required to attend devotional meetings and carry a bible in their bag amongst their nursing equipment, all of which was regularly inspected by the lady superintendents. Looking back in 1960, Stocks comments:

Never again would they be required to look over their shoulders at the strivings of a hard-pressed voluntary committee to raise money for their services. Never again would they feel an obligation to assist at bazaars and local fetes, buy tickets for concerts, or function as uniformed exhibits in support of charitable appeals.

However, this was generally a period when the district nurse enjoyed considerable control over her daily and weekly timetable, frequently fulfilling a much wider, more holistic role than at present (particularly in the more rural areas). So when and why did the public come to perceive the district nurse as an equal to her hospital counterpart? The semantics of district nursing are complex and worthy of more consideration than this chapter has so far been able to give to it. However, research elsewhere (Pitt 1996) has considered the perception of the district midwife by the community using oral history to demonstrate how this has changed over time and current research suggests the same or similar conclusions.

The change appears to centre on an increasing public and professional awareness of professionalisation, largely measured by 'technicalisation', whilst the district nurse's autonomy was simultaneously being subsumed into the medical team and away from the community through more contact with other members of the community health-care team, especially the health visitor, social worker and GP (Merry & Irven 1948). This happened more noticeably in urban areas, probably because the centrality of the district nurse in her multiple role was associated more with the village nurse/midwife.

Traditionally the working relationship between GP and district nurse has been one of cooperation and mutual trust (Vignette 5.13). Whether in the days of local nursing associations with the nurse reporting to the committee or after 1948, when local authorities took control of the service, the district nurse retained a high degree of autonomy on a day-to-day basis. Notified of required visits by the GP, the nurse would prioritise cases and structure her own day. Working within the confines of patient need and with due respect for the doctor, she was not accountable to him. Although most district nurse/GP

relationships were cooperative and friendly, in some cases the doctor remained distant except where discussion of a case was necessary. The GP would diagnose and prescribe but the treatment in the home was administered by the nurse with room to exercise her own discretion.

The superintendent of district nursing services was usually geographically remote but could offer a sounding board for problems and undertook administrative details. The medical officer of health was ultimately responsible for the service and in most cases is reported as being well informed and cooperative. Perhaps as little as once or twice a year, the nurse would have a supervisor accompany her on a day's rounds, giving a chance to express any outstanding difficulties. The hierarchy was thus limited and in rural areas the nurse was left to her own devices for much of the time. Although most nurses seemed to value this as being essential to their sense of autonomy, the lack of professional contact has also been described as isolating. In any case, autonomy was limited to the local sphere as, during debates on the proposed health service in the 1940s, it was the voice of the medical profession, i.e. the doctors, which was loudest and this continued throughout the following decades as calls for reorganisation increased.

To the nurse who first travelled to all patients, then operated small clinics from her spare room, the increase in local authority spending on dedicated clinic buildings was a great leap forward. Her work was halved by the reduced travelling and for many patients, the central locations provided a more convenient point to go for an injection, etc., especially when working. In some areas the old district boundaries were replaced by schemes of GP attachment whereby the nurse would be attached to a GP or group of GPs and attend only their patients regardless of district. Initially preferred by the doctors, this scheme was instituted with no consultation with the nurses. It had positive aspects: a room was often available within the surgery for the district nurse to see ambulant patients; time for case discussions was easy to organise as health visitors and other health-care workers were brought together in the surgeries. But essentially the nurse

Vignette 5.13	Leg ulcer management

I once healed a varicose ulcer with honey. It was a huge ulcer on this old lady's leg and I had tried absolutely everything and I thought well, I think I'll try honey, and I spread it onto a dressing and put it onto her leg and I left it for a whole week and each time I went back, there was new skin growing round about and I eventually healed it. It was really amazing. The doctor didn't interfere in this kind of procedure, leaving the dressings to the nurse.

'belonged' to a particular doctor or surgery as opposed to a district consisting of patients. Even the name of the scheme, GP attachment, suggests an affiliation to the medical profession rather than to the patient.

In short, this system altered the relationship between patient and nurse as the districts were carved up according to doctors' surgeries and the nurse removed from her central role within them. It was possible to have to travel well beyond previous district boundaries to see patients and some nurses perceived themselves as becoming more distanced from their patient community. Furthermore, the predicted cost saving in working from one practice was frequently offset by the additional travelling outwith the district.

TRAINING AND PROFESSIONALISATION

We have so far considered hierarchical and elitist values and judgements as they relate to professionalisation of nursing and how the parameters changed, creating changes in self, professional and public image and status for district nurses. The other contributory factor in the professional equation is training. Oral testimonies suggest little evidence of nursing and/or medically related family backgrounds, quite different from the typical family history of the GP where there often appear to be much closer links with more direct family connections and inspirations (Digby 1999). This doesn't appear to vary between 1930 and 1960. Neither does the comparative social background to which Lisbeth Hockey's research into district nursing in 1966 refers (Hockey 1966), in which 177 district nurses were interviewed, finding 'only a handful of nurses had fathers from the professional class and 77% of husbands were of social classes 2 and 3'.

Similarly, few interviewees describe having felt a clear sense of vocation initially and a few even describe being actively discouraged from becoming nurses by their parents. Training, however, seemed to instil considerable self-respect and a strong and lasting loyalty to their training hospital. This seems increasingly true amongst district nurses who were Queen's or Ranyard nurses where a code of practice and sense of tradition and elitism were encouraged by the institution responsible for their post-registration training and subsequent practice. This was often despite desperately hard and unpleasant working conditions, poor pay and a fiercely authoritarian hierarchy vividly described by those who trained in the prewar and early postwar periods.

Their general training was spent entirely in hospital, often only entering community nursing by accident rather than by design. More than half married and of those who remained single, most were in the early group, qualifying before 1939 (Hockey 1966).

District nursing experience was not included in the general training experience of any interviewees. Neither was there much encouragement to take their careers in that direction when they first qualified, something that was also expressed by the GPs, where medical specialisation was preferred to generalisation and training was similarly 'on-the-job' experience for many years. Yet training is central to interprofessional and public affirmation of professional status and omission of recognised district training at basic and postbasic levels would therefore seem highly significant.

In 1946–47 a working party was appointed to consider the training of nurses and in 1948 the Queen's Institute urged the Minister of Health to grant statutory recognition to its training. Subsequently, in 1953 two more working parties were set up, one of which looked at health visitors while, the other, under the chairmanship of Sir Frederick Armer, Deputy Secretary of the Ministry of Health, looked at district nurse training. He reported (Ministry of Health 1955) a need for district nurses to be trained to a national standard and an advisory council to the Minister was set up in 1957. In 1959, a report (Ministry of Health 1959) provided for 4 months' training operated by local health authorities but carrying a national certificate issued by the Ministry of Health with the Ministry's advisory committee acting as supervisory body. However, much of the decision-making process about training still rested with local authorities.

In fact, many nurses who had been working as district nurses, often for many years, had to attend these training sessions. Several commented that they were delighted to discover that they had actually been doing the right things, having previously learnt 'on the job' with minimal or no instruction. Under direct local authority control, it is significant that the district nurses were more specifically being run by a sector of the medical profession, having to compete for resources against other health and welfare services.

Studies during the 1960s (Hockey 1966, 1968, Skeet 1970) revealed that district nurses were underused and underacknowledged, whilst some training was no longer appropriate to requirements. A revision of the syllabus and examination was recommended, but not implemented, as was a three-tier career system which might have produced a more balanced professional structure and was intended to anticipate and minimise the autonomy dilemma by providing career opportunities for specialists and generalists in this field.

Nevertheless a form of statutory training was imposed from 1960, provided by the local authorities, whilst pay and conditions were now brought in line with those of hospital nurses. Another working party resulted in the Briggs Report of 1972 (DHSS 1972) which included provisions for more specific training although a statutory body for community nurses similar to the midwives' and health visitors councils was not included, again despite pressure from the Queen's Institute then and again 4 years later.

THE PRIMARY HEALTH-CARE TEAM

The development of the health centre had been outlined as an integral part of the new health service in 1948 but even from the early stages, it was postponed due to lack of funds. It was not until the late 1960s that the building of health centres began in earnest despite several earlier experimental health or medical centre projects such as Woodberry Down built at Stoke Newington (Greater London) in 1948 and Swindon in Wiltshire in the 1930s.

The first in Scotland, Sighthill in Edinburgh, built in 1953, was designated as the site for one of four 'experimental units' in health centre building in the country. Initially viewed with scepticism, its first district nurse described it as a 'wonderful new building' offering a radical new facility within the community housing doctors, nurses, dentists, physiotherapists, child welfare and school health services, psychiatric clinic, occupational therapists and pharmacy. Open in the evening, it was more accessible for working patients while providing exceptional facilities for the staff. Its most beneficial feature for the nurse was the opportunity it created to mix both professionally and socially with colleagues (Beatty 1960). Writing in 1958, one district nurse claimed:

Improved social conditions, higher wages, increased employment of women, speed of travelling, have added to, rather than reduced, our responsibilities as district nurses … The establishment of health centres with facilities for group medical practice has done much to increase the cooperation between the various members of the public health team and general practitioners (Dixon 1958)

This was the beginning of the teamwork era where cooperation amongst staff was the key but it created a certain apprehension in district nurses who had always viewed their method of work as cooperative, both with the doctor and patient. Although they welcomed the chance to expand that into the sharing of resources, many also felt a further sense of detachment from their patients. Seeing many more patients in the health centre meant that they spent less time on the district. Effectively this was the beginning of the removal of the nurse from the street (Vignette 5.14).

However, health centres only grew in significant numbers nationally in the late 1960s and

---

Vignette 5.14 Your own people

They didn't rely on you any more. You weren't their nurse any more. There was something about being a nurse in the community that everybody respected you as their nurse. That's gone … I think when we became the health centre, this was an improvement supposed to be … but I did miss the bond that you had with your own people, as I call them…

1970s and then mostly on a smaller format in response to the 1966 review of the family doctor service (Jones 1994, Klein 1995).

CONCLUSION: A COMBINED RETROSPECTIVE AND PROSPECTIVE VIEW

It was during the early 20th century that the long tradition of home nursing culminated in an organised and increasingly professional service, first voluntarily and later under the NHS, as a state scheme to care for the sick in their homes. Many changes have been imposed on the service in the later part of this century: a new administrative authority with the NHS; increased expectations of the welfare state by patients and their relatives; increasing bureaucracy, including major changes in the job description; growing patient awareness of health and legal rights; and the political and media emphasis on provision of community health care as a high priority set against the realities of resources and practical support.

Differences between the rural and urban experience as a district nurse prevail but the popular image of the nurse as firmly rooted in and committed to her patient community has persisted in the public mind and remains the image preferred by the nurse of the 1940s and 1950s. Other, perhaps less surprising comments that occur with significant regularity point to a changing self-image amongst present district nurses, as well as a wider, still evolving public and professional image.

Although the professional status of district nurses is no longer in doubt, they are now closely associated with the medical team aspect of health care while patients are said to have become more critical and less appreciative or cooperative. The nurse is no longer recognised as 'nurse' or 'our nurse' but is one of the district nurses working from the doctor's surgery or health centre in a more institutional and hierarchical system alongside other grades of district nurse, indicating a loss of communitarian image.

In addition, hospital policy changes have dramatically reduced inpatients' length of stay and resulted in a significant increase in the number of acute patients now regularly being nursed at home, making the job more demanding in knowledge of medical and surgical advances and corresponding changes in nursing procedures (DHSS 1993, Timmins 1996). Early discharge of patients following open heart surgery or day surgery may necessitate quite complex dressings or therapies. Patients (for example, postsurgery or terminally ill) are sometimes nursed at home despite requiring intravenous or nasogastric feeding therapy when they would previously have required hospital admission.

Recent developments in health policy have also forced a number of fundamental changes in role and workload and working day routine, redefining the job description and thereby changing the relationship with other health-care professionals, with specialist nurses and practice nurses increasingly present.

It is through these changes and the way the past is described that we can understand the popular perception of the district nurse. Through the fragmentation and change in the role of the district nurse, the importance of the historical context emerges. In a changing environment we can appeal to history to show whether a continuity of function and definition exists or whether the district nurse of the past is simply that: a thing of the past.

Throughout, this chapter has aimed to contextualise district nursing historically within the nursing and wider health-care professions. As well as outlining the many changes, it has incorporated the views expressed by those who worked through them. The view most consistently expressed was that which defined district nursing in terms of the relationships it encompassed, between the nurse and the patient and professional colleagues. In an environment where the dynamics of teamwork are subject to change, it is the ongoing dilemma of present and future nurses to accept or challenge this.

Acknowledgement

Both authors wish to thank Susan McGann, RCN archivist, whose support and encouragement are unfailing and very much appreciated.

Particular thanks for encouragement, advice and support in writing this are due to Prof. Anne Digby, Oxford Brookes University and to Susan McGann, RCN Archivist. Thanks are also due to the staff of the Queen's Institutes for England and Wales and for Scotland and archivists at the Wellcome Institute CMAC. All resulting interviews will be deposited with the RCN archive's oral history collection.

REFERENCES

Abel-Smith B 1960 A history of the nursing profession. Heinemann, London

Baly M 1977 Nursing past into present. Batsford, London

Baly M 1986 Florence Nightingale and the nursing legacy. Croom Helm, London

Beatty D 1960 On the internal phone. All in a day's work. No 14 A district nurse in a health centre. District Nursing 3(7): 154–155

Boddy F A 1969 General practitioners' view of the home nursing service. British Medical Journal II: 438

Crowther M A 1986 Medicine and the end of the Poor Law. Bulletin of the Social History of Medicine 38: 74–76

Department of Health and Social Services 1972 Report of the Committee on Nursing (London) (Chairman Professor Asa Briggs). HMSO, London

Department of Health and Social Services Inspectorate 1993 Regional Health Authority Community Care Monitoring: national summary. HMSO, London

Digby A 1994 Making a medical living: doctors and patients in the English market for medicine, 1720–1911. Cambridge University Press, Cambridge

Digby A 1999 Challenge and change: the evolution of the British general practitioner, 1850–1948. Oxford University Press, Oxford

Dingwall R, Rafferty A M, Webster C 1988 An introduction to the social history of nursing. Routledge, London

Dixon N M 1958 Changes in district nursing. Queen's Nurses' Magazine February: 24

Gordon J E 1948 Scottish journey 6. With the nurses of the Western Isles (III). Nursing Mirror July 10: 235

Hardy G 1981 William Rathbone and the early history of district nursing. GW&A Hesketh, Ormskirk

Hawker J 1995 Parish nursing in Dorset 1700–1915. Unpublished paper presented at the Ailments and Archives Conference at Dorset County Records Office

Hockey L 1966 Feeling the pulse. Queen's Institute of District Nursing, Edinburgh

Hockey L 1968 Care in the balance. Queen's Institute of District Nursing, Edinburgh

Jones C 1989 Sisters of charity and the ailing poor. Social History of Medicine 2 (3): 339–348

Jones H 1994 Health and society in twentieth century Britain. Longman, London

Keywood O 1985 It used to be so different. RCN History of Nursing Group Bulletin 9: 26–28

Klein R 1995 The new politics of the NHS, 3rd edn. Longman, London

Loudon I 1986 Medical care and the general practitioner 1750–1850. Clarendon Press, Oxford

McIntosh J B 1985 District nursing: a case of political marginality. In: White R (ed) Political issues in nursing: past, present and future. John Wiley, Chichester

Merry E, Irven I 1948 District nursing: a handbook for district nurses. Baillière, London

Ministry of Health 1955 Report of the Working Party on the Training of District Nurses. HMSO, London

Ministry of Health 1959 Report of the Advisory Committee on the Training of District Nurses. HMSO, London

Pitt S 1996 Midwifery and medicine: discourses in childbirth 1945–1975. Unpublished PhD thesis, University of Wales, Cardiff

Searle C 1965 The history of the development of nursing in South Africa. Durrant and Viljoen, Pretoria

Skeet M H 1970 Home from hospital. Dan Mason Research Committee. Cited in Baly M 1973 Nursing and social change. Heinemann, London

Stocks M 1960 A hundred years of district nursing. Allen and Unwin, London

Summers A 1997 Nurses and ancillaries in the Christian era. In: Loudon I (ed) Western medicine: an illustrated history. Oxford University Press, Oxford

Sweet H 1997 District nurse a proper nurse? Unpublished paper presented at the Cinderella Services Conference, South Bank University, London

Timmins A 1996 Dilemmas of discharge: the case of district nursing. Department of Nursing and Midwifery Studies, University of Nottingham, Nottingham

Walby S, Greenwell J 1994 Medicine and nursing: professions in a changing health service. Sage, London

White R 1978 Social change and the development of the nursing profession: a study of the Poor Law nursing service 1848–1948. Henry Kimpton, London

White R 1985 The effects of the National Health Service on the nursing profession 1948–1961. King's Fund, London

Williamson L 1996 Soul sisters: the St. John and Ranyard nurses in 19th century London. International History of Nursing Journal 2: 2

District nursing within the professional context

6

Research

Lisbeth Hockey

Key points

- In defence of research
- Basic principles of research and some common approaches
- Involvement in research
- The future

INTRODUCTION

The purpose of this chapter is to bring research as a concept and as an activity right into the domain of district nursing. It is argued that research can no longer remain outside or even at the periphery of professional district nursing practice but that it must be central to it. This statement is not intended to imply that every district nurse has to undertake research but rather that every member of the district nursing profession should have an awareness and a basic understanding of the meaning of research.

IN DEFENCE OF RESEARCH

It is suggested that a chapter on research is justified for four main reasons.

1. Quest for evidence
2. Quest for excellence
3. Quest for professional recognition
4. Encouragement of critical thinking.

Quest for evidence

The term 'evidence-based practice' must now be in every nurse's vocabulary. It is a precursor to another concept which is working its way into all aspects of nursing – clinical governance. There appears to be general agreement that the clinical needs of patients should be the driving force behind treatment and care and the appropriate administrative framework for their delivery. However, such agreement is not in itself adequate to determine the type of care needed. The missing link is evidence capable of defending a particular line of action. There is often, though not always, a choice of interventions at the disposal of health professionals, calling for different levels of resources in terms of time, skills, equipment, medication, dressings, etc. What is needed is a rational defence of one type of care over another which may, on the face of it, be less demanding of resources and therefore cheaper. Of course, one's personal experiences as well as intuition may influence one's choice of intervention but they would not stand up to independent scrutiny. For this, evidence must be available which comes from rigorous research. It is worthy of note, however, that evidence from a variety of sources should be considered and that the nature of evidence needed and accepted may be elusive (Kendall 1997).

Cost-benefit and cost-effectiveness are common terms in modern health care. Economists are being employed at many levels to produce such calculations and on the cost side of the equation, they are the indisputable experts. However, it would seem inappropriate, if not dangerous, to allow economists to make statements about benefits or effectiveness. The contribution of economics to health care is further discussed in Chapter 14.

Understandably and traditionally, nurses have insisted that they know more about beneficial and effective nursing interventions than anyone else, but evidence for such assertions is now demanded and for this, research is essential. The quest for evidence was fully endorsed by the Scottish Executive. In its report *Designed to care* (1997) evidence-based care is identified as a major ingredient of 'good-quality' health care. Chapter 13 brings greater clarity to the all-important concept of 'effectiveness'. It is no coincidence that the journal *Clinical Effectiveness in Nursing*

was launched in 1997 (Churchill Livingstone). In its first edition the editor reminds his readers that the promotion of clinical effectiveness is considered a major challenge facing health care and the Chief Nursing Officer, Department of Health states that nurses frequently lack the required sound evidence for the potential effectiveness of intervention (Moores 1997).

Quest for excellence

Readers of this book are likely to be nurses who want to do an excellent job. They aim to be excellent district nurses. Excellence implies awareness of the latest available knowledge generated by research. Such knowledge is bound to include evidence regarding the most effective care in specific situations. Therefore, it paves the way to excellence.

Excellence is important not merely as vocational aspiration, important though this is. It is possible for a situation to arise which leads to complaints by patients or their carers. Society is becoming increasingly litigation conscious and it may be necessary for a district nurse to defend her actions in a court of law. The court is likely to invoke the judgement of the professional body controlling nursing, who will use the latest available knowledge as a yardstick to assess the standard of care given. As stated above, such knowledge is likely to have been generated by research. Therefore, excellence in care presupposes some familiarity with recent research. Individual excellence contributes to overall excellence and the continuous refinement of the yardsticks to assess it.

Quest for professional recognition

Professional recognition requires not only formal membership of a recognised professional body but also individual adherence to the respective professional code. District nursing, as a branch of general nursing, is therefore inextricably linked with the criteria used by nursing to claim professional status and it is incumbent on each district nurse to act in support and furtherance of those criteria.

It is generally recognised that a profession requires a foundation of science as well as a vocational motivation. Research is essential for the building and growth of the scientific foundation. On a practical level, the professional code which guides an individual nurse's practice dictates that she is personally accountable for her practice. This, in turn, requires the use of the latest available knowledge. The vocational requirement of a profession is a necessary but not sufficient condition for professional status.

Nursing is the art of applying nursing science. The art and the science are part of the same concept of nursing and cannot be separated. As pointed out by Closs (1997), the need to develop an interest in and an understanding of science is becoming ever more urgent because of its close connection with the concepts of evidence and effectiveness. Three years earlier, the same author identified a lack of enthusiasm for science, and even a dislike of it, in many nurses (Closs 1994).

Encouragement of critical thinking

In district nursing, a field of relative autonomy and individual responsibility, the faculty of critical thought is not only desirable but essential. Each patient and each situation encountered bring individual challenges and suggest new questions. If individualised holistic care is given more than lip service, routine tends to be elusive. Therefore, it becomes incumbent on district nurses to become involved in research by asking questions and evaluating research reports.

It must be stressed that not all critical thinking is related to research but that any involvement in research, at whatever level, requires critical thinking.

BASIC PRINCIPLES OF RESEARCH AND SOME COMMON APPROACHES

Often, research in nursing is dismissed as an academic exercise with little, if any, relevance for nursing practice, education or management. Such an attitude may be caused by lack of understanding of the nature and potential of research.

Basically, research attempts to increase available knowledge in any field, including nursing, by the discovery of new facts and/or relationships through a process of systematic enquiry (Macleod Clark & Hockey 1979, 1989). The precise nature of the process varies, depending on the type of new knowledge sought and the discipline in which the investigation is undertaken. In all cases, however, the steps constituting the process must be scientifically defensible and follow a credible design.

It would be impossible to do justice to the topic of research designs and methods within the confines of one chapter. The reader is referred to the rapidly proliferating literature which is freely available, a small selection of which is presented at the end of this chapter. The approach taken here is to give a broad and necessarily superficial introduction to the main principles and designs of research with some examples of relevance for district nursing. The examples have been chosen to illustrate different designs and methods, not for any other reasons. Referring to the definition of research quoted above, it will be appreciated that the methods of enquiry are bound to differ depending on the questions to which answers are sought.

There are many ways in which research approaches can be classified. For the purpose of this chapter, an initial and somewhat superficial division into quantitative and qualitative approaches, especially in the field of nursing research, had been considered 'mutually exclusive', that is, 'either/or'. It is now recognised that many research questions can best be answered by a combination of both approaches. Brief descriptions of both approaches, outlining the main differences, follow.

Quantitative research

As the term implies and as alluded to above, quantitative approaches have their focus on numbers. The researcher asks standardised questions, either by interviewing people or by self-completion postal questionnaires. The answers are counted and tabulated and can be subjected to various statistical manipulations. The usual expectation is that the information gained, the data, might be generalisable over a wider group of people than those questioned and/or that certain patterns might emerge. Not all quantitative research has generalisability of findings as its major aim and numbers alone do not guarantee such an aim. Other factors enter into the picture and statistical advice on the design is essential.

As pointed out by Porter (1996), the first difference between the two approaches is the focus of their analysis. Quantitative research has its focus on numbers, whilst qualitative research concentrates on words. Another important difference lies in the expectation of the quantitative researcher to attain maximum objectivity by the use of standardised means of data collection, while the qualitative researcher stresses the importance of subjectivity.

Experimental research, usually contrasted with descriptive research, also tends to use quantitative designs. The researcher attempts to make precise comparisons between information obtained from two groups: an experimental group, which is subjected to a certain intervention, and a control group, as alike as possible in composition but without the added 'experimental' factor, the intervention of whatever kind. This method is used to identify cause–effect relationships. Clinical trials of various kinds tend to employ such an approach.

The establishment of the Cochrane Centre (named after the main initiator and protagonist of randomised controlled trials) as a way to establish effectiveness illustrates the importance attributed to this approach by the scientific community (Cochrane 1989). The Centre, established in 1992, aims to collate, analyse and disseminate the results of such trials worldwide. The Cochrane Library, an important adjunct to the Cochrane Centre, provides summaries of randomised controlled trials on selected subjects. An example relevant for district nurses is the work on leg ulcers.

Jadad (1998) compiled the adviser's guide to randomised controlled trials. In nursing, such trials are difficult, if not impossible, due to the complex nature of nursing. However, the need to find a credible means to establish evidence remains as urgent as ever. The collaborative network of nursing research centres in Europe, initiated by the World Health Organisation (European Region), represents a powerful attempt to strengthen nursing research, especially in relation to producing evidence.

Surveys

A survey is a frequently used quantitative research tool. For example, West & Poulton (1997) undertook a survey to explore certain aspects of teamwork in primary health care. Several 'team functioning' factors had been identified and teams were scored accordingly. Standardised validated questionnaires were used, which is the most frequently employed method of data collection in surveys.

Surveys tend to be used when relatively simple information is sought about a given group of people. For example, if one wanted to collect data about district nurses in a given geographical area, one could send self-completion standardised questionnaires to all district nurses in that area. Such an approach would be termed a 'census'. The information gained would be applicable to all the nurses who responded to the completed questionnaire. Alternatively, one could select a sample of nurses in the hope that it would resemble the total population as closely as possible. The sample would be randomly selected with additional safeguards to achieve representativeness. For example, a survey of district nurses was conducted more than 30 years ago. It included samples taken from nurses working in industrial areas, in rural areas and in retirement areas because experience had shown that different working patterns would prevail.

Personal interviews, using the same standardised questionnaires, can also be used in surveys. Self-completion questionnaires are cheaper to administer because of the saving of time and transport costs but they tend to result in a lower response rate. It is possible that certain types of nurses are more or less likely to respond to written requests for information and therefore one cannot be certain that the respondents are representative of the total. Early surveys of district nurses in Scotland were undertaken by Carstairs (1966) and of district nursing in England by Potter & Hockey (1975).

Quantitative research requires great care in the choice and wording of questions to be asked. It is all too easy for questions to be loaded or ambiguous. It is advisable to seek skilled advice in the construction of a questionnaire and to test it on a small number of people before using it for a large-scale survey.

Qualitative research

Contrary to frequently held beliefs, qualitative research has little, if anything, to do with the quality of the research. It has a different aim in that it is designed to explore the meaning of specific situations by probing more deeply than standardised questions can do. Personal interviews are most frequently used to collect the information, allowing the respondents to answer open rather than standardised questions. It is possible to combine standardised and open-ended questions in one questionnaire. Hill Bailey (1997) provides a helpful introduction to qualitative methods in nursing research. Qualitative data can also be obtained from observation but scientific rules have to be followed to provide a measure of validity.

An example of a qualitative study highly relevant for district nurses was undertaken by Rapport & Maggs (1997). The researchers sought to elicit the experiences and responses of primary health-care teams to changes taking place in the community.

A qualitative study in the field of district nursing education sought to 'gain an understanding of the learning experiences of district nurse students in the learning environment of the community and to examine learning in the practice setting from the perspective of the student'. The researcher used an ethnographic approach which has its origin in the discipline of anthropology (Mackenzie 1992). This is an example of the use of one of the sciences underlying nursing to illuminate aspects of nursing. Psychology, physiology, ergonomics and sociology are other sciences frequently used for studies of different aspects of nursing.

Within the broad area of qualitative research, there are also different design possibilities. One particular design which is rapidly gaining popularity in nursing research is 'grounded theory'. The method was developed by two American sociologists from their observations of dying patients. They realised that careful documentation of observations and spoken words provided, a potentially fruitful way of capturing real world situations. Detailed analysis of such raw data could lead to the construction of a theory or model which could then be tested in other situations. The theory would be 'grounded' in real world data (Glaser & Strauss 1967, Strauss & Corbin 1991).

An example within district nursing of such an approach in the very early stages of its development was the work by Kratz (1978). She observed that district nurses adopted different caring styles depending on the types of patients they were nursing, ranging from focused to diffuse care. She developed a continuum of care model which has found uses. The principles of grounded theory are examined by Sheldon (1998) who also describes how the approach can influence the way that nurses practise.

Focus groups

Focus groups can be used to obtain free, unstructured and spontaneous comment on certain topics from a group rather than individuals. Morgan (1992) explains how focus group research should be conducted. An assessment of need for district nursing in one inner-city area was undertaken by using focus groups (Brooks & Mackay 1988). Quoting the researchers, 'The focus groups aimed to encourage nurses to explore their views on the district nursing service and how they might use any new investment'. The response rate was 93% and the recommendations made, mostly in connection with recording systems, were accepted by the health authority and the respective NHS trust.

Evaluation research

Evaluation research consists of the systematic collection of data with the aim of making judgements on whatever is being evaluated. Normally, it aims to use predetermined measures or objectives against which the evaluation is made. A framework frequently used for evaluation purposes is that propounded by Donabedian (1966) who advocated a structure/process/outcome approach. He believed that the structure of an organisation or of a programme and the process of carrying out the specific activity to be evaluated could not be ignored in the judgement of any outcome. They were three interdependent dimensions. His model has gained wide acceptance.

Some activities appear similar in character to research but they do not strictly comply with the normally accepted research paradigm, as alluded to in the definition of research above. An example of such confusion is 'audit', a concept which cannot be a stranger to any nurse at present. The differences between research and audit are clearly explained by Closs & Cheater (1994). The authors stress that, while the two processes have much in common, especially in terms of the systematic approach, they have different aims. Research attempts to create new knowledge whereas audit has its focus on setting, raising and monitoring standards.

Similarly, efforts to find formulae for the solution of local management problems are not likely to constitute research although they may well be precursors to it by identifying specific questions which require systematic investigation.

Other research approaches

There are several other research approaches with potential usefulness for district nurses. Examples are action research (Webb 1996), critical incident technique (Cormack 1996) and case study research (Yin 1989).

The approaches mentioned above are empirical in character in that they explore real-life situations. It is also possible to undertake theoretical research which may involve the sciences of philosophy, ethics, linguistics and others. Historical research, which is gaining momentum in nursing, uses the scientific approach of historians in its examination of documents, etc. Examples of

historical research in district nursing were undertaken by Stocks (1960) and by Baly (1987). Rafferty (1996) provides a helpful discussion of historical research. Oral history is an important adjunct to the study of documents. It involves interviews with individuals about their own past.

The collection of data is, of course, not the end of the research process. The data have to be analysed and presented in a written report which will, it is hoped, be published to disseminate the results. For the analysis of quantitative material, computer programs have been available for a very long time. For some years now, sophisticated software packages for the analysis of qualitative data have been available and they are being added to constantly. Thus, the processes of analysis of all kinds of data have been greatly facilitated, although caution is needed in the appropriate use of computer programs.

The above list of research approaches is by no means exhaustive. However, any further expansion within this chapter could easily lead to confusion. The interested reader has a multitude of resources available.

An example

It is possible for a specific question to be approached from different perspectives, using different research methods. An example is the important question of patient satisfaction with the district nursing service. Three studies attempting to address this question were undertaken in 1998.

1. A practising district nurse in an inner-city area, striving for enhanced efficiency, considered it important to elicit the views of users of district nursing service (Cusick 1998). This was a limited 'exploratory' study, which used the postal questionnaire as the main tool for the collection of information.
2. A study which explored the patients' views of the care given by district nurses had a slightly different objective, in its aim to focus more specifically on the care

component of district nursing (Davy 1998). The author used a semi-structured interview technique for the collection of data. Interviews based on structured as well as open-ended questions were conducted in the patients' homes.

3. The third study describes an attempt to develop and validate a measure of patient satisfaction with the district nursing service (Gillard & Reed 1998). This study, also limited to an inner-city area, targeted elderly people who were visited by the local district nursing service and who were living alone and unable to leave their home without personal assistance.

Although the study was limited in sample size, its ambitious aims appear to have been met. The researchers used a structured interview technique and administered four standard questionnaires at the beginning and toward the end of 1991. Based on the assumption that satisfaction with care is a multidimensional phenomenon, the researchers employed the technique of factor analysis to construct their scale. Seven factors emerged. The patients' spontaneous comments were used to judge the concurrent validity of the questionnaire. The analysis of this work called for fairly sophisticated statistical techniques.

This study, like the other two, provides useful pointers for further research on patient satisfaction which, in the present climate of consumerism, is likely to gain public support.

Summary

- Research is a process which follows scientific guidelines.
- There are many types of research approaches depending on the type of questions to which answers are sought. Only a small selection is included in this chapter.
- Any of the sciences underlying nursing can be used to study different aspects of nursing providing its specific perspective is used appropriately.

INVOLVEMENT IN RESEARCH

Reading research reports and assessing their utility

The research report, made accessible to others, is the final stage of a research project, the last stage of a complex process. The report is intended to inform others of any new knowledge that has been created. Clearly, unless the report is read, that intention cannot be met. The careful reading of a research report also affords a valuable learning experience. It should also help the understanding of what the researcher aimed to achieve.

As far as any assessment of utility is concerned, the results of the report as well as the methods used must be considered. Critical reading of a research report requires some basic knowledge and understanding. It is now relatively easy to gain access to research reports through academic and professional libraries who hold extensive databases or through the Internet. In view of the rapidly increasing number of research reports, it may be possible for a group of district nurses or, better still, the multidisciplinary members of a primary health-care team to share the reading and assessment of reports and to stimulate discussion among them. Such a method of coping with information 'overload', which includes government reports, etc., has been tried successfully in several areas in the UK.

Using research findings

It is important to use research findings appropriately. Sometimes, the subject matter is not relevant; sometimes the findings are not generalisable, although they may provide pointers; sometimes the methods used lack validity. Using research is not synonymous with implementing research. It is used if it has been read and deliberately put aside for legitimate reasons. Sometimes, implementation takes the form of synthesising different pieces of research on the same topic and circulating the results to the relevant staff members, as a teaching aid. For example, one NHS trust in Scotland attempted to improve the district nurses' competence in wound care. Their work, which investigated current practice in wound assessment and wound care, led to an ongoing forum to encourage debate on this and other clinical procedures and to the development of a research-based wound assessment tool (Kennedy & Arundel 1998a,b).

Similar utilisation of a cluster of research studies on the same topic resulted in research-based guidelines for the treatment of leg ulcers (Community Nursing Leg Ulcer Link Nurse Team 1998).

Another important way to collate the evidence from different research studies is by systematic reviews of the literature. As the term implies, the reviewer uses predetermined aims and criteria in the critique of the literature. Such reviews contribute to the potential of research for its appropriate use.

An example of how research might help managers was undertaken to measure the workload of an integrated nursing team in general practice (Godfrey et al 1997). Quantitative as well as qualitative methods were used. The limitations of the study are frankly discussed by the authors and, although the results did not achieve the study's intent totally, it provides an extremely useful pointer for further research and for managerial considerations.

In spite of strong pressures for a research base in nursing education and practice, Mulhall (1995) explored possible reasons why the impact of research appeared to have been negligible. She identified a number of constraints, some of which she perceived as inherent in the professional ethos of nursing. Yet Mead (1996) believes that nursing initiatives could be used to encourage the use of research.

The apparent gap between research and its use in practice has been recognised and regretted by researchers as well as clinicians. Blanchard (1996) identified four main factors as being primarily responsible. They include teachers' as well as practitioners' lack of knowledge about research, but some responsibility is attributed to the researcher who does not communicate the research in intelligible language. Since 1996, when her article was published, there has been a marked increase in clinically

relevant research, the lack of which had been highlighted by the author as contributing to poor utilisation.

The Foundation of Nursing was set up in 1991 in order to 'put research into practice'. The Foundation supports projects which disseminate or implement proven research findings in order to change practice in any field of nursing.

Providing research-based teaching

All district nurses are teachers. They are responsible for the teaching of patients and their carers where appropriate; they also teach students in a variety of contexts and, through staff meetings, conferences, study days and similar events, they teach each other. Teaching takes place formally as well as informally, by word of mouth or by silent action. District nurses are influential in many different ways and it is important that their influence is based on knowledge. It is emphasised, again, that knowledge is not static but dynamic, being constantly added to by research.

Facilitating research

Research in district nursing cannot be undertaken without the cooperation of district nurses. They may be requested to complete a questionnaire, to allow themselves to be interviewed or observed. They may facilitate access to patients or clinics or advise on methods to obtain patients' consent. Managers of district nursing may be needed to facilitate research access to practising district nurses. It is important that the research for which the cooperation of district nurses and/or their patients is needed is understood and that the ethical implications are clearly recognised. District nurses need to have some knowledge of the basic principles of research in order to ensure that they are aware of the implications of facilitating specific research. Thus, although their facilitation is important, it should be informed facilitation. Obviously, the responsibility for giving the necessary information rests on the researcher, but the district nurses concerned should be able to discern whether that responsibility has been discharged satisfactorily or not.

Participating in or undertaking research

Often, district nurses are asked to help with research initiated by others. Providing they understand the implications and feel able to support the research, much benefit can be gained in the capacity of a helper. Learning by doing is a recognised, well-researched fact. In such a situation, the helper should be informed of the aims of the research and be given a full explanation of the intended research approach and methods. The ethical issues should be made clear. Moreover, the helper should ensure that the help given is clearly acknowledged in any ensuing publication.

Collaborative research between university departments and clinical staff is welcomed increasingly and has great benefit for both parties by merging academic and clinical expertise. It also contributes to the narrowing of the regrettable gap between academic research and its use in practice.

In the National Working Group Report (Mant 1997) a case is made for an increase of clinical staff with R&D expertise (Recommendation 9) and for local initiatives between researchers outside primary care and primary care clinicians (Recommendation 14).

District nurses who are serious about undertaking research have many opportunities. Their involvement should, most appropriately, begin with a thorough search of the available literature on their topic of interest. As stated above, there are now many data bases available which make such searches relatively easy. This would be a necessary first step for the design of a research proposal. It is not wise for the uninitiated to attempt research without advice and supervision. The burden of this chapter is to underline the scientific nature of the research process and the need to have some understanding of it. Because research requires finance, at the very least in terms of time, it is unlikely that any totally unguided research would be undertaken.

Finance for research

Research is costly and requires appropriate funding. At a time of scarcity of finance and limited budgets, some employing authorities may consider the financing of research as a low priority. However, it is often possible to support the need for research on the basis of expected beneficial outcomes, urgently needed evidence and effectiveness. Efficiency savings are sought in every sphere of health care but health-care providers need to be reminded that efficiency means effectiveness at lowest cost. Thus, research aimed to establish effectiveness can and must be defended. It should be recognised that expenditure on research may, in the long term, lead to savings in care provision. Practising district nurses seeking funding for a specific research project within their area of work are advised to approach their employing authority in the first instance.

However, even at that early point, it is helpful to have a reasonably firm research proposal for submission. The preparation of such a proposal requires considerable expertise, not only for the appropriate scientific approach and data collection methods, including analysis, but also for calculations of expected costs. Therefore, the help of an experienced researcher and, if possible, an appropriate financial expert should be sought. In the UK, it should prove relatively easy to find both kinds of support.

Ethical and financial issues

Ethics and finance are linked as it would be extremely unusual for finance to be made available for a research project which has not been approved on ethical grounds. All research has ethical implications and, for this reason, ethics committees have been established within administrative structures to assess proposed research from ethical perspectives, such as potential harm, respect for confidentiality and anonymity. In the UK, the Royal College of Nursing has produced a helpful guide for nurses involved in research or any investigative project involving human subjects (RCN 1998). The ethical implications of research extend beyond such investigations. As mentioned above, all research has a cost element which has to be balanced against other demands for finance, time or expertise, all of which imply costs of some kind. Therefore, the ethical dimensions of research can never be ignored.

It is difficult if not impossible to undertake research on the cheap. As stated above, it is costly and, at a time of scarcity of resources, research costs have to be carefully weighed up against other expenditure, the benefit of which may seem much more predictable. Any administrative structure funded by public money is accountable to the public for the appropriate use of that money and it is clearly more difficult to defend financial support of activities whose outcome cannot be predicted with any measure of certainty. When seeking financial support, it is advisable to demonstrate an awareness of the political and economic implications and to adopt a diplomatic approach.

The generally accepted need for 'efficiency' savings can and should be used to defend rather than reject research endeavours. Efficiency means 'effectiveness at lowest cost'. Therefore, any research seeking to establish effectiveness, however elusive it may seem, can and should be encouraged. Moreover, exactly because of scarcity of resources, evidence to support their use is demanded. Thus, the quest for evidence, mentioned at the beginning of this chapter, remains a powerful defence of research. The district nursing service itself is, legitimately, under public scrutiny. Therefore, studies seeking to establish public perception of the service are in the public interest and represent legitimate public expenditure. The reader is referred to p 106 of this chapter where three such studies, each using its own unique approach, are mentioned.

In the event of the employing authority not being willing to fund the proposed research, other sources are available. A list of possible funding bodies can be found in the volume *Resources for research* (Clamp and Gough 1999).

There are some voluntary bodies with a specific interest in district nursing, who may provide funding. A notable example is the Queen's Nursing Institute, Scotland which also funds community nursing research in a wider sense, undertaken by the Department of Nursing and Community Health at Glasgow's Caledonian University.

For district nurses within Europe, the European Union may be a fruitful source of funding.

CONCLUSION

It is, of course, impossible to predict the future with any measure of certainty. However, care in the community, in which district nursing plays a major part, is likely to increase rather than decrease.

There are powerful signs, at least in the UK, that research in primary care will receive considerable attention. Government documents provide an extremely strong defence of research, notably *R&D in Primary Care* (Mant 1997), which presents the report of a National Working Group. Most of its 24 recommendations have R&D implications. The very first point made (p. 1) states: 'Decisions made in primary care need to be based on research evidence'. Evidence-based nursing and clinical governance presuppose research. Without it, evidence will remain elusive and no credence will be given to clinicians who base their work on routine and tradition alone. They will have no right to claim clinical governance. Although research cannot guarantee the production of valid evidence which, as stated at the beginning of this chapter, is extremely complex, without research it is not even a remote possibility.

Quite apart from the potential benefits from research for the district nursing service, any practising district nurse, educator or manager would find personal enrichment by acquiring an awareness and basic understanding of research. To be part of a 'research culture' is profoundly exciting, by opening up one's vision to hitherto unimagined possibilities. It is capable of raising interest and increasing job satisfaction. It provides scope for creativity which, in turn, leads to an immensely satisfying path of discovery, a statement based on the author's personal research experience of almost 40 years.

To opt out of the research enterprise represents a negation of all the benefits alluded to above and would seriously threaten the right of such a person to professional status. Conversely, the research-minded and/or research-active district nurse earns professional status and esteem and has an important part in shaping the profession's future.

REFERENCES

Baly M 1987 District nursing. Heinemann, London

Blanchard H 1996 Factors inhibiting the use of research in practice. Professional Nurse 11(8): 524

Brooks A, MacKay K 1998 An assessment of need for district nursing. Nursing Times 94(4): 70–71

Carstairs V 1966 Home nursing in Scotland: report of an enquiry into the local authority domiciliary services. SHHD, Edinburgh

Clamp C G L, Gough S 1999 Resources for nursing research: an annotated bibliography, 3rd edn. Sage Publishing, London

Closs S J 1994 What's so awful about science? Nurse Researcher 2(2): 69–81

Closs S J 1997 Science now more than ever. Clinical Effectiveness in Nursing 1(2): 61–62

Closs S J, Cheater F M 1994 Utilization of nursing research: culture, interest and support. Journal of Advanced Nursing 19(4): 762–773

Cochrane A L 1989 Effectiveness and efficiency: random reflections on health services. Nuffield Provincial Hospitals Trust, London

Community Nursing Leg Ulcer Link Nurse Team 1998 Stepping out together – a research based approach to the management of leg ulcers. Edinburgh Health Care NHS Trust, Edinburgh

Cormack D F S (ed) 1996 The research process in nursing, 3rd edn. Blackwell Science, Oxford

Cusick K 1998 User views of the district nursing service. British Journal of Community Nursing 3(2): 74, 76–81

Davy M 1998 Patients' views of the care given by district nurses. Professional Nurse 13(8): 498–502

Donabedian A 1996 Evaluating the quality of medical care. Millbank Memorial Fund Quarterly 44(3): 166–203

Gillard C, Reed R 1998 Validating a measure of patient satisfaction with community nursing services. Journal of Advanced Nursing 28(1): 94–100

Glaser B, Strauss A 1967 The discovery of grounded theory. Aldine, Chicago

Godfrey E, Rink P, Ross F 1997 Measuring the workload of an integrated nursing team in general practice. British Journal of Community Health Nursing 2(7): 350–355

Hill Bailey P 1997 Finding your way around qualitative methods in nursing research. Journal of Advanced Nursing 25: 18–22

Jadad A R 1998 Randomised controlled trails: a user's guide. BMJ, London

Kendall S 1997 What do we mean by evidence? Implications for primary health care nursing. Journal of Interprofessional Care 11(1): 23–24

Kennedy C, Arundel D 1998a District nurses' knowledge and practice of wound assessment: 1. British Journal of Nursing 7(7): 380–387

Kennedy C, Arundel D 1998b District nurses' knowledge and practice of wound assessment: 2. British Journal of Nursing 7(8): 481–486

Kratz C R 1978 Care of the long-term sick in the community. Churchill Livingstone, Edinburgh

Macleod Clark J, Hockey L 1979 Research for nursing: a guide for the enquiring nurse. H M & M, Aylesbury

Macleod Clark J, Hockey L (eds) 1989 Further research for nursing: a new guide for the enquiring nurse. Scutari, London

MacKenzie A E 1992 Learning from experience in the community: an ethnographic study of district nurse students. Journal of Advanced Nursing 17: 682–691

Mant D 1997 R & D in primary care: national working group report. Department of Health, Wetherby

Mead D 1996 Using nursing initiatives to encourage the use of research. Nursing Standard 10(31): 33–36

Moores Y 1997 Clinical effectiveness. Clinical Effectiveness in Nursing 1(1): 3

Morgan D L 1992 Designing focus group research. In Stewart M, Tudwer F, Bass M, Dunn E, Norton P Tools for primary care research. Sage, Neuburgh Park

Mulhall A 1995 Nursing research: what difference does it make? Journal of Advanced Nursing 21(3): 576–583

Porter S 1996 Qualitative research. In: Cormack D F S (ed) The research process in nursing. Blackwell Science, Oxford

Potter D, Hockey L 1975 District nurses in England. Nursing Research Unit, Department of Nursing Studies, University of Edinburgh

Rafferty A M 1996 Historical research. In: Cormack D F S (ed) The research process in nursing, 3rd edn Blackwell Science, Oxford

Rapport F, Maggs C 1997 Measuring care: the case of district nursing. Journal of Advanced Nursing 25(4): 673–680

Royal College of Nursing 1998 Research ethics. RCN, London

Scottish Office Department of Health 1997 Designed to care: renewing the National Health Service in Scotland. Stationery Office, Edinburgh

Sheldon L 1998 Grounded theory: issues for research in nursing. Nursing Standard 12(16): 47–50

Stocks M 1960 A hundred years of district nursing. Allen and Unwin, London

Strauss A, Corbin J 1991 Basics of qualitative research: grounded theory procedures and techniques. Sage, Newbury Park

Webb C 1996 Action research. In: Cormack D F S (ed) The research process in nursing, 3rd edn. Blackwell Science, Oxford

West M A, Poulton B C 1997 A failure to function: teamwork in primary healthcare. Journal of Interprofessional Care 11(2): 205–216

Yin R K 1989 Case study research: design and methods. Sage, Newburg Park

FURTHER READING

Carter Y, Thomas C (eds) 1997 Research methods in primary care. Radcliffe Medical Press, Oxford

Clamp C G L, Gough S 1999 Resources for nursing research: an annotated bibliography, 3rd edn. Sage Publishing, London

Cormack D F S 1999 The research process in nursing, 4th edn. Blackwell Science, London

Krueger R A 1994 Focus groups. A practical guide for applied research, 2nd edn. Sage Publications, London

Field P A, Morse J 1985 Nursing research: the application of qualitative approaches. Aspen, Rockville, Maryland

Treece E W, Treece J W Jr 1986 Elements of research in nursing, 4th edn. Mosby, St Louis

7

Developing roles which enhance patient care

John Unsworth

Key points

- Role development through socialisation
- Technological advances, professional and organisational influences
- Learning from past experience
- Risk and legal implications

INTRODUCTION

This chapter will explore the changing role of the district nurse with particular emphasis on how this has enhanced patient care. The chapter starts by exploring role perceptions and how these are formed and then goes on to examine the driving and restraining forces which have influenced role development. There are a number of important lessons we can use to shape our thinking around future role development; amongst these are issues around the work of the clinical nurse specialist and the changing boundaries between medical and nursing practice. The chapter goes on to discuss concepts of risk in role development and the legal implications of such work. Finally, the chapter provides practical examples of role development which have altered care delivery through the provision of new services, the expansion of traditional roles and the development of new roles designed to support clinical practice.

The evolutionary development of the district nurse's role has taken on a new pace in recent years, yet some district nurses seek to continue with their traditional role while all around them the world is changing. Over the years district nurses have seen threats to their role come and go, some making major impacts and others making little or no impact. During these changes many nurses have rested on their laurels, decrying how it is possible for nurses without a postbasic community qualification to visit people at home. Many practitioners now realise that their role will not continue in its present form and that they must become proactive in developing their roles and practice to meet the challenges of health care into the millennium.

Role perceptions play an important part in shaping our thinking about our profession and our role as providers of health care. Role perceptions, while a useful way of conveying to others the essence of our role, can also be a two-edged sword, making us think that our role is merely the sum of its constituent parts and not encouraging us to challenge assumptions about the work we do and the way in which we do it. The potential dangers of role perceptions are clearly portrayed in vignette 7.1.

Vignette 7.1 provides insight into the perceived roles of health-care professionals. While such clear role definitions are useful as a way of conveying the bulk of what each professional group does, they can also be restrictive when applied too literally. A much simpler definition of the role for all community nurses would involve the search for health needs and the development

and delivery of programmes of care and education which meet these needs. Gardner (1998) refers to a speech by Trevor Clay in which he said 'Nursing has a wonderful ability to tie itself up in academic and abstract debate about its role, while other groups simply keep their eyes firmly fixed on what is happening in the health service and make themselves essential'.

ROLE THEORY

Role theory goes some way towards explaining how we are socialised into thinking about our roles in a particular way. Katz & Kahn (1966) describe how the process of role sending is one of the ways in which people learn about their work roles.

Everyone who works within an organisation has a defined 'role set', people who perform a similar role or have a vested interest in how an individual performs his role. The role set for most district nurses includes patients, carers, peers, managers and subordinates. Each member of the role set sends important signals to the role holder about his performance and the expectations of his role. Katz & Kahn (1966, p. 190) describe how 'role expectations are by no means restricted to the job description given by the organisation'. Thus those individuals with whom the post holder is in contact early in their career can alter a person's role. People develop techniques to allow them to anticipate the expectations of others with few cues and learn quickly, absorbing a great deal of role sending during the early days of role occupancy (Katz & Kahn 1966).

The forces exerted by a person's role set are not the only factors which influence our perceptions of our role. We are all capable of being 'self-senders', allowing our personalities and past experiences to shape our views of how we should act, think and satisfy the requirements of our posts. Clayton (1984) states that interactionist theorists therefore define role as 'a person's pattern of social behaviour, which seems appropriate to him/her in terms of demands and expectations of others, together with their own self-imposed demands'.

Vignette 7.1   Role perceptions

A colleague and I were asked to teach a session regarding the best use of resources in community nursing. We decided to look at the current use of human resources in relation to the boundaries each professional group had erected regarding their work. To start the session we decided to ask each student to identify the role of the district nurse, practice nurse, health visitor, school nurse, etc. Within a few minutes the groups had identified that district nurses care for people at home, practice nurses care for people in the surgery and health visitors dealt with 0–5 year olds. These descriptions would come as no surprise to most qualified community nurses but here we were faced with clearly defined role boundaries in students who were 4 weeks into their specialist practitioner course.

Finally, our roles are also shaped by the organisational context in which they are performed. Such organisational contexts can be particularly problematic for district nurses because they usually work in more than one organisational culture. Katz & Kahn (1966, p. 197) state, 'Roles become more complex when they require the focal person [*post holder*] to be simultaneously involved in two or more subsystems, since each is likely to have its own priorities and culture'. As such, the subsystem of an NHS trust and the subsystem of a primary health-care team may have different and occasionally opposing views of the district nurse's role.

Such opposing views can lead to the development of role conflict, where the role expectations of one subsystem can make compliance with the other more difficult. Such conflict can also occur between one or more of the role senders from an individual's role set. This can be likened to the conflict that can occur when a student nurse is given one message by his tutor and a different message in a clinical area. Such role conflict can also develop in individuals who attempt to perform more than one role at a time. For example, lecturer practitioners often experience conflict of this nature and describe how the pull of the clinical setting is always greater (Lathlean 1995).

Katz & Kahn (1966) describe the process of role taking and role making. Role takers are socialised into their role by members of their role set and thus take on a received role. Role makers, on the other hand, bring with them their own role perceptions and past experiences that they use to shape their role. Role makers also experience the views of their role set and this can often lead to role conflict but some degree of accommodation is usually reached. Chalmers (1997) found similar role categories amongst nurses in specialist, nurse practitioner and other new roles. In her study, role makers were more certain of their role and demonstrated higher levels of autonomy and decision making. This categorisation is interesting as it may go some way towards explaining why some nurses accept their given role and never contemplate developing it while others seek new challenges and constantly question ways of delivering care and services. Clearly there is a need for further research in this area to help explain these differences and to suggest how such differences can be identified.

Driving and restraining forces in role development

Several forces have driven the development of the district nurse role in recent years. Many of these forces can also be seen as restraining the development of the nurse's role; indeed, some practitioners see some of the changes as a threat to their continued existence. Most influential amongst these has been the introduction of the internal market in health care. The development of market principles led to rapid change in the ways in which many NHS trusts viewed general practitioners, giving them greater influence. This increased influence led to a closer attachment of community nurses to the primary health-care team with a reduction in teamworking on a locality basis. Indeed, some general practice fundholders insisted that the staff they employed (albeit indirectly) worked for their practice only and were not required to help out colleagues from other practices. These restrictions meant that role developments have tended to be micro and specific to the needs of a particular practice, rather than macro, serving a locality or defined population.

The second most significant factor shaping the development of nursing roles was *The scope of professional practice* (UKCC 1992). This document set out principles which require the nurse to ensure that any aspect of practice is directed towards meeting the needs of the patient. He is also required to develop and maintain the skills and competence to meet these needs, acknowledge limitations in skill and competence and ensure that enlargement or adjustment in role does not compromise existing practice (UKCC 1992). *The scope of professional practice* almost revolutionised nursing practice overnight and freed up the small number of practitioners who were certified to perform certain tasks. It was seen by many as the 'removal of the shackles' which not only allowed nurses to be bolder but also encouraged individual assertiveness in identifying professional development needs prior to taking on new roles (Laurenson 1997). Patients benefited because treatment became more timely and unnecessarily long waits were avoided.

While the New Deal (NHSME 1991) for junior doctors' hours brought about considerable change for nurses working in secondary health care, it had little impact for community nurses. However, a continual drop in the number of doctors entering GP training and the difficulty in recruiting GPs to work in inner-city or remote areas have served as the impetus for the development of the nurse practitioner role. Recently, the successive drop in GP trainees over the past six years has been reversed (DoH 1998) and only time will tell what impact this might have on the future development of nurse practitioners. More worrying for the continued development of nurse practitioner roles is the assumption that nurses offer a cheaper alternative when providing certain types of care (Richardson & Maynard 1995). The development of nurse practitioner roles in primary health care is discussed in more depth later in this chapter.

Changes in the provision of secondary health care and the reduction in the number of hospital beds have led to district nurses spending increasing amounts of time caring for more acutely ill people at home (Barret & Hudson 1997). Such changes have also led to hospital at home schemes and facilitated hospital discharge, which either involve community nursing staff or are operated by staff from the acute sector. In many areas district nurses have played a pivotal role in the provision of services to prevent winter bed pressures, setting up rapid response teams to care for people discharged from accident and emergency departments and providing support to early discharge respite services. Such demands are likely to grow into the next millennium as more and more care is provided on a day patient basis and hospital beds reduce still further. The Heathrow Debate (DoH 1993) suggests that by the year 2002, 60% of surgery will be performed on people as day patients. This important document recognises that community nursing may face undreamt-of challenges in trying to prepare traditional acute staff for a new role working in the community. If these predictions are correct we may have only seen the tip of the iceberg in relation to role development for district nurses and others working in primary health care.

The reduction in inpatient beds and transferring of care services into the community is often referred to as the secondary to primary care shift. Many health authorities have strategic plans, which identify the amount of capital and service provision they wish to see NHS trusts move from acute to primary care. The transfer of such services is often problematic, not least because many NHS trusts are not combined acute and community services. As a result, revenue is often not transferred but new services are introduced. These services are often referred to as 'outreach'. Such services are perceived as a considerable threat by many community nurses.

Essentially, there are two ways of looking at this. First, the new service, e.g. hospital at home, is additional work to what is normally provided in the community and as such it should not be perceived as a threat. Second, some new services have been developed in response to perceived unmet need, e.g. outreach ophthalmic nursing. Such services have been developed for one of three reasons: the acute providers wish to offer purchasers a complete package of care; the care provided by district nurses is not seen as optimal; or the care provided by the district nurse is viewed as not specialist enough. The first reason is a rational response to the introduction of the market into health care; a purchaser is more likely to purchase a complete care episode than have to negotiate the care of a patient with more than one organisation. Meanwhile, the other two could be regarded as a failure on the part of the district nurse to develop his role sufficiently to meet the changing face of health care. It is not uncommon to find district nurses reporting that they could not possibly visit more than twice or three times a day to administer eye drops. Additionally, most district nurses would not be able to recognise a hyphaema or other common complication after eye surgery.

Another major influence on role development has been the changing interface between health and social care in many areas. This has meant that the traditional care practices of washing, showering and getting patients up out of bed is now performed by social carers, while district nurses are involved in more complex cases (Barnes 1996, Smith 1997). This change has eroded many of the auxiliary nurse's traditional roles but in many cases the auxiliary nurse has benefited most from the opportunities it has afforded. In many areas auxiliary nurses are now trained to perform venepuncture, ear syringing, lung function tests, ECGs and a whole host of other tasks. The legal implications of such development will be discussed later in the chapter but such opportunities have also meant the release of qualified nursing time and subsequent opportunities for role development.

While there have been many driving forces behind role development there have also been a number of restraining forces. Some of these have been discussed earlier; for example, general practice fundholding and the development of outreach services. One often quoted restraining factor is the nurse's manager, regarded as the person who blocked the development of new services or the nurse's role. *New world: new opportunities* (NHSME 1993) identified that 'Nurses employed by provider organisations have sometimes been hemmed in by nursing bureaucracy, with rules about nursing practices that have cut across the aims and aspirations of the team as a whole'. Tross & Cavanagh (1996) urge managers to 'innovate' or 'stagnate', suggesting that tapping the creative potential of staff is an essential element of survival in a competitive environment.

However, the extent to which managers did block development is open to debate and there are numerous examples where nurses used the alleged non-support of management as an excuse for not developing practice. Clearly, the introduction of the internal market and fundholding changed the manager's perceptions of GPs and the GP's perceptions of managers in many areas and nurses were slow to respond to this newfound freedom.

One of the single biggest restraining forces is time or indeed the lack of it. The changes described above have increased pressure on all members of the primary health-care team. Many teams do not have any spare capacity left for development. This lack of capacity is often not identified in the literature and while nurses are constantly called upon to develop their practice, no mention is made of what happens when we cannot develop anything else.

While time is a major factor it should not be used as an excuse for not moving forward. All nurses should examine what they do and how they do it to see if they can deliver care in a more efficient and effective way. Additionally, staff must consider routine and ritualistic practice; as Ford & Walsh (1994, p. 18) so eloquently put it, 'Might not the reason why nurses feel overworked be that some of what they do is not necessary – it is a ritual, a tradition, but not necessary'.

The second biggest restraining force must be space or the lack of it. Many general practice surgeries and health centres were built in the 1970s and early 1980s at a time before the rapid development of primary care-based services. Many practices were designed with what was thought to be enough space to meet everyone's needs. Since this time the provision of services has grown beyond anyone's wildest dreams and many buildings are now so over utilised that the development of clinics or new services is having to be postponed. This has a major impact on role development for nurses as they often have to share their clinical rooms with other nurses, chiropodists, dieticians, and other health case professionals.

It is hard to imagine but the issues of time and space may become the final frontiers of role development and stifle opportunity for years to come. However, there is hope, at least on the time front. As mentioned earlier, general practice fundholding both restricted and encouraged development. The restrictions centred on nurses only developing services within the specific practice; this obviously restricted the capacity for development and meant that many role developments were small scale. The advent of primary care groups may mean that the capacity for development is increased with teams of nurses sharing workload and developments over a larger locality area. This may provide some of the much-needed time as a member of a practice team may only need to operate one locality clinic per month, sharing the work with others.

When considering the driving and restraining forces behind service and role development, it is important to consider the reasons why nurses wish to develop their role. Katz & Kahn (1966) identify that there are intrinsic and extrinsic rewards related to role development. Intrinsic rewards include job satisfaction and notions of reward associated with a job well done or increased status amongst one's peers. They believe that intrinsic satisfaction is derived from the content of the role; some people are dissatisfied unless their role can continually develop and present new challenges. There is ample evidence that most people who enact work roles with few activities would prefer some additional complexity (Katzell et al 1975, Quinn & Shepard 1974).

Additionally, extrinsic rewards are less likely within the NHS; monetary reward for the development of one's role is not always forthcoming and staff who develop their role for this reason often do not have their ambitions realised. Other forms of extrinsic reward include national recognition and awards and these can enhance motivation and development of the individuals concerned and others throughout the organisation. Managers would do well to note that people do not always seek extrinsic reward but do wish to be allowed to change and receive recognition for their performance (Sathe 1989).

Lessons from the past

There are a number of important lessons we can learn by drawing upon past experiences of opportunities and threats in role development. First, the development of the clinical nurse specialist (CNS), who often worked across the boundaries between secondary and primary care, provides useful insight into how roles developed to fill unmet need and how the development of such roles was perceived as a threat.

The first CNS posts in the UK were established in the 1970s, although it was not until the late 1980s that there was a great proliferation in the range and number of posts. There is a wide spectrum of such posts now in existence and indeed many aspects of district nursing practice have a specialist nurse aligned to them. A number of propositions have been put forward as to why these posts were developed. One view is that they were a direct result of patient needs which were not being met through traditional nursing and medical practice (Thompson 1989). As many of the early posts concentrated on meeting patients' psychological needs as part of a holistic package of care, this argument could be said to have some grounding (Bousfield 1997). It is certainly the case that the posts with the greatest autonomy appear to be those in traditionally neglected medical areas such as continence promotion, stoma care and gerontology.

Another point of view is that as medical and nursing care in these specialist areas advanced, the need for increasing specialisation in nursing was brought to the fore. Early post holders concentrated on the delivery of patient care with secondary aspects of their work dealing with staff teaching and non-clinical work such as ordering supplies, budget management and research. Indeed, the clinical contact with patients was seen as central to the work of the CNS which led to the perception that the CNS was a threat to the role of the 'generalist' nurse. This perceived threat led to accusations about CNSs fragmenting patient care and deskilling the remaining nursing workforce (Williams 1993).

One commonly repeated argument related to non-community qualified CNSs visiting patients at home once they had been discharged from hospital. Many asserted that such practitioners should have a community qualification before they were allowed to visit people at home (Williams 1993). Arguments related to community qualifications are often used as a defence in relation to the district nurse role. Such arguments are unsound as they fail to illustrate the true nature and wide scope of the district nurse role. A post-basic community nursing qualification is not an essential prerequisite to visit a person at home. Indeed, skill mix has demonstrated this. It is, however, an essential prerequisite to the management of complex patient care needs in the community setting (Barnes 1996).

CNSs are providing care for one particular aspect of the patient's condition (hence the accusation of fragmentation) and as such, they should never be the only nurse visiting a patient. There is much to be said for joint visits with CNSs as a way of sharing skills, knowledge and experience for the benefit of patient care. Vaughan (1996) argues just this point and suggests that greater emphasis should be placed upon sharing of skills and consultation so that the range of expertise of the generalist can be extended.

This specialist versus generalist debate is an area worthy of further discussion. Given the diversity of district nursing practice and the increasing knowledge base about specific aspects of patient care, is it still possible to be a generalist? Perhaps, when examining this issue, it may be worth drawing a parallel between nursing and medicine. Medicine has generalists amongst its ranks, i.e. general practitioners, general physicians, as well as those regarded as specialists. Patients see a generalist for most of their care and are referred onto a specialist for advice about treatment or when further treatment is necessary. The gatekeepers to specialist care are the generalists and they are responsible for the continued management of the patient.

Looking at how most CNS posts operate, the gatekeeper is nearly always the specialist. They allow direct referrals from anyone and they refer people back to the generalist for non-specialist care, almost always what is perceived as lower status 'physical' care. Indeed, some CNSs do not refer the patient back to the generalist nurse at all, preferring to keep them within a protective cocoon allowing them to refer themselves back at any time. Thus, in comparison with the medical system, nursing operates in reverse and this leads to a great deal of unrest and fragmented care.

The CNS should act as a resource to generalists, not as a perceived optional care provider. Many CNSs are working towards such a model but when you are faced with reactions from colleagues which range from complete alienation to 'let's just pass all the work over to them', it is an uphill struggle. This issue will be discussed later

when we examine how one CNS worked on reinventing her role in relation to continence care.

Many district nurses will remember how the expansion in the number of practice nurses was seen as a major threat to district nursing. Wood et al (1994) suggest that, 'Practice and district nurses may regard each other as threats due to the overlap in their role, a power struggle may well develop over who does what'. While many general practices employed nursing staff, it was not until the late 1980s, when the GP Contract was altered, that the number of practice nurses mushroomed. Up until this point many attached district nurses had provided regular treatment room sessions within their practices. These sessions involved a wide range of nursing duties including the taking of blood samples, dressings, etc. Some of these duties were taken over by practice nurses and in many areas, a great deal of overlap existed between the work of these disciplines (Obeid, 1997). One particular controversial area of practice was home visiting by practice nurses. However, Atkin et al (1993) state that concern was not justified as practice nurses involved in home visiting rarely offered continuous care, as most of their visits were one-offs requiring no follow-up.

In most cases the threats posed by the development of practice nursing were unfounded and practice nurses have done well to carve themselves out a role in relation to health promotion and education. Atkin & Lunt (1995) describe how the 'growing importance of general practice in health-care services and the contribution that directly employed nurses make to general medical services seem to guarantee the future of practice nursing'. Despite this success, changes in health commissioning suggest that the future of practice nursing may not be as secure as was once thought. Some GP fundholders have used the ability to purchase community nursing services to develop integrated nursing teams where disciplines share common aspects of their work, while others have gone further and have replaced their practice nurses with a larger community nursing team.

While this is perceived as a threat it also serves as a warning. One of the reasons why practice nursing is under threat could be its inability to continue to adapt its role and the lack of professional leadership which has failed to identify that much of what practice nurses do could easily be done by a lower-grade nurse. Handy (1989) states 'that if you put a frog in water and slowly heat the water, the frog will eventually allow itself to be boiled to death'. Paniagua (1995) uses this as a warning to practice nurses and states, 'In common with the frog, some practice nurses have been lulled into a false sense of security as they swim aimlessly in the waters of general practice'. District nurses should also heed such warnings and aim to be at the forefront of developments in primary health care.

The changing boundaries between medicine and nursing present particular problems to some practitioners who decry the erosion of the nurse's traditional caring role through the handing down of medical tasks (Stillwell et al 1987). Many practitioners are concerned that the delegation of such tasks takes the nurse further and further away from the bedside. Such concerns are based upon the assumption that the nurse will hand over some of his aspects of care to less qualified colleagues. Whether or not this is a bad thing is open to debate as skill mix exercises have advocated this division of work in the past. In the community, at least, the development of roles related to delegated medical care has often led to increased staffing and thus it could be argued that the day-to-day nursing care of patients has been unaffected.

The issue of delegated medical tasks or care is coming more and more to the forefront as the reduction in junior doctors' hours has encouraged organisations to delegate certain medical tasks to nurses. Additionally, the increasing number of nurse practitioner-type roles has led to allegations that nurses are being used more and more as a cheaper alternative to medical care. While these changing boundaries are regarded with scepticism by many nurses, a closer analysis of how nursing developed in the past suggests that such changing boundaries are nothing new. Castle (1987, p. 17) describes how 'nursing work has always been defined in relation to the work of other workers involved in

patient care, most obviously and importantly in relation to doctors'. Correspondingly, many now commonplace nursing procedures, such as the taking and recording of observations and the dressing of a patient's wounds, were traditionally the role of the doctor. In many areas, the assessment, treatment and care of a patient's wound is now the sole responsibility of the nurse and the expansion of nurse prescribing is likely to make this the norm.

It is likely that there will always be nurses who are happy to take on delegated medical tasks, just as there are nurses who prefer working in theatre, on wards or in the community. Vaughan (1996) states, 'There are now many examples where nurses have moved in this direction, not shying from taking on additional responsibility and blending all that is best about nursing with some additional skills, which have traditionally been undertaken by others'. I would suggest that those considering developing their role into areas of care traditionally undertaken by medical staff should ask themselves the following question: If this aspect of care is undertaken by a nurse, will the care of the patient be enhanced? Essentially any delegated role should allow the nurse to provide better care to the patient because it is either more timely, accessible or holistic. Viewing the changing boundaries between medicine and nursing as an evolutionary process and not something new and threatening should afford nurses the opportunity to develop skills which both improve patient care and enhance job satisfaction.

Concepts of risk in role development

The notion of risk owes its origin to gambling when it was used to refer to the probability of losses and gains (Hayes 1992). However, as a concept, risk is now regarded as the probability of loss or harm. This concept has lead to healthcare professionals viewing risk very negatively, which has important implications for the way in which individuals practise. Cook & Proctor (1998, p. 278) suggest that 'Health care professionals need to rediscover the original wider connotations of risk and to balance the possibility of negative outcomes against potential gains from risk-taking activities'.

The balance of risk is therefore closely associated with the ethical principles of non-maleficence (avoiding harm) and beneficence (the duty to do good). These two principles must be carefully weighed up in each given situation as part of a comprehensive risk assessment. Nurses take risks almost constantly during their daily work; for example, a district nurse takes a risk when assessing that a patient is able to prepare and consume her breakfast after she has administered an insulin injection. Risks of this type are not simply based upon 'hope' but involve the nurse carefully weighing up the balance of probabilities based upon her assessment at the time. The risks associated with role development must undergo a similar assessment to balance the probability of losses and gains.

Role development carries with it a number of risks, whether these are risks to patients, health professionals or the organisation in which the nurse works. Such risks can be associated with the nurse taking on a role or task which was previously performed by another health-care professional. This may place the patient at risk of harm if the nurse is not competent to perform such a task/role and a risk to the nurse and his employers from litigation if such harm occurs. Reluctance to develop one's role also carries risks; this centres on the notion of 'inertia versus change'. Inertia can place the practitioner, patient and employer at risk on a number of different levels. First, reluctance to develop a new role may result in the purchasers of a nursing service awarding the contract to another provider. Correspondingly, the overdevelopment of a nurse's role may also result in the loss of a contract if the nurse's 'traditional' work is seen to suffer. Additionally, the neglect of the 'traditional' work is likely to reduce the time available for the supervision of other staff within the team and the potential for a reduction in the standard of patient care, both of which could result in legal action.

Finally, another interesting but frequently neglected area in the inertia versus change debate is the notion of legal action if a nurse is not seen to maintain his practice at the level accepted by his peers. This notion is based upon the Bolam principle (see below), which is of interest in this area because the principle alters as standards of care develop. With this in mind the developments in practice presented in this chapter could become the accepted standard in a few years' time and thus a practitioner who has failed to develop his role could find himself open to a charge of negligence. The Bolam and other guiding principles will be discussed further later in the chapter.

Role development or indeed the lack of it has a number of potential legal implications. Legally, the only restrictions on the development of the nurse's role are those provided by statute, i.e. the Medicines Act, the Mental Health Act, etc. and the Statutory Instruments. In practice, the Acts are rarely prescriptive about the role of each health professional and this is left to the statutory bodies such as the UKCC and the General Medical Council. As mentioned earlier, the development of nursing roles is governed by *The scope of professional practice* (UKCC 1992) which sets out the profession's standards for the development of new and expanded roles. Legal liability for malpractice following such role development is guided by case law. Young (1995) describes how case law is a major feature of English law which allows for the testing and refinement of law whether criminal, civil or statutory. Case law is essentially based upon precedent and judges refer back to similar cases when making a decision.

There are a number of precedents from case law which are useful to consider in relation to role development. As mentioned earlier, the Bolam principle (*Bolam* v. *Friern Hospital Management Committee*, 1957) lays down the accepted standard of care, being that of the 'ordinary skilled doctor acting in accordance with a practice accepted by a responsible body of medical men skilled in that particular art'. Although originally related to medicine, this principle is now widely accepted for other professional groups including nurses and members of the professions allied to medicine. One of the key features of the Bolam principle is that it develops as standards of care develop, so as a result what was considered good practice 20 years ago may lead to a prosecution for negligence now.

The Bolam principle raises a number of issues in relation to role development; one main concern centres around people who pioneer a new nursing role. Applying the Bolam principle to such pioneers would result in them being judged not against the standards of their peers but against the standards of another professional group. While initially this could be a cause for concern, it could be argued that where the nurse has taken on a role previously undertaken by another health-care professional, the patient should expect the same level of care. With this in mind, the Bolam principle remains the precedent by which a practitioner should be judged. Dimond (1994, p. 65) states 'Where activities normally undertaken by doctors are delegated to nursing staff, they would be expected to meet the standards that would be required from a doctor were the doctor to perform the task'.

Another important principle is that related to supervision by a more experienced colleague (*Wilsher* v. *Essex Area Health Authority*, 1986). Both the law and the UKCC *Code of professional conduct* require that a practitioner acknowledges his limitations. By doing so and calling for assistance, the nurse's actions will usually offer a defence (Montgomery 1995, p. 84). The *Wilsher* v. *Essex Area Health Authority* case is interesting as it also set a precedent in relation to the liability of a team as opposed to an individual. The Court of Appeal held that there was no concept in law of team negligence. Therefore each practitioner is accountable for his or her actions. The principle of supervision by a more experienced colleague can involve supervision from a practitioner from the same professional background or a different background. A nurse practitioner could therefore use this principle to refer a patient on to a GP if she was unsure of her diagnosis or the appropriate course of treatment.

Finally, it is important to consider causation. This relates to the establishment of a causal link between the breach of a duty to care and the harm which occurred to the patient. One concern often expressed by nurses is that they may miss some-thing when assessing a patient which may turn out to be serious. This is a very real concern, as we will see later in the chapter when we discuss the nurse's role in continence promotion. Using the principle of causation, the plaintiff must show that the breach in the duty to care which resulted in the harm was reasonably foreseeable. Therefore if a patient visited a nurse complaining of particular symptoms which could be associated with a disease and the nurse did not detect these symptoms during his assessment or chose to ignore them, he would be liable. However, if a patient was seen for another medical problem unrelated to the disease and did not identify any of the symptoms, the nurse could not be liable. Lord Wilberforce (*McLaughlin* v. *O'Brien*, 1983) states 'a defendant is not liable for a consequence of a kind which is not foreseeable'. This principle will be illustrated later in the chapter.

Liability can be divided into two forms: direct and vicarious. *Direct* liability is when an individual or organisation was clearly at fault. *Vicarious*, on the other hand, means 'through another' and this type of liability can mean that an employer is liable for the actions of its employees when they act in the course of their employment. Vicarious liability means that organisations should be concerned with professional standards and the training of practitioners who develop their roles. Dimond (1995, p. 20) states that 'An employer is vicariously liable if the practitioner was performing an act authorised by them, the act was not authorised but is performed for the purpose of the employer's business or the act is incidental to employment'. With this in mind, staff developing a new role would be wise to negotiate a change in their job description to include aspects of their new role. Such a change will provide recognition that the employer is aware of and supports the development of the practitioner's role.

DEVELOPING NEW ROLES

Laurenson (1997) states that new roles for nurses fit into two main categories:

- additional skills which are new to existing roles (upskilling)

- new posts which incorporate many new skills and wider decision-making powers.

The development of new roles carries with it benefits for patients, nurses, the organisation and other professions. Patient benefits include improved continuity of care, increased choice, reduced waiting times and more holistic care, while nurses and the organisation can benefit through job enrichment, professional development, the widening of career choices, improved efficiency and effectiveness (Laurenson 1997).

This section will examine the development of new roles within district nursing practice. Each vignette will describe the process of role development and this will be followed by a discussion about the issues raised.

Vignette 7.2 raises a number of issues around role development. It provides a interesting description of how CNSs and district nurses can work in partnership to enhance patient care. While continence care may not be the most glamorous aspect of nursing work, for most district nurses it represents a major component of their caseload. Indeed, many nurses can have over 50 patients with continence problems in their care at any one time. In the vignette the CNS describes how she perceived her role in a different way to the way her colleagues perceived it. These perceptions are most likely to have developed as a result of the way her predecessors worked.

Additionally, there appears to be a degree of role ambiguity in relation to the specialist's role. Role ambiguity can be very demoralising and this could account for the CNS's feelings in relation to having to turn away certain types of referral. Williams (1993) suggests that a lack of consistency in describing the responsibilities of the CNS's role leaves the position open to a vari-

---

Vignette 7.2   Sandra's story – changing the boundaries between the district nurse and clinical nurse specialist

I came into my new role as a clinical nurse specialist from a background in district nursing. My predecessors had concentrated on patient care and I felt that the role should be more about teaching others and enhancing the care that they provided. The truth was that I could not see the wood for the trees and barely had time to turn around, never mind develop coherent educational programmes. Eventually, after an uphill struggle, I managed to find time to move things on by turning away referrals from patients. At the time this was the hardest thing I had done because I knew that the care they would receive from some of the district nurses would be of a poor standard with little assessment and no treatment.

Around this time the British Association of Continence Care said that, given the present number of continence advisors, it would take 10 years for every patient to be seen once by a specialist nurse. I quickly realised that it was necessary to maximise the greatest good for the greatest number and this could only be achieved through education and service development. Luckily the tide of change was with me as the trust was examining ways in which they could develop services in primary care which had traditionally been the role of secondary care. We decided to develop a pilot general practice continence clinic in a large general practice. Physiotherapy colleagues offered to help us run the clinic and this provided the opportunity to share skills and experience; indeed, these colleagues provided training for staff in techniques such as pelvic floor assessment and proved to be an asset to the development.

From the outset we were determined that the clinic would be more than a pad assessment opportunity and we managed to secure funding for some equipment such as a perineometer (to measure pelvic floor muscle contraction) and one neuromuscular electrical stimulator (used to treat stress and urge incontinence). The clinic proved to be very successful and another clinic followed in a smaller practice. Our initial success was notable, with many patients achieving full cure and many more reporting dramatic improvement in their symptoms.

The second clinic was run by Lynn, a very dynamic enrolled nurse from a smaller practice. Some colleagues were concerned that an enrolled nurse should be allowed to assess, diagnose, treat and onwardly refer patients unsupervised. However, the district nursing sister from the practice was unperturbed, stating that 'initial registered qualifications were irrelevant and what mattered was that the individual was competent'. It was Lynn who provided the catalyst for the widespread acceptance of such clinics, as many nurses doubted that they could find the time to develop such services on top of their day-to-day work. Rather than being told about the development by a clinical nurse specialist who had little or no understanding of their work, they were presented with success by one of their colleagues.

Many more clinics followed and the advent of locality commissioning provided much-needed equipment and very quickly the community ended up with more equipment than our colleagues in the hospital. We now have eight clinics treating over 50 patients with more than half of the district nursing teams involved.

ety of interpretations, causing dissatisfaction for the CNS and his patients. Role conflict can also occur when the nurse is faced with competing expectations of the various stakeholders (Bousfield 1997).

The development of district nurse-led specialist clinics raises a number of issues, not least how they were perceived by the role sets of both the district nurses and the CNS, as well as notions of reward and concepts of risk associated with such a development. Let us first examine how the development was perceived amongst the various role sets. In vignette 7.2 the CNS describes how one enrolled nurse became the motivator of others while attempts by the CNS to motivate other district nurses were largely unsuccessful, principally because the CNS was not part of the district nurses' role set and therefore lacked influence in the way the nurses developed their roles. The enrolled nurse, although not directly part of the nurses' role set, demonstrated how she was able to develop her role while at the same time working in a busy general practice.

What is not evident from the vignette is the reactions of the CNS's peers to the development of such clinics. Most of her colleagues disregarded the development and many viewed the training of district nurses to undertake advanced assessment and treatment techniques as misguided and dangerous. Most of the anxiety around the development centred around the performance of pelvic floor muscle assessment by per vaginal examination. Many CNSs felt that this should not be performed by a nurse in case she missed something and the patient subsequently was found to have a more serious condition. Such fears should not be dismissed because nurses working in such clinics may see patients who have not been seen by any other health-care professional. However, it is important to consider that the nurse would be assessing muscle strength and not looking for any other disease. If the patient mentioned a particular problem or symptom then the nurse should refer the patient to her general practitioner for further assessment and investigation.

It is useful in this case to consider the legal precedents which were discussed earlier in the chapter. Taking into account the Bolam principle, the nurse trained to perform pelvic floor assessment would be judged by the standards of others undertaking such assessments for urinary incontinence, i.e. physiotherapists and continence advisors. Such practitioners would be reasonably expected to identify abnormalities which could be easily palpated or which were associated with particular symptoms. If these were present then onward referral would be indicated. The principle of causation is also useful in this incidence as if the patient failed to report symptoms associated with a more serious condition then the nurse could not be held liable for the unforeseeable consequences (*McLaughlin* v. *O'Brien*, 1983).

Many of the CNS's colleagues' fears were based upon the fact that district nurses were being trained to undertake work that they perceived as being the domain of the specialist. As we have seen, when faced with threats to their role nurses become very defensive. It is indeed sad that this occurs in a field where there is more than enough work for everyone.

A useful way to look at work structuring is to consider whether care provision should be centralised or decentralised (APM 1990). Work which is of low volume but which requires high skill should be centralised within an organisation and performed by a specialist person or small team. Thus specialist nursing posts may be required in highly specialist areas which have only a few patients. Other work which is high volume regardless of whether it requires high or low skill should be decentralised and performed by a large number of people within the organisation. Areas such as wound care and continence care would therefore fall into this category. Additionally, work which is low volume and low skill can also easily be performed by a large number of people within the organisation.

Finally, it is useful to consider what drove the district nurses to develop their roles in relation to continence promotion. By far the greatest reward was the increased job satisfaction, which resulted from being able to assess, diagnose, treat and successfully cure or help a patient. Most of the district nurses felt that it was far better to be able to actively do something to help the patient, rather than simply giving out pads and other aids. Reward of this type is likely to be more forthcoming in patients with incontinence because of the debilitating effects it has on a person's life. One nurse described how an elderly lady referred herself with her bladder problem that had become so bad that she could no longer take her dog for a walk. Three months later the lady was cured and waved to the nurse each day as she set off to take her dog for a walk.

Other rewards associated with a development of this type include the recognition it brings to the nurse. Many of the nurses running the clinics are enrolled or staff nurses who have developed their role in this specialist area. The nurses manage their own caseload of patients, seeing the same patients at each clinic and following their progress through treatment. The nurses take referrals from hospital consultants and general practitioners, reporting the patient's progress in letters to the referer after each consultation. These issues may seem small and insignificant but they can provide considerable reward for the practitioners concerned.

Vignette 7.3 provides an interesting insight into role development within an organisation. What is clear from the outset is that Helen is a role maker and she has successfully brought about the need for a post and has decided from the outset the parameters of her role. This was probably made easier because the post was new and thus no one had a preformed perception of what the role was about. While the development of the clinic set out to prevent some of the mis-

---

Vignette 7.3   Helen's story – advancing wound care practice

My interest in wound management started many years ago when I attended a research course. The course encouraged me to examine my practice and examine its evidence base. I very quickly realised that there were a number of changes I would need to make and a great deal more I had to learn about wound care.

Over the next 4 or 5 years I often discussed the possibility of developing a nurse-led wound care clinic with my manager and, while she was enthusiastic, it was usually put on the back burner. As my knowledge and interest developed I began to try out new techniques such as low-level laser therapy and I was lucky enough to be able to get a machine on loan for a few months. Following this, we highlighted our success to the chief executive. To our delight, she agreed to fund the purchase of a laser machine for us and we were then able to continue to treat patients both within the community and in hospital.

Over a short time period the number of patients we were treating grew and we were finding that we were very stretched, having to manage a busy caseload with this additional work. A casual conversation with a colleague resurrected the idea of a specialist clinic and within a matter of weeks the clinic was born. We decided that the clinic would offer district-wide assessment and specialist treatment to patients within the community and hospital. The specialist clinic was run by a small group of district nurses, although I and a colleague were present on each of the twice-weekly sessions.

The clinic was based within a general hospital, which allowed us to utilise ambulance transport, thus enabling us to bring patients to the clinic who would not normally be able to access such services. The clinic would act as a focal point for education, training and patient care and from the outset we planned that the patient's district nurse would remain responsible for the patient's ongoing care. The exception to this was patients who were undergoing laser treatment who needed to attend the specialist clinic twice per week.

In the past I had been very against the development of more and more specialist posts and services as I felt that would lead to a deskilling of the district nurse. As a result, we planned that when patients were referred for specialist assessment or treatment, their nurse should be invited to attend with them. Where this was not possible, patient-held documentation was used to inform the district nurse of the plan for continued treatment.

The clinic proved very successful, healing 87% of venous ulcers within 12 weeks of referral. We were also able to increase the number of patients undergoing laser treatment by 80%. As well as these outcomes, the clinic also provided a number of unexpected benefits and patients found the environment very supportive and enjoyed interacting with other patients in the waiting room. Our initial plan to refer patients back to their district nurses failed because we found that many staff did not have the skills to apply compression bandaging.

Over the months, we provided education to staff in relation to this but our initial plan was thwarted because the patients preferred to attend the specialist clinic. This preference was clearly demonstrated by a patient satisfaction survey in which the patients expressed appreciation for treatment consistency and continuity which, they felt, was sadly lacking in district nursing practice. In the survey one elderly lady remarked that, 'After 3 months of alternating treatment I was amazed at how quickly my ulcer healed after attending the clinic'. Others voiced similar concerns in relation to treatment consistency and one patient said, 'You just think you're getting somewhere and along comes a different nurse

---

Vignette 7.3   Cont'd

who says the dressing is no good and changes it for something different'.

While the clinic proved very successful, it was very costly in terms of staff time and commitment. From the initial development, the work spiralled out of control and this placed considerable pressure on me and my colleagues. Eventually, the trust decided to create a new post of practice development nurse (tissue viability) to provide specialist advice and education and develop clinical services across the organisation. While this meant that I had to move away from my post as a district

nursing sister, I have successfully worked with colleagues to develop wound care clinics within GP practices. I don't see myself as a specialist nurse but rather as a nurse developing the knowledge, skills and practice of others. If someone had said to me 10 years ago that I would have ended up in a specialist post I would not have believed them as I really believed that such posts deskilled district nurses and resulted in fragmented care. I now think that it's not necessarily the post but how you do it that counts.

---

takes of the past, some of these were unavoidable. For example, it was not possible to refer the patients back to their own district nurse for a variety of reasons and this resulted in the clinic being seen by some people as a specialist centre with little or no communication between the 'specialist nurse' and the district nurses.

There is little doubt that some district nurses refuse to refer their patients to the clinic or do so only reluctantly because they feel that this is yet another erosion of their role. While some district nurses bemoan the need for a specialist clinic, it is unclear to what extent they are prepared to develop their own practice to ensure that some of the concerns highlighted by patients are addressed. The issue around treatment consistency and continuity is interesting and while it has been highlighted in some of the research on perceptions of leg ulceration (Walshe 1995), it must impact on the care of other types of wounds. Clearly there is a need for further research in this area. However, it is surely not beyond most district nursing teams to examine their systems of care delivery to ensure that patients have continuity of nursing staff.

Consistency of treatment is another big issue which is often not considered by nurses. It is not uncommon for nurses to change a dressing after 4 days and when he discovers that the wound is showing no signs of improvement, to select an alternative dressing. It remains to be seen whether the widespread implementation of nurse prescribing will impact on these inconsistencies. One would hope that when the district nursing sister is the prescriber, she will require the nurse to

provide a clear rationale for a change in product or, better still, reassess the wound herself.

While the specialist clinic has been very successful in terms of referrals it is unclear whether it would work on anything other than a district-wide model. To date, one or two areas have set up similar wound care clinics but these tend to be based in the larger GP practices. Whether an average-sized practice would have sufficient patients to warrant a clinic is debatable and this clearly highlights the problems of role development for nurses who work in small teams. Similar problems occurred in this development because of the pressure on the two main staff. Both of these staff worked in the same GP practice, which meant that the work of their district nursing caseloads had to be done on days when they were not working in the specialist clinic. Few practices would be happy to allow their attached staff to spend so much time caring for other nurses' patients.

One solution to these problems may lie in the creation of primary care groups, which work on a locality basis, providing greater opportunities for the pooling of resources to develop such services. The challenge must be for the district nursing representatives on these groups to articulate the need and benefits of such sharing so that staff can develop their roles.

Barbara's story (Vignette 7.4) centres around the development of a nurse practitioner (NP) type role within primary health care. Many would argue that Barbara has not developed her district nursing role but moved into a completely different role, although she is clearly going to utilise some of the skills and knowledge she has developed as a district nurse.

To what extent a NP should be viewed as a different role is open to debate and many district nurses are developing this type of role parallel to their day-to-day district nursing practice. For example, some district nurses are developing triage services for GP home visits and others provide out-of-hours nursing services, working closely with GPs and others to provide more comprehensive out-of-hours care (Carlisle 1996). These nurses are not necessarily seeking to carve out a new role for themselves but recognise the need to fully utilise their skills and knowledge to the benefit of patients. In the past district nurses have been frustrated by having to call upon doctors to help them sort out relatively simple problems like constipation. The more widespread introduction of

nurse prescribing should alleviate many of these problems.

Barbara also raises the issue of what will happen to her post when GP fundholding ends. This is an issue which concerns a number of nurses around the country as many GP fundholders established new posts, both clinical and administrative, once they were free to purchase nursing services. It is likely that such posts will continue once the primary care groups are established; indeed, opportunities may exist to extend the range and number of such posts in the future.

The concept of a NP role is not new; it originated in the USA in the 1960s in response to a shortage of primary care physicians. Pearson et al (1995) describe how doctors and managers here, like their colleagues in America before them, have begun to wonder if some more flexible community nurses might be able to

---

Vignette 7.4 Barbara's story – nurse practitioner roles

After 10 years working in the same inner-city practice, I felt that I needed a change; my role had developed as far as I thought it could. The practice was a nice place to work and everyone got on really well together. The four general practitioners had found themselves under considerable pressure over the last couple of years because of the increasing demands of patients. These pressures were putting the appointments system under considerable strain and we had reached the point where you could not get an appointment for about 3 weeks. Emergency patients were simply slotted in at the end of the surgery or they insisted on a home visit. It was not uncommon to have 20 extras at the end of a busy surgery.

One of the partners, Simon, said that he had recently attended a conference at which a GP and nurse had presented their work around the development of a nurse practitioner in general practice. He had suggested to the others that they consider this as a way of relieving some of the pressure on the appointments system and, despite their initial reservations, they had agreed to investigate the possibility further. I said that I was interested in such a development. Simon and I visited two other practices in the region who had developed such practitioners. I managed to find the time to undertake a literature review and found a number of interesting evaluation studies of this type of role. I also discovered that the local university ran a course for nurse practitioners which looked ideal as it covered areas such as clinical assessment, pharmacology, decision making, risk management and reflective practice.

Simon and I put together a presentation which we made to the other partners, trust managers and

representatives of the health authority. The presentation went very well and the partners agreed to a 1-year trial of a nurse practitioner role. It was decided that they would reorganise the appointments system so that I would see all emergency or urgent appointment requests, working closely with Simon. The trust agreed to second me from my post and fund replacement staff.

The course passed very quickly and I was able, with Simon's help, to develop clinical assessment skills. At first I was very unsure about whether I had done the right thing; decision making about treatment was initially very anxiety provoking. It's not that I hadn't made decisions about treatment in the past, most nurses do these things as part of their work, it was the gradual realisation that I was now on my own and responsible. In hindsight, of course, I should have realised that I always had been responsible for my own decision making. These reservations quickly settled as I became increasingly assured of my ability. The module on decision making really helped in this respect because it clarified the sources of knowledge I was using to make the decision and suddenly I realised that I was not simply plucking an answer out of the air.

It's now 2 years since I started and I feel I'm an accepted part of the team. Some patients book appointments specifically with me because they feel that I am easier to speak to. My only concern now relates to what the future holds when GP fundholding ends. It's difficult to see how the other practices in the primary care group will be happy to fund additional services in the two practices with nurse practitioners.

cost-effectively take on some of the roles they are unable to fulfil adequately. The first NP posts in the UK were established in 1982 and, as discussed earlier, the number of posts continues to grow because of the shortage of GPs in some areas and the increasing pressure on primary health-care services.

While in secondary care NP and CNS roles have concentrated on development in clearly associated medical specialties, the NP in primary care has developed in a more general capacity. The role is characterised by the ability to assess, make a differential diagnosis, onwardly refer, treat in accordance with agreed protocols, health educate and counsel. Stillwell et al (1987) describe how research in the USA suggests that NPs can have a positive effect on patient behaviour, including better blood pressure control in patients with hypertension, more effective weight loss and that patients were better at keeping appointments and complying with recommendations. NPs in primary care have demonstrated that they are able to manage minor or chronic illness and successfully integrate the traditional medical model with health promotion, education and patient support. Pierson (1997) clearly supports this assumption, arguing that NPs do not do it better but do it differently and this clearly benefits patient care.

A metaanalysis carried out by the American Nurses Association suggests that NPs provided more health promotion activities than physicians and that, although they ordered more tests than doctors, the total costs of the tests ordered were lower. Prescribing practices between the two groups were found to be equal while the average cost per NP visit was 39% lower than the cost of a physician visit (Sharu 1997). However, others have argued that far from being a cheaper alternative to general practitioners, NPs actually see fewer patients, taking considerably longer over consultations, thus driving up costs (Pearson et al 1995). This criticism must be viewed in the light of the small but compelling number of studies which have suggested that NPs achieve better outcomes (Ramsey et al 1982, Watkins & Wagner 1982). Further research in this area is needed before more NP posts are established.

Finally, there has been considerable debate over the status of NPs following the UKCC's PREP proposals (UKCC 1994) which outlined the framework for specialist practice and described the nature of advanced practice. Since then, the UKCC has been reluctant to make the NP qualification a registerable or recordable one. This failure, coupled with the mystery surrounding the notion of advanced practice, allowed practitioners to speculate about their status. Such speculation can be likened to the situation which arose after clinical grading when nurses were given the rather vague criteria long before their individual grades were announced. It was not uncommon to find nurses who felt they met the criteria for a grade far beyond that they were subsequently awarded. Such confusion adds little to the professional status of nursing and, indeed, as the number of NPs grows the situation of allowing anyone to call themselves a NP regardless of the level or content of their education/training could result in unsafe practice. Given that the UKCC (UKCC 1994) states that its primary function is to protect the public, one could question its inability to act on such a major issue.

Roles which enhance patient care

There are a number of role developments which enhance the care of patients. These include learning new tasks such as male catheterisation or the management of total parenteral nutrition in the community. In this section we will examine two specific areas of role development: the district nurse's role in health improvement and nurse prescribing. These have been selected because they are areas of current development in district nursing practice.

Health improvement

District nurse involvement in health improvement is nothing new and most nurses are involved in health promotion and education to a greater or lesser degree. However, the recent drives towards health improvement brought about by the publication of the Green Papers by each of the UK health departments and the establishment of health action zones have added increased impetus to the expansion of such roles by all health-care professionals.

Traditionally, district nursing practice has involved secondary or tertiary health promotion and many authors believe they are ideally placed to offer health education to individuals at home (Baly et al 1987, Ewles & Simnet 1996). While this traditional role is likely to continue there will also be increased opportunity for the district nurse to establish a greater public health role. This will involve practitioners moving beyond their largely individual patient or family focus towards a more macro community focus. Clearly such a move will mean a major paradigm shift for some practitioners, as they have for a number of years been encouraged to develop services around a specific practice population. The attachment of district nurses to GP practices has in many ways proved to be reductionist and has prevented practitioners from focusing on the health care of a neighbourhood or community. It remains to be seen whether the planned closer cooperation between GP practices in a locality, through the advent of primary care groups, will go some way towards redressing the balance.

In the meantime there are a number of ways in which district nurses can become more involved in health improvement. Most are in an ideal position to assess the health needs of the community and then target frequently neglected groups. One example would be people living in residential care or sheltered housing schemes; such homes allow for the development of health promotion activities because they have a sense of community spirit and many organise frequent residents' meetings. On a locality basis, it is possible for district nursing teams to share the workload providing advice and education to residents of such homes across a wide geographical area. Additionally, district nurses could capitalise on their own special interests and develop health promotion activities around these; for example, activities which raise awareness of common leg problems such as ulceration and aim to advise at-risk individuals on how these can be avoided. Other examples of a developing public health role for district nurses include the provision of free first aid training for residents of an inner-city area, supporting national health promotion campaigns such as National No Smoking Day and by manning a health stand in a local shopping area. Fieldgrass (1992) believes that 'community health care nurses are in a prime position to be practically involved in this development either through their role as a professional or as an individual, they may influence both the community and work place settings'.

The possibilities for health improvement are endless and because district nurses are easily recognisable and their role is understood by the general public, they are in a position to generate considerable interest in health promotion activities.

Nurse prescribing

The introduction of the nurse prescribing pilots following the production of the Crown Report (DoH 1989) was one of the major changes to impact on district nursing in the last decade. The report recommended that 'suitably qualified nurses working in the community should be able, in clearly defined circumstances, to prescribe from a limited list of items and to adjust the timing and dosage of medicines within a set protocol'. This acceptance of the idea of nurse prescribing followed an ongoing campaign since the early 1980s to legitimise what many believed was already happening (Pickersgill & Clarke 1990).

The Crown Report identified a number of benefits which could arise from the introduction of nurse prescribing. These included an improvement in patient care, better use of time and clarification of responsibilities. Prior to the nurse prescribing pilot projects, the Department of Health commissioned Touche Ross (DoH 1991) to conduct a study identifying the costs and benefits of nurse prescribing. The report concluded that although there would be some saving of time, this could not be translated into financial savings and thus the financial costs exceeded any initial benefits. This report failed to consider any potential savings which might occur as a result of nurses being more accountable for the items they recommended/prescribed. This is particularly relevant given that the total cost of the items in the Nurse Prescriber's Formulary accounted for 10% of the drugs bill (Luker et al 1996).

The recommendations of the report dealt a cruel blow to the advocates of nurse prescribing and delayed the widespread introduction of the concept for 7 years. The government of the day did, however, press ahead with a small number of pilot sites which were subsequently evaluated. The evaluation suggested that the main advantages of nurse prescribing were savings in time, increased job satisfaction and an increased awareness of costs which may have brought about cost savings (Luker et al 1997). However, the evaluation was unable to quantify savings in prescribing costs. The authors were able to conclude that 'there is no evidence to suggest that prescribing costs in the eight demonstration sites increased more than they would have done in the absence of nurse prescribing'.

The widespread introduction of nurse prescribing over the next year will have a considerable impact on the district nurse's role. Many of the role developments described in this chapter can be enhanced by the nurse's ability to prescribe. It is anticipated that care will improve because it will become much more seamless, allowing nurses to manage the complete care of the patient with a chronic wound or a continence problem. Whether the nurse's formulary is comprehensive enough to meet the rapidly developing roles of some nurses only time will tell. The issues surrounding the implementation of nurse prescribing are dealt with in more depth in Chapter 8.

Roles which support clinical practice

Recent years have seen a plethora of new roles which are designed to support practitioners either with their clinical practice or leading teams who deliver patient services. Such roles provide essential infrastructure at a time when the scope and nature of practice are rapidly changing. It would be beyond the scope of this chapter to examine each role in detail and we will therefore focus on two specific roles: that of the practice development facilitator and a leadership role within a primary health-care team.

The recent emergence of practice development facilitation roles is hardly surprising given the rapid changes in care delivery and practice which have impacted on both organisations and

---

Vignette 7.5   Jackie's story – facilitating the development of practice

Taking up a new role as a practice development facilitator is a rather daunting experience. Everyone seemed to have worked out what my role was about before I had even started. Many people said that my role was about introducing skill mix because we had finances available to support developments in practice by employing other staff; others thought I was coming along to tell them what services they needed to implement and how to do things differently. The truth was that I had little or no idea about what I was going to do, except help people develop their practice. The initial reservations were quickly overcome once we started to look at the areas they felt needed development. We did this through a process of joint working and the brainstorming of ideas. The initial ideas generated ranged from the simple changes to major organisational change. Most of what was presented was nothing new and I had to reassure myself that innovation was something which was new to the individual (Rogers 1983, p. 11).

Once we decided what to work on, I set about doing the background work. This involved preparing bids for funding, sorting out proposals, meeting stakeholders, undertaking literature reviews and developing documentation for the developments. Some of the innovations were small-scale developments which were quickly achieved, like teaching the auxiliary nurses to do venepuncture, ECGs and clinical observations. I did wonder why such developments needed facilitation at all and why these things had not simply been implemented by the district nurse.

As work with the teams progressed, I learnt that after I had taken a team through the change process once, they quickly took the running on the other projects. I would negotiate deadlines for each stage with them and set a time scale and I often found that when I returned, they had moved on to the next stage. I learnt a great deal from working with these teams and developed my own role perception which allowed me to explain to others what my role was all about. Quite simply, 'I'm not there to tell you what to change; I'm simply there to hold the torch and guide the way!'

practitioners. The roles can be very diverse and usually reflect the prevailing needs within the organisation (Mallet et al 1997). It could be argued that the overall aim of the role is that of change facilitator who works to ensure that practice meets the needs of patients, purchasers and other stakeholders. Although there is a dearth of research in this area, the establishment of such posts could be considered as a statement about existing practitioners' ability to initiate and manage innovation. However, this is unlikely to be the whole story and the organisation and its past or current culture may have directly influenced the practitioner's ability to manage change.

Mason et al (1991) state that 'Health care institutions are highly complex organisations where change does not come easily. Many nurses have been frustrated in their attempts to bring about change that would improve and facilitate their everyday practice'. Organisational change requires a practitioner to be politically astute if he is going to be able to negotiate the minefield of the large bureaucratic organisation. Manion (1993) believes that 'Individuals must be empowered before innovation will occur ... and not all individuals who are empowered in their daily practice accept responsibility for innovation. In some cases, the individual may not have the specific skills needed or the bureaucratic system they are in has too many barriers to innovation'. This may shed some light on the scenario Jackie describes in Vignette 7.8 where the first innovations were driven by her but, as practitioners developed the skills required to function in a politically astute way, they took more of a lead in future developments. This raises important issues for the future preparation of specialist practitioners. If they are going to lead clinical practice they not only require a theoretical grounding in the management of change but they need to be able to try out these concepts in a protected environment.

Jackie's perception of her role as a guide is useful in that it clearly allows the practitioners to select and focus on the area of practice they wish to change. This in turn allows the practitioners to develop a sense of ownership which should ensure their continued involvement and the

success of the development. Cauthorne Lindstrom & Tracy (1992) suggest that active involvement is the key to success as a 'lack of meaningful involvement can easily lead to festering resentment on the part of the people who have to make the design work, without ever having any input into it'.

The way in which Jackie has developed her post has allowed her to become the champion of other people's ideas. This is not to say that she is seeking to associate herself with the hard work of others but that she is able to represent other people's ideas to relevant stakeholders and ensure that developments stay on course. Champions are useful because they are able to generate enthusiasm amongst others, work within the organisation to access much-needed resources and take care of all the little details which are necessary to ensure that the change is successful.

Organisations may employ practice development facilitators for a variety of reasons and, as we have seen from Jackie's story, many employees may regard the appointment of such a person with scepticism. Such facilitators should be wary of hidden agendas and be aware that the most amazing myths can spring up overnight during their work. Clarke (1998) has identified that change facilitators need the following characteristics and skills: the ability to cope with uncertainty, intellectual curiosity, openness to change, commitment to the project, respect for others, access to authority and credibility.

Sally's story in Vignette 7.6 demonstrates how the boundaries between the different nursing disciplines can be altered to reduce overlap and provide more effective health care for the community served. The concept of integrated nursing teams is new and such teams have been defined as 'a team of community-based nurses from different disciplines, working together within a primary care setting pooling their skills, knowledge and ability in order to provide the most effective care for the patients within a practice' (Health Visitors Association 1996). Such teams provide a unique opportunity to develop innovative and effective services which cut across traditional boundaries between primary and secondary care and to pool resources, thus avoiding the difficulties associated

---

Vignette 7.6 Sally's story – leadership

When our practice became fundholders I felt very threatened as the idea of the market economy in health care was very alien to me. The first year saw a rapid rise in the range of services provided in the surgery and I felt this was benefiting the patients who could now get chiropody, physiotherapy and psychology services locally rather than having to travel to the local hospital. When the practice was able to purchase nursing services, I was understandably very keen that they purchase from my employing trust. They were, however, very concerned about the high management costs which were included in the contract as they were bewildered about what they were getting for their money. Tough negotiations followed but eventually the trust was awarded the contract. The compromise had been that the trust would develop a team leader to lead the nursing team.

Around the same time, one of the practice nurses left and we had offered to cover her work in return for some bank nurse help. I was approached by Peter, the senior partner, to ask what I thought about developing a nursing team which covered all of the work within the surgery and on the 'district'. I agreed that this would be possible provided the district nursing team was made larger and the necessary training was provided to ensure that the staff had the skills to undertake the many and varied

practice nurse duties. The team was expanded following the appointment of E and F grade staff nurses and we quickly integrated the team to provide cover for the two practice nurses. The staff nurses valued the opportunity to lead their own clinics and to specialise in specific areas like asthma care. A few months later the new team leader post was advertised; the incumbent would lead all the nursing services attached to the practice and would coordinate the other services provided by the trust. I applied for the post and was successful and started a week later.

At first, the health visitors were a little perturbed that their new leader was a district nurse but I reassured them that I was there to provide liaison with the practice and not to direct their health visiting work. Through closer working, we initiated integrated care with the health visitors developing skills in family planning, bereavement counselling and asthma care. This allowed us to share skills and knowledge to the benefit of our patients. Many practice nurses were very angry that their traditional role had been taken over by district nurses and health visitors and were concerned that such erosion would become commonplace. I felt that the model was just one that worked for us and probably developed because of circumstances rather than any plot to oust the practice nurses.

---

with small teams. The initial reactions from some of the staff in Sally's team are not uncommon and relate to attitudes and professional jealousies (Mackenzie & Ross 1997). These attitudes must be overcome so that practitioners and practice can develop to meet the challenges of the primary care-led NHS.

CONCLUSION

Much has been achieved in relation to role development over the last 5 years and district nurses appear to have harnessed the potential afforded by the internal market and GP fundholding. Whether or not the lessons from the past have been learned is open to debate as the number of specialist posts continues to grow in response to increased specialisation in medicine. It is not possible to predict whether district nursing has done enough to avoid the threats to its role in the future. However, at the present

time the future remains bright and the advent of primary care groups will hopefully provide more opportunities for nurses to take a lead role in the development and planning of services.

At the same time it is likely that there will be an increasing drive towards integration of nursing roles over the next few years and this can only be of benefit to the patients we serve. The opportunity to share common nursing skills at the same time as celebrating our special skills sounds like a good idea. However, interprofessional jealousies and fixed role boundaries will threaten this. The road to the blurring of role boundaries in community nursing is a bumpy one but it remains one of the major professional highways we should aspire to travel along. Young (1997) sums up the potential for role development by describing the only limits to practice as being *The scope of professional practice*, the needs of the community and, most importantly, imagination.

REFERENCES

A P M Inc 1990 Decision to centralize/decentralize. APM Inc, New York

Atkin K, Lunt N 1995 Nurses in practice: the role of the practice nurse in primary health care. Social Policy Research Unit, University of York

Atkin K, Lunt N, Parker G, et al 1993 Nurses count: a national census of practice nurses. Social Policy Research Unit, University of York

Baly M, Robottom B, Clarke J M 1987 District nursing, 2nd edn. Heinemann, London

Barnes M 1996 Assessing need for district nursing: study findings. Nursing Standard 10(31): 32

Barret G, Hudson M 1997 Changes in district nurse workload. Journal of Community Nursing 11(3): 4–8

Bousfield C 1997 A phenomenological investigation into the role of the clinical nurse specialist. Journal of Advanced Nursing 25: 245–256

Bolam v. Friern Hospital Management Committee 1957. Butterworths Medico-Legal Reports 1, Butterworth, Sevenoaks

Carlisle D 1996 Open all hours. Nursing Times 92(12). 16–17

Castle J 1987 The development of professional nursing in New South Wales, Australia. In: Maggs C (ed) Nursing history: the state of the art. Croom Helm, London, ch 3

Cauthorne-Lindstrom C, Tracy T 1992 Organizational change from the 'mop and pop' perspective. Journal of Nursing Administration 22(7): 61–64

Chalmers H 1997 Educational requirements for new nursing roles. Unpublished MPhil thesis, University of Newcastle-upon-Tyne

Clarke C L 1998 Developing health care practice: a facilitated seminar programme. University of Northumbria at Newcastle, Newcastle

Clayton C M 1984 The clinical nurse specialist as leader. Topics in Clinical Nursing 6(1): 17–27

Cook G, Proctor S 1998 Risk: a nursing dilemma. In: Heyman B (ed) Risk, health and health care. Edward Arnold, London, ch 15

Department of Health 1989 Report of the Advisory Group on Nurse Prescribing (the Crown Report). Department of Health, London

Department of Health 1991 Nurse prescribing final report: a cost benefit study (the Touche Ross Report). Department of Health, London

Department of Health 1993 The challenges for nursing and midwifery in the 21st century (the Heathrow Debate). HMSO, London

Department of Health 1998 Milburn welcomes first rise in trainee GPs for six years. DoH press release 98/210, 28 May

Dimond B 1994 Legal aspects of role expansion. In: Hunt G, Wainwright P (eds) Expanding the role of the nurse: the scope of professional practice. Blackwell, Oxford, ch 4

Dimond B 1995 Legal aspects of health care. The Open Learning Foundation, Churchill Livingstone, Edinburgh

Ewles L, Simnet I 1996 Promoting health: a practical guide, 3rd edn. Baillière Tindall, London

Fieldgrass J 1992 Partnerships in health promotion: collaboration between the statutory and voluntary sectors. Health Education Authority, London

Ford P, Walsh M 1994 New ritual for old: nursing through the looking glass. Butterworth Heinemann, Oxford

Gardner L 1998 Leading primary care: time for action. Health Visitor 71(11): 21–22

Handy C 1989 The age of unreason. Arrow Books, London

Hayes M V 1992 On the epistemology of risk: language, logic and social science. Social Science and Medicine 35: 401–407

Health Visitors Association 1996 Integrated nursing team – initial information. Professional Briefing 1, HVA, London

Katz D, Kahn R L 1996 The social psychology of organizations. John Wiley, New York

Katzell R A, Yankelovich D, Fein M et al 1975 Work, productivity and job satisfaction. Psychological Corporation, New York

Lathlean J 1995 The implementation and development of lecturer practitioner roles in nursing. Ashdale Press, Oxford

Laurenson S 1997 Changing roles of nurses in Scotland. Health Bulletin 55(5): 331–337

Luker K A, Ferguson B, Austin L et al 1996 Evaluating nurse prescribing. Unpublished report, Department of Health, London

Luker K A, Austin L, Hogg C, Ferguson B, Smith K 1997 Nurse prescribing: the views of nurses and other health care professionals. British Journal of Community Health Nursing 2(2): 69–74

Mackenzie A, Ross F 1997 Shifting the balance: nursing in primary care. British Journal of Community Health Nursing 2(3): 139–142

McLaughlin v. O' Brien 1983. Butterworths Medico-Legal Reports

Mallet J, Cathmoir D, Hughes P, Whitby E 1997 Forging new roles. Nursing Times 93(18): 38–39

Manion J 1993 Chaos or transformation: managing innovation. Journal of Nursing Administration 23(5): 41–48

Mason D J, Costello-Nickitas D M, Scanlan J M, Magnuson B A 1991 Empowering nurses for politically astute change in the workplace. Journal of Continuing Education in Nursing 22(1): 5–10

Montgomery J 1995 Negligence: the legal perspective. In: Tingle J, Cribb A (eds) Nursing law and ethics. Blackwell, Oxford, ch 5A

National Health Service Management Executive 1991 Junior doctors: the new deal. NHSME, London

National Health Service Management Executive 1993 Nursing in primary health care. New world: new opportunities. NHSME, London

Obeid A 1997 The district/practice mix. Nursing Management 2(9): 17–18

Paniagua H 1995 Practice nursing: will it survive? British Journal of Community Nursing 4(20): 1173–1174

Pearson P, Kelly A, Connolly M, Daly M, O'Gorman F 1995 Nurse practitioners. Health Visitor 68(4): 157–160

Pickersgill F, Clarke S 1990 A prescription for nursing. Nursing Standard 4(44): 10–11

Pierson C A 1997 Do nurse practitioners do it better? Nurse Practitioner Forum 8 (4): 129–130

Quinn R P, Shepard L 1974 The 1972–1973 Quality of Employment Survey. AAA Survey Research Centre, University of Mitchigan

Ramsey J, McKenzie J, Fish D 1982 Physicians and nurse practitioners: do they provide equal health care? American Journal of Public Health 72: 55–57

Richardson G, Maynard A 1995 Fewer doctors, more nurses? A review of the knowledge base of doctor–nurse substitution. Centre for Health Economics, University of York

Rogers E M 1983 Diffusion of innovations, 3rd edn. Free Press, New York

Sathe V 1989 Fostering entrepreneurship in a large diverse firm. Organizational Dynamics 18(1): 20–32

Sharu D 1997 Advanced nursing practice in the USA: new directions for nurse practitioners. British Journal of Nursing 6(16): 934–938

Smith J P 1997 Editorial: the challenge of providing primary health care for all. Journal of Advanced Nursing 26: 1057–1059

Stillwell B, Greenfield S, Drury M, Hull F M 1987 A nurse practitioner in general practice: working style and pattern of consultations. Journal of the Royal College of General Practitioners 37: 154–157

Thompson L 1989 Caught in the crossfire. Nursing Times 85(48): 51

Tross G, Cavanagh S J 1996 Innovation in nursing management: professional management and methodological considerations. Journal of Nursing Management 4(3): 143–149

United Kingdom Central Council for Nursing, Midwifery and Health Visiting 1992 The scope of professional practice. UKCC, London

United Kingdom Central Council for Nursing, Midwifery and Health Visiting 1994 The future of professional practice: the Council's standards for education and practice following registration. UKCC, London

Vaughan B 1996 The role of the specialist: time to reflect. British Journal of Community Health Nursing 1(6): 371–372

Walshe C 1995 Living with a venous leg ulcer: a descriptive study of patient experiences. Journal of Advanced Nursing 22: 1092–1100

Watkins L, Wagner E 1982 Nurse practitioner and physician adherence to standing orders criteria for consultation and referral. American Journal of Public Health 72: 22–29

Williams A 1993 Steps to develop a working relationship: an evaluation of the community-based clinical nurse specialist. Professional Nurse 8(12): 806–812

Wilsher v. Essex Area Health Authority 1986. All England Law Reports 801

Wood N, Farrow S, Elliot B 1994 A review of primary health care organisation. Journal of Community Nursing 3: 243–250

Young A 1995 The legal dimension. In: Tingle J, Cribb A (eds) Nursing law and ethics. Blackwell, Oxford, ch 1

Young L 1997 Improved primary health care through integrated nursing. Primary Health Care 7(6): 8–10

FURTHER READING

Hunt G, Wainwright P 1994 Expanding the role of the nurse: the scope of professional practice. Blackwell Science, Oxford

Reed S 1995 Catching the tide: new voyages in nursing. Occasional Paper 1. SCHARR, University of Sheffield

8

Nurse prescribing

Jane Harris

Key points

- Impetus for change
- Implications for patients
- The prescribing process
- Professional aspects
- Interprofessional relationships and teamwork

INTRODUCTION

District nurses develop close professional relationships with patients whom they visit on a regular basis, often over a long period of time, and are well placed to assess accurately the patients' needs. However, they have relied on general practitioners to supply prescriptions for items which are an integral part of nursing care but may be of limited relevance to the medical management of the patient's condition. This chapter focuses on the issues surrounding the introduction and impact of prescribing authority for district nurses. It explores and analyses the relevant literature and uses the experience of prescribing district nurses to highlight some of the implications of their change in role.

Many of the publications cited are theory papers and opinion pieces, including editorials. Research evidence is limited due to the early stage of development of nurse prescribing. A study referred to repeatedly is the evaluation of the English nurse prescribing pilot programme commissioned by the Department of Health (Luker et al 1997). This remains the only comprehensive work undertaken following the introduction of nurse prescribing and therefore reports on actual rather than anticipated effects of nurse prescribing.

For many years, nurses have been frustrated by limitations to their practice which the inability to prescribe has imposed. Nurses in family planning settings recognised 20 years ago the potential for a more responsive and flexible service to clients if nurses were able to prescribe contraceptives (RCN 1980).

The Medicinal Products – Prescription by Nurses, etc. Act (DoH 1992a), the primary legislation which permitted nurses to prescribe, was passed on 16 March 1992. There followed an apparent delay before the secondary legislation defining the categories of nurses eligible to prescribe and the commencement order were finalised in October 1994. This enabled a specific group of community nurses, namely those with the qualification of either district nurse or health visitor, to prescribe from a limited formulary, the Nurse Prescribers' Formulary (NPF), which appears in the British National Formulary (BNF). It is anticipated that prescribing will not be an integral part of the role of all district nurses, both experienced and newly qualified, until 2001.

BACKGROUND

Traditional roles of doctor as prescriber, pharmacist as dispenser and nurse as administrator of medicines were not formally challenged until nurse prescribing was first proposed in the Cumberlege Report (DHSS 1986) which reviewed the organisation of community nursing services in England. Nurse prescribing proposals were hailed by some as the recognition of community nurses' ability to make autonomous clinical decisions. However, they would appear also to have resulted from concerns, highlighted by Cumberlege, about the complex arrangements that had developed to enable nurses to gain easier access to prescription items which they required in the course of routine patient care. The Crown Report (DoH 1989a) recommended that district nurses and health visitors, whom it was felt were the only nurses with clear responsibility for care and management of patients, should be given prescribing authority. It was not seen to

be necessary for nurses working in secondary care settings or with secondary care involvement, such as the community psychiatric nurses and other specialists, to have prescribing rights.

Shepherd et al (1996) note that prescribing is the only area of practice in which the law defines the nature of the work carried out by health professionals. It was therefore clear, following the Crown Report (DoH 1989a), that a process of legislative change would be necessary if the recommendations were to be accepted.

Jones & Gough (1997) document the role of the Royal College of Nursing in gathering support and lobbying for the introduction of nurse prescribing. Following the failure of a private member's bill presented by Dudley Fishburn, the Nurse Prescribing Bill, presented by Roger Simms in 1991, made a successful passage through Parliament and The Medicinal Products – Prescription by Nurses, etc. Act received Royal Assent in 1992. This led to amendment of the Medicines Act 1968 and the NHS Act 1977 (Dimond 1995). Finally, in 1994, the Pharmaceutical Services Regulations were passed to allow pharmacists to dispense items prescribed by nurses. However, current legislative changes only enable initial prescribing for certain categories of nurses from the NPF. The two other classes of prescribing recommended in the report (DoH 1989a) were not included.

In 1994 the Department of Health in England established eight demonstration sites, based at one fundholding general practice in each regional health authority, and commissioned a team at the universities of Liverpool and York to evaluate initial prescribing by nurses (Luker et al 1997). The results of the evaluation supported the anticipated outcomes of nurse prescribing highlighted in the Crown Report (DoH 1989a), benefits such as the saving of time and patients receiving treatment more promptly being notable examples. Anticipated disadvantages, for example, restrictions imposed by the limited range of items included within the NPF, were not confirmed. However, the small size of the study made the generalisation of findings difficult. A total of 58 nurse prescribers were involved at the outset (27 district nurses, 24 health visitors and seven practice nurses) with 49 remaining for the duration of the evaluation. Nurse prescribing was considered to be a success by patients, nurses, general practitioners and other health professionals and there was general support for it to be 'rolled out' on a national basis. In spite of this, the government was cautious and suggestions that there was inadequate evidence to proceed appeared to result in an extension to the pilot programme in 1996, rather than a national implementation programme.

The government's commitment to fully implement nurse prescribing was confirmed in the White Paper *Primary care: delivering the future* (DoH 1996). The frustration caused by the apparent delay in the introduction of nurse prescribing has been well documented (Hancock 1996, Jones & Gough 1997). However, it was not until 1998, following an announcement in April by the Secretary of State for Health Frank Dobson, that a national 'roll-out' got under way with completion anticipated by 2001. In addition, nurse prescribing was included in the initial programmes of preparation for district nurses and health visitors from September 1999. Consequently, nurses successfully completing these programmes will be eligible to record the nurse prescribing qualification along with their specialist qualification with the UKCC. They will then be able to prescribe once the nurse prescribing scheme is implemented within their employing authority.

Primary care: delivering the future (DoH 1996) also contained plans for a thorough review of prescribing practices and the supply and administration of medicines, including the use of protocols by nurses. The review commenced in 1997, under the chairmanship of June Crown, and finally reported in March 1999 (DoH 1999), with an interim report on group protocols (DoH 1998a).

The report on group protocols (DoH 1998a) included a definition and standard for the use of protocols and recommended legal clarification of their use. Despite the issue of a health service circular (DoH 1998b) requiring trusts to review their existing arrangements, according to Gooch (1999), many group protocols still fail to meet the criteria set out in the report.

Thirty nine recommendations were included in the Crown Report (DoH 1999). As in the 1989 report, improved patient care and assured patient safety are the stated objectives of the proposed change. Current prescribing authority is recommended to continue with new groups of prescribers to be introduced. The report proposes that there should be two groups of prescriber: independent prescribers responsible for the initial diagnosis and authority to prescribe as part of the treatment plan and dependent prescribers authorised to prescribe certain items within an agreed treatment plan for patients already assessed by an independent prescriber. Crown also proposes that a UK-wide advisory body, the New Prescribers Advisory Committee, will be set up under Section 4 of the Medicines Act. This will review applications from professional organisations seeking new prescriber status for their members.

The response to the report, following a consultation period which ended in June 1999, was submitted to UK ministers. However, a long wait, estimated to be between five and 10 years, lies ahead which includes changes in legislation before any real changes in practice will be seen.

Meanwhile the RCN and others continue to campaign for nurse prescribing to be developed. There have been calls to include all specialist nurses following the relevant training in pharmacology and diagnosis together with the authority to prescribe from all items listed in the BNF. Both the UKCC and the BMA continue to support nurse prescribing and its expansion but advocate the imposition of a limited formulary.

IMPETUS FOR CHANGE

Central to the issue of nurse prescribing is change, from a tradition where one professional group has near monopoly over the performance of a particular function to a situation where another professional group is given authority to perform the same function, albeit in a limited way. Nurse prescribing has implications for patients, the individual nurse and the nursing profession, the process of care, teamwork and interprofessional relationships. The rationale for change must therefore be convincing and the anticipated benefits clearly positive. But, convincing and positive for whom?

The Crown Report (DoH 1989a) was clear that foremost among the anticipated benefits of nurse prescribing was a significant improvement in patient care, in terms of both clinical effectiveness and convenience to patients and their carers. Indeed, the new Crown Report (DoH 1999) only proposes new groups of prescribers in clinical areas where improved patient care and safety would result. It is useful to remember that the report's recommendations are based on the evidence collected from nurses, other professional groups and statutory bodies that may be affected by or have been exposed to nurse prescribing. Most importantly, the views of patients themselves are included.

However, ulterior motives have been suggested for the introduction of nurse prescribing. McCartney et al (1999) propose that nurse prescribing was used as a tool by the Conservative government to save time and money, delegate routine medical work to nurses and challenge the authority of the medical profession. There seems little evidence to support this proposal. Interestingly, the two attempts to evaluate the economic aspects of nurse prescribing, the cost benefit analysis undertaken by Touche Ross (DoH 1991) and the economic evaluation of the English pilot, failed to demonstrate saving. Luker et al (1997) admitted difficulty in identifying costs and benefits directly attributable to the introduction of nurse prescribing but concluded that there was no evidence to suggest that costs had either increased or decreased since its introduction. However, prescribing appeared to make the nurses in the study by Luker et al (1997) more cost conscious. They felt that they were cost-effective prescribers because they were aware of the costs of the items they were prescribing, tailored the volume of the items prescribed to the patients' needs to avoid wastage and stockpiling and used generic prescribing. There was some evidence suggesting time savings for health-care professionals, as in the original cost-benefit analysis (DoH 1991), it could not be confirmed that a net financial saving would result. The act

---

Vignette 8.1 Delegation

Before the district nurses in our practice could prescribe, we used to enter requests for prescriptions for our patients in a book at reception. At this point, we had visited and assessed the patient, decided on a treatment plan and made a decision as to the most appropriate product, for example for wound care, to meet the patient's needs. The prescription was generated by the office staff, signed by the doctor when he had time and finally available for collection. We found this both time consuming and unnecessarily complicated and often delayed the onset of appropriate treatment for the patient. The doctor's task was not onerous and he was perhaps caused the least inconvenience of all.

---

of delegation suggests an advantage to the delegator and disadvantage to the delegate. However, consider the scenario depicted in Vignette 8.1.

In the absence of nurse prescribing, it is generally accepted that diagnosis and selection of the item have already been made by the nurse and the doctor's role is merely to rubber stamp this decision with a signature so it is difficult to accept that the actual signing of the prescription is of any great consequence to either. The nurse's authority to complete the prescription herself is most convenient to all concerned. In addition, many district nurses' patients have chronic conditions requiring limited medical intervention or contact with the doctor anyway. The ability to prescribe therefore enhances the district nurses' capacity to provide comprehensive nursing care with fewer unnecessary interruptions.

Finally, nurse prescribing is a weak challenge to medicine for the following reasons. There has already been a shift away from the supremacy or monopoly of the doctor in general practice, which has been doctor driven. For example, many general practices actively encourage patients in certain circumstances to consult the nurse rather than the doctor. This can be viewed as acknowledgement that the nurse can, at times, be an appropriate alternative. The example can be taken further to suggest that patient independence and ability to self care with an ever-expanding range of over-the-counter medicines have again been encouraged by doctors. Therefore, it is difficult to view nurses' authority to prescribe from the NPF, consisting primarily of over-the-counter medicines, as a threat to the medical profession.

Practices such as general practitioners signing blank prescriptions to be completed as required by nurses were, strictly speaking, illegal but reflected the frustration many community nurses felt in being prevented from providing comprehensive care responsive to the needs of their patients. Processes to enable nurses to supply items according to protocol developed in order to overcome some of the problems associated with the lack of prescribing authority. As Leifer (1997) points out, the law clearly covers protocols for individual patients but is less clear where the responsibility lies where group protocols are concerned. This, in effect, called into question the legality of established practices such as the use of group protocols to cover nurses' supply of immunisations in clinic settings and led to appeals for clarification by commentators such as Casey (1996) and Williams (1998).

IMPLICATIONS FOR PATIENTS

It was anticipated that nurse prescribing would result in a number of benefits for patients (DoH 1989a, 1991). However, one of the problems associated with evaluating an intervention such as nurse prescribing, which is part of a treatment plan, is identifying the outcomes which are a direct result of that particular intervention. It would be wrong to assume that these all relate to the generation of a prescription. Implicit in the qualification to make safe and effective prescribing decisions is an enhanced level of knowledge of all treatment options available to the client. Nurse prescribers are therefore ideally placed to provide sound and appropriate advice to patients whether or not an item is prescribed.

Convenience to patients

Evidence from the study by Luker et al (1997) evaluating the eight English pilot sites supports the patient benefits anticipated by the government. A number of patients were interviewed prior to the introduction of nurse prescribing (n=157) and again following its introduction

(n=148). They reported advantages relating to time saving, convenience in obtaining their prescription and more prompt access to the item prescribed. Interestingly, patients' comments depended on the occupation of the nurse prescriber involved. For example, some district nurses' patients were able to avoid dependence on others to obtain their prescription and direct access to the prescription enabled them to obtain the item up to 48 hours earlier. Health visitors' clients also reported easier and more prompt access to the prescribed item as they did not need to visit the general practitioner following a consultation with the health visitor. These benefits were not as noticeable for practice nurses' patients visiting the surgery, due to more direct access to the general practitioner.

Clinical effectiveness

Several aspects of clinical effectiveness cited as outcomes of nurse prescribing in the Crown Report (DoH 1989a) relate to areas which were not included in nurse prescribing legislation; for example, increased continuity of care resulting from nurses' ability, in certain circumstances, to alter the dosage and timing of drugs. Earlier commencement of treatment has been proposed as an aspect of clinical effectiveness that could be attributed to initial prescribing (Moreton 1992, Harrison 1993, Smith 1990); patients in the English evaluation did report receiving treatment more quickly as a result of nurse prescribing.

Information giving, in the form of practical advice about the item at the time of prescribing, and patient teaching/health education as a therapeutic treatment option, either as an adjunct to prescribing or as an alternative, make an important contribution to clinical effectiveness. Tones & Tilford (1994) and Downie et al (1996) view teaching as the role of the health-care team member closest to the patient. Where nurse prescribers assume responsibility for comprehensive nursing care, they may be the patient's main contact with the health service and in this context, their teaching role becomes more important. This is a situation well known to district nurses.

In Luker's study (Luker et al 1997), the majority of nurses interviewed felt that they gave more information to patients when issuing the prescription than the general practitioner did (13% of the patients and almost half of the general practitioners agreed). They felt that they had more time than general practitioners and a closer relationship with the patient. They also felt that giving more detailed information was more likely to promote compliance with the treatment and that they were in a better position to evaluate this than the general practitioner. Patients in the study reported that they found it easier to talk to the nurse as she was more approachable and knew them better than did the general practitioner.

Time saving

The Cumberlege Report (DHSS 1986) first proposed that nurse prescribing would result in better use of community nurses' skills and improved quality of care for patients. One reason for this, suggested in the Crown Report (DoH 1989a), was the additional time available which nurses would not have to spend in travelling and waiting to ask doctors to write prescriptions on their behalf.

However, a spokesman from Touche Ross, cited by Tattam (1992), warned that time saving would depend on how nurse prescribing was introduced and there was a danger that time-consuming procedures could negate some prescribing gains. This problem had been anticipated in the original cost–benefit analysis (DoH 1991). Interestingly, some of the nurse prescribers in the English evaluation, notably some of the health visitors, reported having to make a specific journey to the surgery to record prescribing details in patients' case notes. Luker et al (1997) concluded that the type of time saving initially anticipated may indeed be cancelled out by the additional time spent on prescribing-related activities such as administration and record keeping.

The importance of adequate documentation and of sharing information with other team members as appropriate is undeniable and was stressed in the Crown Report (DoH 1989a). Experience suggests that primary care teams develop mechanisms for record keeping which satisfy legal and professional requirements while at the same time are best suited to the needs of the practice.

A further anticipated concern, documented in the literature (Luker et al 1997), was the self-referral of patients and the subsequent additional workload. Although the English evaluation did report nurse prescribers experiencing increased self-referral of patients and also referral from non-prescribing nurse colleagues, this did not appear to constitute a problem in terms of time.

THE PROCESS OF PRESCRIBING
The Nurse Prescribers' Formulary

The recommendations of the Cumberlege Report included: 'The DHSS should agree a limited list of items and simple agents which may be prescribed by nurses as part of a nursing care programme' (DHSS 1986, p.33). The NPF covers a wide range of therapeutic areas, including items such as laxatives, wound management products, catheter care products and skin preparations. However, the three categories of licensed medicines defined in the Medicines Act (1968) are not equally represented. Few prescription-only medicines (POMs) are included and, with an increasing number of items being deregulated to pharmacy status (P) or available in retail outlets (GSL), patients are able to buy many of the items over the counter.

But does this matter? Some consider (Bradley et al 1997) that these factors threaten the value of the nurse prescribing scheme. However, as shown in vignette 8.2 the categorisation of the catheter care products used by the district nurse in the care of an elderly housebound man with urinary problems is immaterial to both the man and the district nurse. The man relies on the district nurse's expertise at all stages of the management process, including selection and use of the product. The district nurse welcomes any opportunity to improve the service that can be provided, which includes easy access to the resources required.

Vignette 8.2   Meeting client needs

Mr Jones, a 93-year-old man living 2 miles out of town, had to be catheterised at home by the district nurse for urinary retention. Following catheterisation and an introduction to the management of his urinary catheter, the nurse prescribed the leg bags and night bags that the man preferred and was able to drain. In view of this man's independent nature and social isolation, it was crucial that he could competently care for his catheter.

Prior to the introduction of nurse prescribing, the provision of catheters and associated appliances was often haphazard. Patients often received items from stock available within the community nurse's store or those prescribed at random within the practice due to insufficient prescribing information being made available. This variety of supplies often added to the confusion for the patient as they attempted to independently manage their catheter.

Vignette 8.3   Scope of the NPF

I visited 43-year-old Mrs Sinclair postoperatively. She had recently had a hysterectomy for a cancerous tumour. I discovered that the wound was infected and although I could remove the sutures, advise the patient and prescribe appropriate dressings, I could not prescribe an antibiotic to treat the infection. Instead, I had to follow the time-consuming procedure of finding a GP, discussing the case and arranging the issue of a prescription with the surgery. This not only meant that Mrs Sinclair had to organise its collection, but the prolonged process drew attention to the fact that there was a problem and caused added strain on the patient and her family.

Another criticism of the NPF is that it is limited and restrictive (Gunn 1997, Luker et al 1997, Wedgwood 1995). On analysis of the roles of the three disciplines of community nursing eligible to prescribe, it appears that the value of the formulary varies. For example, district nurses write more prescriptions than their colleagues and find the NPF more appropriate to the needs of their client groups. Luker et al (1997) found that the contents of the NPF limited the prescribing role of the health visitors and practice nurses in their study and they were still reliant on general practitioners to sign prescriptions for items commonly used by their clients. Clegg (1995) highlights concerns that prescribing health visitors may lose their prescribing skills due to the inappropriate content of the formulary.

Not surprisingly, clients requiring wound and catheter care have benefited most from nurse prescribing. Easy access to the items required has streamlined their care and often avoided problems such as lack of supplies on hospital discharge and delayed commencement of treatment. This is particularly important considering the increase in early discharge and subsequently the demand for more acute care in the community by district nurses. In this case, though, the scope of the formulary may prevent district nurses from providing a full range of care to the patient, allowing them to prescribe some of the items which they require. An example of this is demonstrated in vignette 8.3.

However, extending nurse prescribing across a greater range of items is controversial, with international examples contributing to the UK debate. Interestingly, proposals for nurse prescribing in New Zealand described by Gunn (1997) include a formulary which is appropriate to the scope of nurse specialists' practice rather than being limited to a number of specific items. A similar argument is proposed by Mayes (1996) who, in discussing the prescribing practices of nurse practitioners, suggests that the formulary should reflect the profile of their caseloads. This would appear to be a sensible development. The Crown Report (DoH 1999) recommends that authority to prescribe and supply should be extended but limited to items within specific therapeutic areas which fall within the prescriber's range of experience and competence.

For some, this does not go far enough. Gunn suggests that if nurses are to be accountable for their own practice which is based on thorough educational preparation, then they should be able to access the national formulary in the same way as doctors. Jones & Gough (1997) advocate an unlimited list for nurse prescribing in the United Kingdom. Evidence to support independent prescribing from an unlimited list is unconvincing and the issues surrounding education and monitoring, to name just a few of the implications, are extremely complex.

Review of American nurse practitioner literature documents the lack of autonomy in decision making, with many states imposing strict regulations and mandatory supervision by physicians

(Craig 1996, Meyer 1994). Doctors in Ontario were reported by Spurgeon (1995) to be concerned about patient safety following government plans to expand the nurse practitioner role to include diagnosis and treatment of uncomplicated diseases and injuries, including prescribing. Although nurse practitioners are well established in Canada and the USA, prescribing authority is generally supervised and in many instances protocols are in place. In Sweden all district nurses have prescribing authority but again, lack independent prescribing status. They can prescribe approximately 230 listed products for 60 specific indications but are not expected to make a decision about differential diagnosis (David & Brown 1995).

Decision making

Andrews (1994) describes two elements of decision making in nurse prescribing: primary decision making, being a process involving the diagnosis of a condition and, secondary to this, deciding on the course of action. This distinction is a useful basis for further discussion.

Diagnosis, as an activity traditionally associated with the medical profession, is controversial in nurse prescribing terms. This is evident in both nursing and medical literature. Bradley et al (1997) writing in the *British Medical Journal* state that nurses have no basic training in diagnosis or therapeutics and will therefore have limited effectiveness as prescribers. An editorial by Gledhill (1994), a nurse, includes nurses' differential diagnosis in a list of risks associated with nurse prescribing. However, it depends on the context and definition of the term 'diagnosis'. Dictionary definitions include phrases such as 'an opinion reached through the analysis of facts', 'a thorough analysis of facts or problems in order to gain understanding' (*Collins dictionary* 1991). This can easily be applied to a comprehensive nursing assessment followed by identification of the patient's problem. The context is also important. Cumberlege (DHSS 1986) recommended that a list of items should be developed that nurses could prescribe as part of a nursing care programme.

Medical diagnosis and intervention may have very little to do with the nurses' assessment and care plan in many instances but an important aspect of the nurse prescriber's role is to refer to colleagues when necessary and naturally a medical opinion or diagnosis would be sought in some circumstances. The English evaluation (Luker et al 1997) reported that nurses expressed anxiety over the prescribing of items such as laxatives and analgesics for which they felt a medical diagnosis was required.

Theorists such as Voss & Post (1988) differentiate between social science problem solving, which involves planning and is very familiar to community nurses, and the problem-solving activity in medicine which leads to the medical diagnosis. This is not to say that the two processes are mutually exclusive. Barrows & Feltovich (1987) question the reality of the structured problem-solving approach depicted in medical diagnosis and support the concept of a temporal unfolding of information as a consequence of unstructured clinical situations which are more realistic. Bryans & McIntosh (1996) highlight the relevance of this in community nurses' patient assessment and cite the observation of Cowley et al (1994) that this is a continuous process rather than a one-off event.

In support of diagnosis by nurses, it was the Cumberlege Report (DHSS 1986) that focused attention on the process whereby general practitioners endorsed nurses' decisions by effectively rubber stamping the treatments they proposed for their patients. Underlying this practice is evidently a diagnosis by the nurse, accepted and acknowledged by the doctor through the signing of the prescription. Other literature endorses the claim that nurses were already diagnosing problems and making prescribing decisions as part of the nursing management of clients, nurse prescribing merely clarifying professional responsibility (Carlisle 1989, Pickersgill & Clarke 1990).

An abundance of literature from North America discusses and develops the concept of nursing diagnosis, a term beginning to be used more widely in the United Kingdom.

Nursing diagnosis is a clinical judgement about individual, family or community responses to actual or potential health problems/life processes. Nursing diagnoses provide the basis for selection of nursing interventions to achieve outcomes for which nursing is accountable. (Carpenito 1991, p.65)

Carpenito's definition makes a distinction between nursing and medical diagnosis, with nursing diagnosis being the basis for nursing intervention. This is clearly reflected in the Crown Report (DoH 1989a) which recommends that nurses would prescribe as part of nursing care and not medical care and as such would be accountable for their decisions.

A study by Peate (1996), which the author admits was motivated by the concern that high-level decision making would be required by nurse prescribers, looked at how nurses make decisions about administration of medicines. A range of qualitative techniques, including grounded theory and participant observation, were used to identify the decision-making processes of seven qualified nurses. Although a substantial amount of qualitative data was generated, the author tentatively concluded that nurses find it difficult to describe the cues and knowledge base upon which they make decisions.

Theories of decision making are evident in the literature and contribute to the debate on how nurses make decisions about prescribing. These include a rational or scientific approach which is based on knowledge and involves analysis of the situation (Harbison 1991), with nursing diagnosis as an example of this process (Hardwick 1998, Wooley 1990), and intuitive knowledge associated with experience which has been discussed in detail by Benner (1982). Benner's model describes the nurse moving through five stages of experience from novice to expert with decision-making processes being linked to the level of experience. Both of these theories can account for uncertainty and anxiety in decision making. For example, Harbison (1991) describes how incomplete objective knowledge can lead to uncertainty and difficulty in making decisions and a study by Watson (1994) showed that lack of previous experience made decisions more

difficult. Other factors cited as affecting decision making by nurses include their relationship with the patient (Radwin 1995) and their relationship with doctors and other colleagues (Jenks 1993), with nurses reporting feeling less confident about their decisions where relationships with doctors were not good.

Secondary decision making, in terms of selecting the appropriate treatment, has received less attention. However, an American study by Mahoney (1994) compared the prescribing decisions of nurse practitioners and physicians using standardised case vignettes and found that nurse practitioners scored higher on an index of appropriateness than physicians. None of the general practitioners in the English evaluation had concerns about the appropriateness of prescribing decisions by the nurses prescribers. However, they also believed the NPF to be too limited to result in serious errors. The nurse prescribers reported that the difficulty in prescribing treatment lay more in whether to write a prescription or advise the patient to buy the item over the counter, rather than which item to prescribe (Luker et al 1997).

PROFESSIONAL ASPECTS

Role development

The subject of role development and expansion in nursing is not new but has received more attention at government level in recent years (DoH 1992b, 1997, UKCC 1992a). The role development and reprofiling debate may be viewed from a number of perspectives depending on the outcome desired. Economic and professional incentives appear to command more attention in professional debate and the literature than clinical effectiveness and user satisfaction. Role development is discussed in more detail in Chapter 7 but some of the issues have particular relevance to nurse prescribing and are included here.

As the emphasis on cost effectiveness in health care gathers momentum, initiatives aimed at substituting cheaper providers for more expensive ones have become accepted practice, with doctor–nurse substitution receiving most attention (Richardson & Maynard 1995). Rapid and substantial change in primary health care, for example, the GP Contract (DoH 1989b) with its increased workload for general practitioners, encouraged redefinition of roles and concomitantly delegation of doctors' duties to community nurses, usually practice nurses (Gilhespy 1993, Robinson 1990, Robinson et al 1993). Interestingly, practice nurses have become nurse prescribers more by default than design so the delegation argument applied to prescribing is weak in their case.

Role development of nurses in order to provide more comprehensive care and a sharing of patient management with doctors is an alternative viewpoint. Conflicting views are evident in the literature based on the motives underlying professional aspects of role development. Delegation implies a task-oriented approach, which nursing as a profession has been trying to renounce, or it implies an opportunity for more independence and autonomy, hallmarks of professional status.

Strauss (1985) contends that when doctors find a task dissatisfying they delegate it to other health workers. However, because these other workers lack medical knowledge and expertise, the doctor usually imposes regulation and control to ensure safe and effective practice. There is a strong argument against the notion that nurse prescribing was introduced as a delegated function. Cumberlege (DHSS 1986) reported on methods that practices had already developed to overcome the problems associated with prescribing and supply of items for district nurses. Inconvenience appeared to be encountered by district nurses and their patients rather than the general practitioners and the methods described by Cumberlege and later Crown (DoH 1989a) were designed and implemented to minimise their inconvenience. In addition, regulation imposed on nurse prescribers to ensure safety and effectiveness is clearly legislative and enacted and monitored through the UKCC. In fact, the influence of the medical profession can only be viewed as positive to date, with general practitioners contributing to nurse prescribing

courses and supporting their nurse prescribing colleagues in practice. Furthermore, far from being a task-oriented activity, nurse prescribing is part of a nurse-managed comprehensive programme of care delivered to an individual patient.

Shepherd et al (1996) also argue that prescribing is merely a form of role extension, with nurses working under the direct delegation and financial control of the provider practice. Again, nurse prescribers would claim that, far from being an act of delegation and control, prescribing authority gives them more freedom and independence in caring for their patients. UK nurse prescribers have independent prescribing status which is unusual compared with schemes in other countries. There may be examples where practices have placed budgetary restraints on nurse prescribers but these are rare and perhaps relate to the early days of nurse prescribing when caution was being exercised. It is generally accepted that prescribing by nurses is substitute prescribing and does not incur a financial burden on the prescribing budget.

There is general support, particularly in the nursing literature, for the change in nurses' role to prescriber. However, as already stated, the effects of nurse prescribing are either speculative (DoH 1989a, 1991) or based on the evaluation of a small cohort of nurse prescribers over a limited time scale (Luker et al 1997). It would appear that the long-term effects of this role change, which clearly bisects the boundary between medical and nursing work, have been given little attention.

Shepherd (1998) suggests that the traditional role of the nurse may indeed be threatened and envisages a situation where nurses become more involved in the diagnostic procedures required for prescribing decisions. Subsequently, the more caring elements of their role would be delegated to less qualified and experienced staff.

Skidmore (1999) discusses nurse prescribing from the perspective of the nursing profession. He suggests that confining prescribing to certain categories of nurses is discriminatory and divisive and damaging to the profession as a whole. This begs the question, whose interests does nurse prescribing seek to serve? The profession or the client? Surely, those familiar with the district nurse's role could not fail to see the benefits of prescribing as part of a nursing care plan, particularly when many of the items contained within the NPF are ideally suited to meeting the needs of patients with chronic, nurse-managed problems.

There is some evidence from earlier research which suggests that nurse prescribers may not necessarily be accepted by patients. Bevan (1979) reported that patients saw nurses in a caring role and were reluctant to accept them in a decision-making role unless doctors said it was appropriate. Luker et al (1997) reported that patients were positive about the nurses' role as prescriber and in some circumstances, such as wound management, district nurses were considered to be more appropriate prescribers than general practitioners, due to their familiarity with the patient and expertise in that area of practice.

Accountability and responsibility

Butterworth (1990) observes that nursing in the UK has had a tradition of collective (shielded) responsibility rather than individual responsibility for action. However, one of the basic premises of nurse prescribing is the notion of individual responsibility and accountability. *The scope of professional practice* (UKCC 1992a) and *The code of professional conduct* (UKCC 1992b) formally reaffirmed the profession's view that nurses were indeed accountable for their own actions. In relation to nurse prescribing, the literature clearly reinforces the point that nurse prescribers are wholly professionally and legally responsible for the prescriptions they sign (Elliot Pennels 1997).

However, the issue of a prescription is just one part of the process. The nurse prescriber is accountable for the decisions made to either prescribe or not prescribe, the recommendation of alternative treatment or over-the-counter purchases, advice giving and instruction to the patient and carers and monitoring and recording of her actions. In addition, there is accountability for the prescribing decision to the person for whom the prescription is issued or not issued, to

---

Vignette 8.4 Experienced prescribers

We have now been prescribing for over 3 years. When it was announced that we, very experienced district nurses, were to be among the first prescribers we had mixed feelings. We were genuinely excited, but somewhat daunted and nervous about the responsibility that prescribing would entail. Following the nurse prescribing course, we were reassured that we had the clinical knowledge to competently prescribe from the current nurses' formulary. Equipped with the information and guidance about prescribing itself, we tentatively filled out our first prescriptions. With time, prescribing experience and, along with it, confidence developed. Now we view prescribing as part of our everyday role as district nurses. We are as aware of issues of responsibility and accountability in our role as prescribers as we are in any other aspect of our role.

---

the public in general, to the employer and to the profession. Anxiety associated with the responsibility and accountability of the prescribers' role is commonly anticipated and often experienced by new nurse prescribers. An example is given in vignette 8.4. However, as prescribing experience develops and becomes an accepted element of the district nurse's role, responsibility and accountability for prescribing appear to be more easily accepted (Harris 1998, Luker et al 1997). In reality, district nurses accept accountability for the care they give, whatever care that may be.

Educational preparation

Crucial to the success of district nurses as safe and effective prescribers is their educational preparation and knowledge base. Indeed, the recommendations of the Crown Report (DoH 1989a) assumed a level of knowledge and expertise of the practising district nurse and health visitor which would only require to be supplemented by an additional 3 days training in preparation for prescribing. In practice, this became a 15-hour distance learning package and a 2–3 day taught component which is formally assessed. It was envisaged that the process of prescribing would be a large component of the taught course, as this is a skill new to nurses. It was assumed that potential prescribers would be at least familiar with items in the NPF and would not require specific instruction in the use of every item as part of the course.

Given the complex nature of prescribing, there is surprisingly little research evidence to support nurses' proficiency in undertaking this new role. One study frequently cited in the nurse prescribing debate, (While & Rees 1993) surveyed the knowledge base of a small non-randomised geographically selected sample of health visitors and district nurses. The results indicated that their knowledge of the full potential and side effects of items included in the NPF was incomplete. Obviously, this study predates nurse prescribing but many of the nurses involved had been advising general practitioners about the use of products for their clients. Despite the limitations of the study in terms of sample size and selection method, the findings are a cause for concern in the absence of any contradictory evidence. Indeed, the knowledge base of district nurses has been found to be low in other studies (Bell 1994, Koh 1993, Roe et al 1994).

These results have been used to suggest that community nurses are not well equipped to prescribe. In the absence of the additional training which nurse prescribing necessitates, this could well be true and not just of community nurses. The current success of nurse prescribing has, however, demonstrated that community nurses have been well prepared for their role and do prescribe safely and effectively (Luker et al 1997). It has also been suggested that the authority to prescribe sharpens the prescriber's focus on all aspects of the patient's treatment regimen. It draws attention to other medications, whether prescribed or bought over the counter, which the patient is taking and elicits a more analytical and critical approach to decision making. This is described in vignette 8.5.

In order to comply with the standard, kind and content of nurse prescribing preparation laid down by the UKCC, the educational packages provided by the institutions of higher education have been very similar in terms of programme and content. This standardisation has in effect failed to acknowledge the diversity in the professional profiles of potential prescribers and overlooked the educational needs of individuals. The

---

Vignette 8.5   Knowledge sharing

I work within a team of five district nurses, only two of whom are nurse prescribers. As prescribers, our knowledge not only of NPF items has increased immensely since the introduction of nurse prescribing but also other items within the BNF prescribed by the GPs and items bought by our patients at the chemist. In addition, the introduction of nurse prescribing has generated a completely new level of discussion and knowledge sharing within the entire nursing team regarding NPF products and their uses.

---

same performance has been expected of district nurses with many years of experience but limited exposure to recent academic study and the rigours of formal assessment and newly qualified, inexperienced district nurses. This may have led to unnecessary anxiety amongst some of those undergoing prescribing preparation and even resistance in others to become prescribers. Organisers of nurse courses and managers of potential prescribers should not underestimate the amount of support and encouragement which some nurses require at this time.

Despite the standardisation of the preparation for prescribing, consolidation and further development of prescribing skills has been diverse and patchy across the UK. A number of factors could be responsible for this. First, however, nurses are aware of the statutory requirements for effective registration (UKCC 1994). An element of this is that they are accountable for their practice and must maintain a profile of their personal and professional development and updating of skills and knowledge. Interestingly, requirements for the content of the personal professional profile have never included specified links to the parts of the professional register for which the nurse seeks to maintain registration. It is therefore the responsibility of individual practitioners, and in this case nurse prescribers, to direct continuing professional development activities appropriately. In some areas, employers have invested in further training and education for nurse prescribers or supported the development of informal networking. In others, existing methods of clinical support have been used, including clinical supervision. In fact, Luker et al (1997) recommended that clinical supervision should be an important method of developing effective prescribing practice following completion of the course.

In the absence of a model of clinical support and employer-initiated strategies for further education, nurse prescribers have been left to their own devices to ensure development of their skills. Examples include nurses arranging local tutorials with the community pharmacist to discuss issues such as wound care products, practice lunchtime meetings with prescribing team members using case studies as the basis for discussion and more formal workshops arranged with the local course provider to enable updating and networking.

One of the problems in the early days of nurse prescribing was that in many pilot schemes, individual nurses were selected from the practice to undergo preparation for prescribing, rather than all those eligible. This meant that on completion of the course, nurse prescribers were often isolated and lacked the support and encouragement that day-to-day contact with other nurse prescribers can provide. Now that the roll-out is almost complete, nurses are much more likely to benefit from the support of experienced colleagues.

This is one reason why the timing is right for the introduction of prescribing into initial programmes of preparation for district nurses as most assessors will be qualified and fairly experienced prescribers. Students will have the opportunity to relate theory to practice as they witness nurse prescribing first hand during placements and are able to discuss prescribing practice with their assessor as the course progresses. In addition, they will be assured of beginning their district nursing career in an environment in which nurse prescribing is familiar to all concerned. As nurse prescribing preparation is integrated into initial programmes, it is more likely to be viewed as a natural part of the district nurse's role rather than the high-profile addition and focus of attention which it has been up to now.

Job satisfaction

It had been envisaged that nurse prescribing would increase job satisfaction as nurses were

---

Vignette 8.6   Job satisfaction

Before I became a nurse prescriber, I anticipated benefits such as getting access to prescribed items more easily and being able to start treatment with the most appropriate products more quickly. But I completely underestimated the sense of satisfaction and fulfilment that the role would bring. I feel that the quality of care which I can offer many of my patients has improved immensely.

---

able to manage the patient's condition more effectively (DoH 1989a). However, there is more evidence in the literature to support enhancement of professional identity and increased status resulting in increased job satisfaction.

A study by Wade (1993) surveyed the job satisfaction of district nurses, health visitors and practice nurses working in four community NHS trusts. The findings indicated that practice nurses were the most satisfied group and health visitors the least. The author suggested that there were links with job satisfaction theory (Hackman & Oldham 1980, cited by Wade 1993) which states that feedback, variety, task identity and autonomy are highly related to job satisfaction. Feelings of increased status and autonomy were mentioned by nurse prescribers now that they were seen to be taking responsibility for their decisions and working independently (Luker et al 1997). They reported an increase in job satisfaction as a result of nurse prescribing. Vignette 8.6 supports this view.

Interestingly, Shepherd (1998) and Butterworth (1990) both express concerns that nurses may be more motivated to advance their professional standing rather than to respond to patients' needs and improve patient care. In the context of nurse prescribing, all available evidence allays this concern.

INTERPROFESSIONAL RELATIONSHIPS AND TEAMWORK IN PRIMARY CARE

The Crown Committee considered the practice of doctors signing prescriptions for nurses for items which they needed as part of nursing care to be undesirable and professionally demeaning to those involved (DoH 1989a). It therefore proposed that nurse prescribing would clarify professional roles and responsibilities. Pickersgill & Clarke (1990) suggested that role clarification would extend to patients also, with nurses having more credibility if they are given the authority to act on treatment decisions rather than seeking the endorsement of a doctor. Role clarification and demarcation are important components of the skill mix debate. Heath (1994) supports the view that skill mix enables health needs of local populations to be met more effectively and appropriately, providing there is teamwork and sharing of common goals.

The Crown Report (DoH 1989a) also anticipated that as a result of role clarification, professional relationships would be strengthened with each member being able to exercise their skills more effectively. In addition, communication within the primary health-care team, as an important component of quality health care, could be improved as a result of nurse prescribing. This would result from increased collaboration not only between doctor and nurse but also between nurse and pharmacist. An example of this is given in vignette 8.7.

Many community pharmacists see nurse prescribing as an opportunity to develop existing relationships with district nurses and contribute to improvements in the primary health-care service. In many institutes of higher education,

pharmacists have been involved in the development and delivery of nurse prescribing courses. This has not only enabled nurses to gain a greater understanding of the role of the pharmacist but also the direct contact with local pharmacists during the course enhances future relationships and networking opportunities. Pharmacists also play an important role in supporting novice nurse prescribers in practice and are well placed to help nurses to identify and meet continuing professional development needs.

However, lack of communication and poor relationships between nurses and doctors have been cited as possible barriers to the successful introduction of innovation. In a study by Mackay (1989) it was found that the relationship between doctors and nurses was marred by poor communication, with nurses' biggest complaint being the failure of doctors to listen to what they had to say. Nurse prescribers will be aware of preexisting difficulties within their practice and have a professional responsibility to confront factors which threaten the successful introduction of nurse prescribing.

The effective management of change, as an essential component of the process of introducing nurse prescribing, further endorses the importance of supportive professional relationships. Moffatt & Dorman (1996) and Vaughan (1997) stress the value of multiprofessional collaboration in the current climate of change in health care. They suggest that change in practice is not always welcome and a conscientious and collaborative approach may help to dissipate anxiety and uncertainty. Oughtibridge (1998) contends that most discussions which take place between doctors and nurses relate to patient care and interprofessional issues are rarely discussed. This therefore limits the opportunity to discuss new ideas and the implementation of change. However, primary care groups and local health-care cooperatives will provide a forum for multidisciplinary debate which may enable or, in some circumstances, necessitate consideration of interprofessional issues.

Successive government publications have stressed the importance of teamwork and collaboration in primary health care in order to provide

---

Vignette 8.7 Benefits

One of the benefits that nurse prescribing has brought to us as a team is the increased openness and focus for discussion. These discussions frequently revolve around clinical and cost effectiveness and regularly involve not only district nurses but also other professionals such as the practice-based pharmacist and the general practitioners. Cost effectiveness especially was rarely discussed in the past and we were often unaware of the costs of treatments we initiated, although obviously did not prescribe at that time. Although we would not compromise on quality, we often find that we can prescribe a similar item for less. We all feel that our increased knowledge and the forum for discussion which this has inspired has a positive effect on the quality of care which we give.

efficient and effective services (DoH 1990, 1992, 1993, 1996, Scottish Office 1997). However, evidence to support the widespread existence of effective teams is difficult to find. On the contrary, much of the literature focuses on the problems that exist in primary health-care teams and proposes team-building strategies (Øvretveit 1990, Poulton & West 1993). These include mutual understanding of team members' roles, communication and shared goals. Problems associated with teamwork are not only interdisciplinary but also intradisciplinary. The Cumberlege Report (DHSS 1986) followed up concerns first documented in a study of nursing teams in general practice (Gilmore et al 1974) that shortcomings in the organisation of the community nursing services led to lack of coordination and cooperation and underuse of nurses' skills. Despite developments such as integrated nursing teams, some community nurses still appear to find teamwork problematic. Mackenzie & Ross (1997) cite professional jealousies and lack of role demarcation as the source of problems between community nurses. In addition, there are fundamental differences associated with traditional management structures brought about by employment of practice nurses by GPs and district nurses and health visitors by NHS community trusts. Given the complexities of successful team functioning, it seems difficult to envisage how the introduction of nurse prescribing could make an impression on teamwork. On the contrary, as mentioned earlier, it has been proposed that nurse prescribing is divisive rather than uniting (Skidmore 1999). Interestingly, practice nurses involved in the English pilot programme did report an improvement in teamwork, with a stronger, closer team than before prescribing.

Crown (DoH 1989a) identified another objective for good communication between the professional groups involved in prescribing. It was felt that this was not only vital to ensure the effectiveness of clinical audit processes in place to monitor and evaluate nurse prescribing but also, as highlighted by Andrews (1994), to avoid the duplication or issue of conflicting prescriptions. There is probably less risk of this under current legislation than there may be in future,

assuming that prescribing authority is extended and the NPF expanded.

CONCLUSION

The future for nurse prescribing seems very bright. District nurses would admit that it has had more impact on their practice and subsequently more positive outcomes for their clients than those of nurse prescribing colleagues, namely health visitors and practice nurses. This has as much to do with the clinical orientation of their work as the content of the NPF. However, evaluation of the impact of nurse prescribing remains limited. Research into issues such as educational needs and decision making would provide useful data to inform future developments. There are still many unanswered questions. Continuing professional development and updating are vital to the development of the role. Nurse prescribers should be constantly reviewing and updating their prescribing skills and knowledge within a framework of clinical governance.

There is every likelihood that Crown (DoH 1999) proposals will be enacted and the role and remit of the nurse prescriber will extend further. The result would be some nurses having dependent prescribing status, others independent status and some a combination of the two depending on their area of clinical practice. This suggests that a more elaborate mechanism for recording, monitoring and regulation by the professional body for nursing will be necessary in order to ensure safe and effective practice. Continuing professional development will become even more important and there may be moves for a more structured process requiring specific learning outcomes to be demonstrated. There are also incentives for the development of collaborative approaches which enable dependent, independent and nonprescribing nurses to work together to meet the needs of their clients.

As the implementation of nurse prescribing nears completion and all new district nurses and health visitors will be qualified to prescribe, a more critical approach to practice needs to be adopted. Prescribing will no longer be perceived as a new skill or novelty with which a chosen few are getting to grips but an established part of the professional role of all district nurses. Under scrutiny, they have demonstrated their competence to prescribe but the level of scrutiny will justifiably now shift to issues of quality and expansion. This is where nurse prescribing really starts.

REFERENCES

Andrews S 1994 Nurse prescribing. In: Hunt G, Wainwright P (eds) The expanding role of the nurse. The scope of professional practice. Blackwell, London

Barrows H S, Feltovich P J 1987 The clinical reasoning process. Medical Education 21: 86–91

Bell M 1994 Nurses' knowledge of the healing process in venous leg ulceration. Journal of Wound Care 3(3): 145–150

Benner P 1982 From novice to expert. American Journal of Nursing 82(1): 402–407

Bevan J 1979 Doctors on the move. Occasional Paper No. 7. Royal Society of General Practitioners, London

Bradley C P, Taylor R J, Blenkinsopp A 1997 Developing prescribing in primary care. British Medical Journal 314: 744–747

Bryans A, McIntosh J 1996 Decision making in community nursing: an analysis of the stages in decision making as they relate to community nursing assessment practice. Journal of Advanced Nursing 24: 24–30

Butterworth T 1990 Patient's needs or professionalism? Nursing Standard 4(21): 36–37

Carlisle D 1989 Prescribing change. Community Outlook 85: 45

Carpenito L 1991 In: Carroll-Johnson R M (ed) Classification of nursing diagnosis. Proceedings of the 9th conference. J B Lippincott, Philadelphia:

Casey N 1996 The issue of nurses prescribing under protocols. Nursing Standard 11(9): 1

Clegg A 1995 Stretching the limits. Health Visitor 68(10): 39–40.

Cowley S, Bergen A, Young K, Kavanagh A 1994 The changing nature of needs assessment in primary health care. Paper presented at the 4th International Primary Health Care Conference, Kensington Town Hall, London, June

Craig E J 1996 A review of prescriptive authority for nurse practitioners. Journal of Perinatal and Neonatal Nursing 10(1): 29–35

David A, Brown E 1995 How Swedish nurses are tackling prescribing. Nursing Times 91(50): 23–24

Department of Health 1989a Report of the Advisory Group on Nurse Prescribing (Crown Report). DoH, London

Department of Health 1989b General practice in the National Health Service: the 1990 contract. DoH, London

Department of Health 1990 The NHS and Community Care Act. DoH, London

Department of Health 1991 Nurse prescribing final report: a cost benefit study. (Touche Ross Report). DoH, London

Department of Health 1992 The extended role of the nurse/scope of professional practice. DoH, London

Department of Health 1992a Medicinal Products Prescription by Nurses Act. DoH, London

Department of Health 1993 New world, new opportunities. DoH, London

Department of Health 1996 Primary care: delivering the future. DoH, London

Department of Health 1997 The new NHS: modern, dependable. DoH, London

Department of Health 1998a Review of prescribing supply and administration of medicines: a report on the supply and administration of medicines under group protocols. DoH, London

Department of Health 1998b Review of Prescribing Supply and Administration of Medicines. A report on the supply and administration of medicine, under group protocols. HSC 1998/OSI DoH, London

Department of Health 1999 Review of prescribing supply and administration of medicines. DoH, London

Department of Health and Social Security 1986 Neighbourhood nursing: a focus for care (Cumberlege Report). HMSO, London

Dimond B 1995 The legal aspects of nurse prescribing. Primary Health Care (special supplement) 5(1): 2–12

Downie R S, Tannahill C, Tannahill A 1996 Health promotion: models and values. Oxford University Press, Oxford

Elliot Pennels C J 1997 Nursing and the law. Nurse prescribing. Professional Nurse 13(2): 114–115

Gilhespy N 1993 Practice nurses. British Journal of General Practice May: 219

Gilmore M, Bruce N, Hunt M 1974 The work of the nursing team in general practice. Council for the Education and Training of Health Visitors, London

Gledhill E 1994 Implications of nurse prescribing. British Journal of Nursing 3(9): 439–440

Gooch S 1999 Nurse prescribing and the Crown review. Professional Nurse 14(10): 678–680

Gunn D 1997 What's in the way of nurse prescribing? Kai Tiaki: New Zealand Nursing 3(4): 12

Hancock C 1996 Nurse prescribing's time has come. Nursing Standard 11(8): 20

Harbison J 1991 Clinical decision making in nursing. Journal of Advanced Nursing 16: 404–407

Hardwick S 1998 Clarification of nursing diagnosis from a British perspective. Assignment-Ongoing Work of Health Care Students 4(2): 3–9

Harris J 1998 Nurse prescribing in primary care: examining the views of Scotland's nurse prescribers on its introduction and impact. Unpublished Msc thesis, University of Aberdeen

Harrison A 1993 Job prescription. Nursing Times 89(24): 50–51

Heath I 1994 Skill mix in primary health care. British Medical Journal 308: 993–994

HMSO 1968 The Medicines Act, HMSO, London

Jenks J M 1993 The pattern of personal knowing in nurse clinical decision making. Journal of Nurse Education 32(9): 399–405

Jones M, Gough P 1997 Nurse prescribing – why has it taken so long? Nursing Standard 11(20): 39–42

Koh S 1993 Dressing practices. Nursing Times 89(42): 82–86

Leifer D 1997 Get a move on. Nursing Standard 11(48): 14

Luker K A, Ferguson B, Austin L et al 1997 Evaluation of nurse prescribing: final report. University of Liverpool/University of York

McCartney W, Tyrer S, Brazier M, Prayle D 1999 Nurse prescribing: radicalism or tokenism? Journal of Advanced Nursing 29(2): 348–354

Mackay L 1989 Nursing a problem. Open University Press, Milton Keynes

Mackenzie A, Ross F 1997 Shifting the balance: nursing in primary care. British Journal of Community Health Nursing 2(3): 139–142

Mahoney D 1994 The appropriateness of geriatric prescribing decisions made by nurse practitioners and physicians. Image: The Journal of Nursing Scholarship 26(1): 41

Mayes M 1996 A study of prescribing patterns in the community. Nursing Standard 10(28): 34–38

Meyer B M 1994 Prescribing authority for non physicians. American Journal of Hospital Pharmacy 51: 308–311

Moffatt C, Dorman M 1996 Changing clinical practice. Journal of Community Nursing 10(3): 20–26

Moreton J 1992 Nurse prescribing: how and when? Health Visitor 65(3): 90

Oughtibridge D 1998 Under the thumb. Nursing Management 4(8): 22–24

Øvretveit J 1990 Making the team work. Professional Nurse 5(6): 284–288

Peate I 1996 How nurses make decisions regarding patient medication. British Journal of Nursing 5(7): 433–437

Pickersgill F, Clarke S 1990 A prescription for nursing. Nursing Standard 4(4): 410–11

Poulton B, West M A 1993 Effective multidisciplinary teamwork in primary health care. Journal of Advanced Nursing 18: 918–925

Radwin L E 1995 Knowing the patient: a process model for individualised interventions. Nursing Research 44(6): 364–370

Richardson R, Maynard A 1995 Fewer doctors, more nurses: a review of the knowledge base of doctor–nurse substitution. Discussion paper 135. Centre for Health Economics, University of York

Robinson G 1990 The future for practice nurses. British Journal of General Practice 40: 132–133

Robinson G, Beaton S, White P 1993 Attitudes towards practice nurses – survey of a sample of general practitioners in England and Wales. British Journal of General Practice 43: 25–28

Roe B H, Griffiths J M, Kenrick M, Cullum N A, Hutton J L 1994 Nursing treatment of patients with chronic leg ulcers in the community. Journal of Clinical Nursing 3(3): 159–168

Royal College of Nursing 1980 Nurse prescribers of contraceptives for the well woman. RCN, London

Scottish Office 1997 Designed to care. Renewing the National Health Service in Scotland. Scottish Office, Edinburgh

Shepherd E 1998 I prescribe, therefore I am. Nursing Times 94(14): 34–35

Shepherd E, Rafferty A M, James V 1996 Prescribing the boundaries of nursing practice: professional regulation and nurse prescribing. Nursing Times Research 1(6): 465–478

Skidmore D 1999 Do not go gentle … In: Humphries J L, Green J (eds) Nurse prescribing. Macmillan, London

Smith S 1990 Take with caution. Nursing Times 86(24): 26–31

Spurgeon D 1995 Expanded role planned for Ontario's nurses. British Medical Journal 310: 80

Strauss A 1985 The social organisation of medical work. University of Chicago Press, Chicago

Tattam A 1992 Time-consuming procedures may negate prescribing gains. Nursing Times 88(46): 7

Tones K, Tilford S 1994 Health education – effectiveness, efficiency and equity. Chapman and Hall, London

United Kingdom Central Council for Nursing, Midwifery and Health Visiting 1992a The scope of professional practice. UKCC, London

United Kingdom Central Council for Nursing, Midwifery and Health Visiting 1992b The code of professional conduct for nurses, midwives and health visitors. UKCC, London

United Kingdom Central Council for Nursing, Midwifery and Health Visiting 1994 The future of professional practice: the Council's standards for education and practice following registration. UKCC, London

Vaughan B 1997 Future developments in nursing practice. Nursing Standard 12(2): 68–70

Voss J F, Post T A 1988 On the solving of ill structured problems. In: Chi M T H, Glaser R, Farr M J (eds) The nature of expertise. Lawrence Erlbaum, New Jersey

Wade B 1993 The job satisfaction of health visitors, district nurses and practice nurses working in areas served by four Trusts: Year 1. Journal of Advanced Nursing 18: 992–1004

Watson S 1994 An exploratory study into a methodology for the examination of decision making by nurses in the clinical area. Journal of Advanced Nursing 20: 351–360

Wedgwood A 1995 The case for prescribing the pill. Nursing Times 91(50): 25–27

While A, Rees K 1993 The knowledge base of health visitors and district nurses regarding the proposed formulary for nurse prescribing. Journal of Advanced Nursing 18(10): 1573–1577

Williams A 1998 Multidisciplinarity and the idea of profession. Assignment-Ongoing Work of Health Care Students 4(2): 1–2

Wooley N 1990 Nursing diagnosis: exploring the factors that may influence the reasoning process. Journal of Advanced Nursing 15: 110–117

FURTHER READING

Humphries JC, Green J (eds) 1999 Nurse Prescribing. Macmillan, London

Courtney M, Butler M 1999 Nurse Prescribing Principles and Practice Greenwich Medical Media, London

9

Educational issues

Sue Hickie

Key points

- Changes in nurse education and regulation
- Specialist and higher level practice
- Lifelong learning
- The learning environment and practice education

INTRODUCTION

It is now recognised that learning must continue throughout the working life of each individual in order to meet the challenges of advances in technology and changes in society. The fields of both education and health care have seen immense change in the latter part of the 20th century and community nurses have a professional obligation to both keep abreast of developments and contribute to the educational growth of new nursing practitioners. This chapter will discuss current issues in nurse education and continuing professional development and the implications for district nurses.

DEVELOPMENTS IN NURSE EDUCATION

Nurse education has undergone dramatic changes in the last decade. These changes can be linked to the respective policies of different governments and demographic changes and also correspond to developments in higher education and health-care provision.

During the 1980s, nurse education was completely reviewed and the UKCC set new

---

Box 9.1   The UKCC Professional Register

Part 1:   First-level nurses – general
Part 2:   Second-level nurses – general (England and Wales)
Part 3:   First-level nurses – mental illness
Part 4:   Second-level nurses – mental illness (England and Wales)
Part 5:   First-level nurses – mental handicap
Part 6:   Second-level nurses – mental handicap (England and Wales)
Part 7:   Second-level nurses (Scotland and Northern Ireland)
Part 8:   Nurses trained in the nursing of sick children
Part 9:   Nurses trained in the nursing of persons suffering from fever
Part 10: Midwives
Part 11: Health visitors
Part 12: Nurses – adult
Part 13: Nurses – mental health nursing
Part 14: Nurses – learning disability nursing
Part 15: Nurses – children's nursing

---

standards (UKCC 1986) for nursing education programmes which led to initial registration on the professional register. This new programme, often referred to as Project 2000 (P2000), consisted of a common foundation programme lasting 18 months and then a choice of four branch programmes each leading to a recording on a different part of the register (Box 9.1).

The academic level of this programme is Diploma in Higher Education although, of course, many centres offer the programme with additional academic content which results in the award of a degree as well as the professional qualification. There is ongoing dialogue about the advantages or otherwise of all first-level nursing education programmes being offered at degree level. The decision is in many ways a political one because of the resource implications, but the UKCC Commission for Nursing and Midwifery Education report *Fitness for practice* (UKCC 1999a) proposes that there should be an increase in nurses being prepared at degree level.

Major innovations in the diploma programmes include the change in status of the student nurse from being part of the clinical workforce to a student receiving a non-means tested bursary and being supernumerary to normal staffing

requirements. Another radical change is the initial emphasis on health and health promotion within the curriculum and also the assumption that newly qualified practitioners will be competent to practise in both community and acute settings. The standards for this first-level qualification also meet the requirements of European Directive (77/453/EEC) Training Programme for Nurses Responsible for General Care and therefore cannot be changed without general agreement between member countries.

There has been debate in the profession and in the general press about the merits of the diploma programme, which commenced in the late 1980s in England and Wales and 1992 in Scotland. Some initial responses from existing practitioners and nurse managers identified a lack of clinical skills and confidence in the newly qualified staff nurses. Formal evaluation of the implementation and outcomes of P2000 is ongoing. Elkan & Robinson (1995) provide a comprehensive overview of many of the initial evaluations. Studies commissioned by the English National Board (ENB) by White et al (1993, 1994) and the National Board for Nursing, Midwifery and Health Visiting for Scotland (NBS) by May et al (1997) all describe similar findings. Some of the above researchers identify a different type of nurse at the end of the programme, a knowledgeable staff nurse with the ability to solve problems and see the big picture in health care but needing structured support during the first months to consolidate case management and practical skills. Nearly all the researchers describe some issues in the varying quality of the clinical learning experiences of students and these will be discussed in more detail in a later section of this chapter.

As a result of these various evaluations of P2000 education programmes, the recruitment difficulties in certain areas of nursing provision and the increasing tendency for the roles of different health-care professionals to blur, in 1998 the UKCC agreed to the establishment of a Commission for Education. The Commission, chaired by Sir Leonard Peach, was charged with 'proposing a way forward for pre-registration education that enabled fitness for practice based on health care need'. The methodology used by the Commission was wide ranging and included a large-scale attitudinal survey of 84 000 final-year nurses and midwives, written evidence from 450 organisations and an extensive literature search. The findings were also informed by a specially commissioned report, *Health care futures 2010* (Warner et al 1998), which looks at the generic issues of present and future health care and describes possible scenarios for nursing and midwifery in 2010.

The final recommendations, based on a number of key issues that were quite consistently reported by all sources, were divided into three sections. The first deals with ways in which flexibility can be increased in programmes of nurse education. Proposals include more flexible means of entry into nursing programmes and modes of delivery which will ensure fairness and accessibility for a wider range of individuals and are in keeping with general trends in adult education for wider entry gates, clearer frameworks of qualifications and lifelong learning patterns.

The second section deals with issues around achieving fitness for practice. These recommendations discuss how core and specialist competencies can be clearly identified, taught and assessed in nursing and midwifery programmes and how 'the sequencing and balance between university and practice-based study should be planned to promote an integration of knowledge, skills and attitudes' (UKCC 1999a). The report recommends that each student develop a portfolio of practice experience which should be extended to demonstrate fitness for practice and provide evidence of rational decision making and clinical judgement. The use of portfolios as a means of demonstrating competence is now widespread in many areas of education and training and provides a very useful introduction to notions of reflection on practice and methods of learning in which the student takes an active role in defining learning needs and assessing outcomes. This style of learning is an important foundation for continual review of professional practice and identifying future personal development needs.

The second section also addresses reported difficulties in accommodating the increasing numbers of students in clinical areas by proposing that students experience the full 24 hour per day and 7 day per week nature of health care instead of the present arrangement, which often results in large numbers of students being present in clinical areas for restricted periods of time and competing for learning experiences. More importantly, it may also mean that patients and/or clients have more choices with regard to involvement in teaching and learning opportunities for student nurses and that qualified staff have less juggling to perform in terms of allocating attention and time to the differing responsibilities of patient care and support of students.

Another theme of this section is the transition from student status to that of qualified practitioner in nursing or midwifery. To aid this transition and to give students an opportunity to gradually take more responsibilities in terms of care management and consolidating practical skills, it is recommended that all students have a period of supervised practice of at least 3 months' duration at the end of their education programme, which should be managed by specifically prepared nurses and midwives. It is also recommended that all newly qualified nurses and midwives should receive a properly structured period of induction and preceptorship when they begin their employment. This initial support of newly qualified nurses is essential to prevent loss to the profession of many who leave because of the difficulties and stresses of those transition months.

The third section of the recommendations relates to the important subject of partnership working which can enhance educational experiences and learning opportunities. This includes partnerships between educational providers and the service providers to provide high-quality learning environments and ensure consistency between theoretical input and clinical experiences. It also includes recommendations on interprofessional teaching and learning, collaboration between the NHS and the private sector to improve workforce planning for nursing and also joint working between social work and health service agencies in each of the four UK countries to ensure that the preparation of health-care assistants and social care assistants is based on common standards (see Box 9.2 for more details of *Working in partnership* recommendations).

Many of the recommendations of the Commission for Education are already in place to lesser or greater degrees in the different parts of the UK and some reflect current educational practice of post-registration programmes of nurse education such as the community nursing qualifications. Several recommendations propose further exploration and research in order to find an appropriate way forward and all nurses and midwives should contribute as much as possible to the debates on the future of our profession which is very much on the current political agenda as we enter the new millennium.

First-level qualifications are the gateway into professional nursing practice and the foundation

---

Box 9.2 *Fitness for practice:* recommendations 23–33 (UKCC 1999a)

23 Service providers and HEIs should continue to develop effective, genuine partnerships to support:
- their respective commitments to students
- curriculum development, implementation and evaluation
- joint awareness and development of service and education issues
- delivery of learning in practice
- defining responsibilities for underpinning learning in practice
- monitoring the quality of practice placements.

24 An accountable individual should be appointed by purchasers of education to liaise with the service providers and HEIs to support:
- the provision of sufficient suitable practical placements
- staff and students during placements
- the development of standards and specified outcomes for placements
- the delivery and effective monitoring of the contract to ensure that the contractual requirements are met.

25 Recognising that no one individual can provide the full range of expertise required by students, service providers and HEIs should work together to develop diverse teams of practice and academic staff who will offer students expertise in practice, management, assessment and mentoring and research.

26 Service providers and HEIs should provide dedicated time in education for practice staff and dedicated time in practice for lecturers to ensure that practice staff are competent and confident in teaching and mentoring roles and lecturers are confident and competent in the practice environment.

27 The good practice of formalised arrangements for access to practice for lecturers and to education for practice staff should be adopted by service providers and HEIs.

28 Service providers and HEIs should formalise the preparation, support and feedback to mentors of pre-registration students. This should be continued by service providers, in line with best practice, for preceptors of newly qualified nurses and midwives.

29 Funding to support learning in practice should be reviewed to take account of the cost of mentoring and assessment by practice staff and the cost of lecturers having regular contact with practice.

30 To improve workforce planning for nursing, NHS requirements should increasingly be informed by comprehensive information from the private and independent sector.

31 Taking into account changes in health and social care delivery, education and government departments of health, social care and social services, education and employment, in each of the four countries, should work together to ensure that the preparation of health-care assistants and social care assistants is based on common standards.

32 The health-care professions should be actively encouraged to learn with and from each other by:
- purchasers of education including interprofessional teaching and learning – as appropriate – as a criterion for evaluating the quality of education
- explicit encouragement for interprofessional learning in the planning of all pre-registration curricula
- the development of the shared use of learning resources and technology in practice placements
- the UKCC leading joint initiatives with relevant professional bodies.

33 We recommend that consideration should be given to the most appropriate method of funding students of nursing and midwifery in the future. The forthcoming government review of nursing, midwifery and professions allied to medicine (PAMs) student funding in England should consider the professed willingness of the private and independent sector to participate in funding students.

for ongoing professional development. District nursing or community nursing in the home, as it is now officially termed, is a post-registration qualification and the next section will examine the ongoing developments in specialist and higher level practice.

SPECIALIST AND HIGHER LEVEL PRACTICE

Post-registration education and practice

Building on the revised pre-registration programmes introduced in the late 1980s and early 1990s, the UKCC designed a framework which aimed to meet changing health care needs and protect the public by regulating post-regulation practice. PREP, the post-registration and education framework, was introduced in 1994. The framework included descriptors of specialist practice, set standards which all registered nurses must meet in order to renew their registration and made return to practice programmes compulsory (from April 2000) for nurses who had not worked in some capacity, by virtue of a nursing, midwifery or health visiting qualification, for at least 750 hours in the previous 5 years.

PREP (CPD) standard

In order to maintain and develop professional knowledge and competence, all nurses, midwives and health visitors are required to undertake continuing professional development, referred to as PREP (CPD). The standard for PREP (CPD) is that each practitioner must 'undertake at least five days (35 hrs) of learning activity relevant to present practice during the three years prior to renewal of registration' (UKCC 1999b). Each practitioner is required to maintain a personal professional profile (PPP) recording all learning activity and comply with any request from the UKCC to audit compliance with these requirements. These requirements have existed since 1995 and since 1998 all registrants have had to declare on their notification to practice form that they have met

the requirements. Piloting of the audit of this standard is taking place at present.

Nursing has been at the forefront of developments in CPD activity and many other health-care professionals, including medicine, pharmacy and the professions allied to medicine, are now developing models similar to the PREP framework. This requirement for professionals to demonstrate continuing fitness for practice is very much in response to increased scrutiny of professional practice by government and users of services and is an integral part of the clinical governance agenda. Recent high-profile litigation cases support the demand for evidence of continuing competence to practise. The introduction of portfolio compilation in pre-registration nurse education sets the foundation for the lifelong professional activity of reflection on practice and planned continuing development which is now a fundamental element of nursing practice.

The learning activities undertaken as part of the PREP (CPD) requirements have to be relevant to each practitioner's working commitments (or non-working commitments if not working). However, the definition of learning activity is flexible, something which some practitioners and employers have found difficult to understand at first, tending to focus on formal, academic programmes. The learning undertaken may be in the form of formal education programmes or may equally well consist of activities such as time spent in the library or on a computer database researching an area of interest. Shadowing a colleague or observing practice in another area is an excellent way to stimulate changes in practice, especially when followed up with some analysis and reflection on the activity with a mentor or clinical supervisor. There is no such thing as approved PREP (CPD) learning activity. The essential aspect of any PREP activity is that the practitioner can demonstrate in what way the learning was related to her work and influenced and informed that work.

Responsibility for CPD activity does not lie solely with the individual. Employers have a part to play also. In *Making a difference* (DoH 1999a), it is stated that when planning or providing CPD, organisations should ensure that it is:

- purposeful and patient centred
- targeted at identified educational need
- educationally effective
- part of a wider organisational development plan in support of local and national service objectives
- focused on the development needs of clinical teams, across traditional and professional and service boundaries
- designed to build on previous knowledge, skills and experience
- designed to enhance the skills of interpreting and applying knowledge based on research and development.

District nurses have a wide range of responsibilities and will therefore have to consider carefully what priorities they have in terms of learning needs. It could be updating on aspects of clinical care or it could relate to management or committee skills which would enhance team leading or participation on boards or committees such as the primary care group or local health-care cooperative board. Resources for education activities are scarce and increasingly managers are expecting that all supported learning activities will be able to demonstrate outcomes in terms of enhanced performance and patient care. The recent human resources policy documents *The new NHS – working together* (DoH 1998) and *Learning together* (SEHD 1999) both describe the NHS workforce as a valuable resource and discuss ways in which individuals can participate in lifelong learning and professional development. The rights and responsibilities of both individual practitioners and employers are explored in relation to this theme.

Also within the HR policy documents are details of local learning plans, which each NHS trust will have to formulate annually. These learning plans will articulate the learning needs of all members of the organisation in relation to ongoing and new developments in health care and will form the basis of discussion and negotiation with universities, colleges of further education and other education providers. The learning plans may also include a strategy for in-house education programmes aimed at developing expertise in very specific areas of practice. Since 1997, the National Board for Scotland has been working in partnerships with NHS trusts to develop a quality assurance framework for such in-house training initiatives which established agreed standards and increases transferability (NBS 1998).

Specialist practice

Together with the standards for re-registration and return to practice, the PREP framework contained standards for specialist practice. The rationale for setting these standards was again protection of the public. The UKCC argued that specialist health care and specialist patient requirements call for additional education to ensure safe and effective practice. It was proposed that:

Specialist practitioners should be able to demonstrate higher levels of clinical decision making and be able to monitor and improve standards of care through the supervision of practice; clinical audit; the provision of skilled professional leadership and the development of practice through research, teaching and the support of professional colleagues. (UKCC 1994)

To qualify as a specialist practitioner, a first-level nurse has to successfully complete a National Board approved programme at degree level and record that qualification on the UKCC professional register. Council decided not to describe specific areas of specialist practice except within the community. The rationale for this decision is not explained within the Registrar's letter of 1994 which gave the initial information about standards for specialist practice but is possibly due to some lobbying of the UKCC by established nursing disciplines. Within community nursing practice, eight areas of practice were described: general practice nursing, community learning disability nursing, community mental health nursing, community children's nursing, occupational health nursing, school nursing, community nursing in the home – district nursing and public health nursing – health visiting. Health care in primary care and community settings is continuing to evolve within the revised organisational structures and policy changes initiated by the new Labour government and this calls into question the wisdom of setting specific areas of nursing practice. New models of practice are developing which call for transferable skills and integrated teamwork and these will invariably impact on education programmes.

Between 1995 and 1998, specialist practitioner programmes were developed and replaced the previous education programmes for community nursing. Initial concern was expressed by existing practitioners as to the worth of their qualification within this new framework. However, the UKCC made it clear that existing practitioners would not be disadvantaged by the changes and would be able to use the title 'special practitioner' as long as they could demonstrate ongoing professional development and were supported by their employer. During this transition period there was also opportunity for nurses who had not previously been able to record a qualification on the register to do so if they could meet specific criteria. This included completion of a post-registration educational programme of at least 4 months or, in some cases, a portfolio of evidence. Practice nurses and school nurses were the community nursing groups which used this option the most.

The new specialist practitioner qualification (SPQ) programmes consisted of a common core of preparation and then specific specialised modules for each discipline of nursing. The standards described by the UKCC for these programmes were broad statements of principle and there was freedom for individual educational institutions to develop programmes in different ways to meet the needs of local health-care providers and students, many of whom undertake these programmes on a self-funding basis. The differences between levels of preparation for different community nursing practitioners disappeared and for the first time, general practice nursing and children's nursing in the community became recordable qualifications on the professional register. Students who complete the public health nursing (health visitor) pathway of a SPQ

programme continue to register on Part 11 of the professional register, whilst other community nurses who complete the SPQ programme record the qualification. It is possible this situation may change when the Nurses, Midwives and Health Visitors Act is revised and the professional register is rationalised (JM Consulting 1998).

Community nurse education programmes have been implemented in different ways around the UK. Some are offered at unclassified degree level and others at Honours degree level. Most offer part-time options as well as full-time programmes and some can be accessed by distance learning with the practice element usually negotiated locally. All consist of 50% practice and 50% theory. There has been little rigorous evaluation of these programmes to date to show if sharing common modules really does increase understanding of colleagues' roles, enhance teamworking and impact on practice. However, informal evaluation does appear to show advantages of this approach and programmes which involve shared learning with other disciplines are also being encouraged (DoH 1999a). Hugman (1995) takes these ideas further and explores the idea of generic community workers with a range of health and social care competencies and Bell et al (1997) provide a useful overview of interprofessional education in health and social care in the community.

Higher level practice

Following on from the PREP framework and the setting of standards for specialist practice, there has been a lot of debate in nursing as to the need for and the nature of advanced or higher level practice. Some argue that higher level practice should be linked directly to higher level academic awards but the UKCC is not prescriptive about this. In many ways, this debate has been reactive rather than proactive, in an effort to rationalise and clarify the many new nursing role developments which have already taken place in practice settings and also, importantly, to ensure protection of the public. Despite the lengthy debates, there remains a lack of clarity for many nurses and employers of the differences between specialist and higher level practice and how these levels should be articulated in terms of job descriptions and career pathways.

Changes in health-care practice, such as the reduction of junior doctors' hours, the search for cost efficiencies and an increase in crossboundary working, have resulted in a proliferation of new nursing roles across all health-care sectors. Many of these roles exist in community and primary care settings and have evolved within the new structures and developing public health agenda. For example, there are district nurses who offer expert services and advice to colleagues on palliative care, wound care or coronary rehabilitation. Some nurses are employed by social work departments and offer specialist services to the elderly or those with learning disabilities. Others offer nurse-led services to vulnerable groups who often have difficulties accessing traditional health-care services. The nurses who have developed these new services have a range of educational and professional qualifications and also an array of job titles such as nurse consultant, nurse practitioner, nurse specialist or advanced practitioner. Some of the new roles cross professional and organisational boundaries. There is confusion within the profession about this varied nomenclature and even more confusion outwith the profession amongst colleagues in medicine and social work and the general public.

Both the government and the UKCC have responded to this confusion. A working group coordinated by the UKCC has set standards and descriptors for a higher level of practice and also suggested assessment processes by which higher level practice can be identified. Following consultation with the profession and health service organisations, in the year 2000 there will be a pilot study of the standard and the assessment process to test the standard's robustness and applicability across all health-care settings in the UK. Council has also agreed a set of core principles for the assessment process. This will focus on what individuals are able to achieve in practice and the responsibility for collecting evidence will rest primarily with the practitioner seeking recognition. An individual assessment of the evidence presented will be undertaken by the UKCC or others acting on its behalf. The work is ongoing on systems of support for those seeking recognition of higher level practice and also the necessary quality assurance and appeals systems for the process. It is not anticipated that great numbers of nurses will reach this level of practice. Most nurses will choose to contribute to health care working at first or specialist levels of practice and maintaining and developing competencies as required reflecting changes in health-care delivery.

In July 1999, the Department of Health in England published a strategy for nursing, midwifery and health visiting (DoH 1999a). This document, *Making a difference*, explains the government's strategic intentions for nursing, midwifery and health visiting and its commitment to strengthen and maximise the nursing, midwifery and health visiting contribution to health care. To date, no similar strategy has been produced by the Health Department of the Scottish Executive, (although there are plans for the publication of a Scottish strategy late in 2000) but it is reasonable to expect similar policies in principle. The agenda for action set out within the document is important reading for all nurses and includes sections on:

- recruiting more nurses
- strengthening education and training
- developing a more flexible career structure
- improving working lives
- enhancing the quality of care
- strengthening leadership
- modernising professional regulation
- supporting new roles and new ways of working.

In the discussion on how nurses are working in new ways, the government clearly states a wish to extend the remit of the nursing profession to make better use of nursing skills, including making it easier for nurses to prescribe. It also wishes to see more nurse-led primary care services to improve accessibility and responsiveness. The onus is put onto NHS organisations to support role development for nurses, midwives and health visitors and to identify opportunities for nurse consultant posts. The term 'nurse consultant' is defined in

Box 9.3   New roles, new ways of working from *Making a difference* (DoH 1999a)

The development of new and expanded nursing, midwifery and health visiting roles needs to be a managed process. NHS organisations should ensure where they occur:
- the development is based on a thorough needs assessment and is consistent with government policy and is designed to benefit patients and clients
- the purposes and responsibilities can be clearly specified and the role invested with professional and organisational autonomy and authority which matches the purpose and expectations
- the professional competencies and additional knowledge and skills can be identified and appropriate education, training, competence assessment, continuing support and supervision put in place
- an assessment of risks and professional and legal liabilities is made and appropriate indemnification arranged

- new or additional job titles properly reflect the role, experience, qualifications and professional status of the post holder so that patients and colleagues can be in no doubt that the individual is a registered nurse, midwife or health visitor
- the role can be clearly located in the wider health-care team, complementing and working collaboratively with others
- any substitution for medical, technical or other roles does not obscure professional accountability for the fundamental nursing, midwifery or health-visiting function
- there are arrangements to monitor the contribution made and to make adjustments to minimise risks and maximise benefits
- the post holder can be properly supported through clinical supervision, leadership development and continuing professional development.

Department of Health guidance to trusts and specifies a strong element of clinical practice within the remit. It is strongly emphasised that the NHS organisations have a responsibility to ensure that the introduction of all new roles is carefully managed and properly supported. Box 9.3 gives more details of how this should occur.

The opportunities for new roles defined in *Making a difference*, such as the nurse consultant role, have in general been well received by professional nursing organisations as creating a career pathway for nurses who wish to demonstrate higher levels of expertise whilst remaining active in clinical practice. Time will tell if this strategy succeeds in recruiting and retaining nurses. It must be acknowledged that whilst these strategies present some opportunities for the nursing profession, they have also come about because of political expediency and the need to provide health care for an ageing population with finite financial resources.

THE DISTRICT NURSE AS SUPPORTER AND ASSESSOR OF STUDENTS

District nurses play an important part in the support of both pre-and post-registration students and most of them enjoy this demanding but often satisfying aspect of their role. However, changes in pre-registration education have resulted in students spending greater periods of time with nurses in community settings and this puts great pressure on the qualified nurses there who struggle with the competing demands of teaching and assessing students and offering high-quality care to their patients.

This section will explore this aspect of district nursing practice and the framework in which it occurs. It will begin with the role of the statutory bodies in nurse education and then explore some of the factors necessary for the provision of good-quality learning environments in clinical placements.

Role of the UKCC and the national boards

The UKCC and the four National Boards for Nursing, Midwifery and Health Visiting have been in place since 1982. They were set up following the revision of the Nurses, Midwives and Health Visitors Act in 1979 and replaced a number of professional statutory bodies which regulated nursing, midwifery and health visiting. At the time, the UKCC was charged with maintaining the professional register, matters of professional conduct and setting standards for nurse education. The National Boards have responsibility for implementing the education standards in each of the four countries by approving courses and monitoring the provision of those courses in both academic and clinical settings.

Over time, as nurse education has transferred into higher education institutions and existed within higher education frameworks of quality assurance, the National Boards have evolved new ways of working. This includes delegating some aspects of quality assurance to the universities. For example, audit and approval of clinical areas for the placement of student nurses used to be conducted by National Board Officers. It is now a responsibility of each nursing department who must, however, demonstrate at the time of course approval that they have appropriate systems in place to carry out this activity. The Boards are now also beginning to work in partnership with organisations like the Quality Assurance Agency (QAA) which monitors quality assurance in higher education, to coordinate and synchronise quality assurance activity for vocational programmes and prevent duplication which is wasteful of time and resources for all concerned.

The National Boards also provide careers information for both prospective and existing nurses and, especially in England and Scotland, commission and manage research and development projects which evaluate educational provision and provide an evidence base for professional education and regulation. The research and development programmes undertaken by the Boards include aspects of competence to practise and curriculum development support. Another part of this research activity aims to enhance the research capacity of nurses by providing small research grants for novice researchers and widely disseminating research reports. Information on all these activities is widely available as publications from the Board offices in each country and/or on their websites.

In 1997, the Nurses, Midwives and Health Visitors Act was again reviewed and a report was prepared and presented to government ministers by JM Consulting Ltd in 1998. There was a

---

Box 9.4 A new regulatory framework for nursing, midwifery and health visiting: government plans in *Making a difference*, (DoH 1999a)

Subject to consultation and legislation, we will:
- establish a new, smaller, UK-wide council to replace the UKCC and the four National Boards to sharpen accountability and streamline regulation
- lay a duty on the new council to treat the interests of patients and clients as paramount in carrying out its functions
- ensure the new council collaborates with other stakeholders and consults appropriate interests
- ensure there is a simplified register to make it easier for the public and employers to establish the status of registrants
- require the new council to set standards for education leading to registration in terms of outcomes, to accredit institutions and quality assure courses either directly or indirectly
- give the new council additional powers so that it can deal more effectively with misconduct, poor performance and health issues.

---

government response to this (DoH 1999b) and the main points of the response were reported in *Making a difference* (DoH 1999a) and are shown in Box 9.4. The main change is that a new regulatory framework is to be set up with a smaller, UK-wide body to replace the present Council and the four National Boards. As health is a devolved responsibility, the new arrangements for replacing the Boards will be decided by the health departments in each country. There are already change management groups in place to decide on the shape and remit of the new structures and some changes can be expected by the year 2001.

THE CLINICAL LEARNING ENVIRONMENT IN PRIMARY CARE

Nursing is a practice-based profession and all preparation for practice therefore involves learning in practice. This is evidenced by the fact that 50% of all nurse education programmes leading to registration or a recording on the professional register is practice based. As discussed earlier in this chapter, this means that quality education of all types of nursing is therefore dependent on close partnership working between nurse educators and health-care service providers.

This partnership working must be evident at a strategic level as well as between individual lecturers and practice areas if there is to be elimination of the legendary theory–practice gap and quality assurance of educational experiences. In primary care settings, the situation is complicated by the fact that different professional groups have differing financial arrangements for the support of students in practice and this fact sometimes leads to lack of understanding of the teaching responsibility that is part of every nursing role. Strategic issues which require clarification at national or regional level include workforce planning, the setting up of joint clinical/academic career pathways and commitment to supporting clinical learning environments.

In the early 1990s there was a huge dip in the numbers of nurses who were recruited in the UK and this in part has resulted in the shortage of qualified nurses which has been causing problems over the last few years. Also, many nurses were leaving the profession for a variety of reasons, including low pay and difficult working conditions. These problems vary in different clinical and geographical areas, generally being greater in densely populated parts of England than in Scotland. Demographic profiles of the nursing workforce show that certain groups of nurses have increased numbers reaching retirement age over the next 10 years and that short ages can be expected unless action is taken. Community nurses, including district nursing and health visitors, form one of these groups. Sophisticated workforce planning is required to inform the process of establishing appropriate numbers of nurses entering education programmes to maintain a well-balanced workforce. It could be argued that this planning also needs to take place within a renewed framework for the financial support of nurse education if it is to be successful. Many district nursing teams now operate within a skill mix situation which can provide opportunities for succession planning and development of specialist skills to meet local health needs. It is possible that succession planning needs to be considered in more systematic ways if skill shortages are to be avoided in the future.

Workforce planning is required on a national scale to provide the big picture but more local negotiations between senior managers of NHS trusts and other providers and the educational institutions are required to meet local needs and establish the numbers of specific students that can be accommodated in well-supported practice placements. The UKCC report *Fitness for practice* (UKCC 1999a) fully supports the setting up of systems to facilitate such communications and suggests a senior role within trusts which would have a coordinating and liaison function. The partnership forum of the health-care providers and the university representatives should also be used for discussion of how clinical skills can best be taught to students and agreement of career pathways for nurses who wish to be involved in both education and clinical practice. This could include, for example, joint appointments of lecturer/practitioner posts, teaching fellow posts and honorary contracts for lecturing staff who wish to maintain clinical skills by part-time work in practice. There also need to be agreements at this level on how clinical staff can contribute to programme development and course management committees to ensure that curriculum developments reflect current practice. These professional activities can take busy practice staff away from direct patient care but, it can be strongly argued, in the long term will enhance patient care.

The development of clinical skills and confidence in practice is most likely to take place in clinical areas where there is a positive educational ethos characterised by professional leadership, motivated and enthusiastic practitioners and access to educational resources. Often these areas have staff who are participating in ongoing professional development and present positive role models for students. In primary care, clinical areas often offer placements to a range of students from the various health and social care professions. Many of these areas have established systems of clinical supervision. An NBS-commissioned research project (Watson 1999) reports from the perspectives of students, mentors and nurse lecturers on the support of students in a wide range of practice placements in Scotland. The study includes students from both pre-and post-registration programmes of nursing and midwifery, including those on community SPQ courses. The report identifies a number of issues which underpin good experiences for students and makes recommendations about standards for high-quality learning environments. Included in the issues identified are length of mentor preparation, quality of communications between university and practice staff, length of student placement and the nature of the support offered to students by mentors and university lecturers. Many of the findings and corresponding recommendations reflect those of the UKCC Commission report.

Nurses who support and assess students in practice are known by a variety of titles and this can confuse discussion of the subject. A common nomenclature may enhance understandings of differing roles. The UKCC suggests that those who teach, support and assess pre-registration students should be called mentors. Formal support of newly qualified staff nurses for the first few months following qualification should be conducted by specifically prepared preceptors and the support of nurses on specialist practitioners level programmes is usually undertaken by those who have undertaken more substantial preparation for the role and may be called practice educators.

The preparation for mentoring pre-registration students varies considerably (Watson 1999) from 2-day courses to degree-level modules within post-registration frameworks of education. The evidence appears to show that longer courses of preparation are more likely to prepare mentors who are confident in the role, have a fuller understanding of assessment of competence issues and support learning. Traditionally district nursing students were supported by practical work teachers (PWTs), later to be named community practice teachers (CPTs). Preparation for both these roles was substantial and consisted of both theoretical learning and initial supervision and reflection on the teaching and assessing role. Most community nurses would argue that this is a very satisfactory model of student support.

All specialist practice programmes now contain a module on the theories of teaching and learning, reflective practice and notions of ongoing professional development which is an excellent foundation for all teaching and support activities undertaken by experienced practitioners. In order to support students on different programmes, practitioners who have undertaken the basic preparation then need to participate in short update programmes offered by programme leaders which give information on curriculum developments and assessment procedures and allow the practice educators the opportunity to share experiences and give feedback to educational staff on their experiences. It has also been found beneficial for university departments to feed back in a systematic way to clinical areas the evaluations of students and the results of educational audits. When viewed positively, such information can form the framework for discussion for further quality initiatives and is a good example of productive partnership working.

Clinical supervision

Tony Butterworth, in the introduction to a text on clinical supervision (Butterworth & Faugier 1992), describes it as embracing 'a range of strategies in nursing which include preceptorship, mentorship, supervision of qualified practice, peer review and the maintenance of identified professional standards'. Pateman (1992) discussed how managers and practitioners were responding to recommendations about implementation of clinical supervision in district nursing practice.

It is not possible within this chapter to fully explore models of clinical supervision and the extent to which they are now utilised within district nursing. However, previous sections have discussed the support of students which includes elements of mentorship and preceptorship. In the section on PREP, the requirements for demonstrating continuing professional development and lifelong learning were explored. Other chapters within this book also discuss how professional practice is developed and enhanced by audit and other quality assurance activities. All nurses have a responsibility to undertake professional development as they proceed along the continuum between indexing as a student nurse and eventual retirement. Clinical supervision in all its many forms facilitates this process.

CONCLUSION

What does the future hold for nursing education and regulation as we move into the 21st century? Some aspects we can anticipate, others must be speculation.

First, the review of the Nurses, Midwives and Health Visitors Act will result in a new model of nurse regulation which will exist in a world of increased scrutiny of professional practice by both politicians and the public. Models of profession regulation may be developed across health and social care disciplines which share core values and principles.

Second, fundamental changes in first-level nurse education will have an increased emphasis on the achievement of core clinical competencies and will reflect the trend in many areas of professional education towards flexible competency-based education and training. There may be a move towards an all-graduate profession of nursing. The educational process will take place in a context of increasing partnership working between health-care providers from both the public and the independent sectors and the educational institutions. Education and health-care policy documents also indicate that both

education and professional practice will be expected to take place across professional and organisational boundaries.

Third, lifelong learning will become an established part of professional nursing practice and refinement of the notions of specialist and higher level practice will take place. The role of nurse consultant will be piloted and evaluated and possibly extended. New roles for nurses will emerge as the public health agenda of social inclusion and the addressing of health inequalities is addressed. Preparation for these new roles will have an impact on the education of community nurses.

Fourth, the provision of nurse education will evolve to reflect current educational practice including further development of problem-based learning methods and increasing use of technology. These changes will affect all levels of nurse education and will aim to provide flexible, accessible provision to meet customer needs. Resource centres and skills laboratories will increase and may be used to teach clinical skills to students and by experienced practitioners to maintain competence. Career pathways should be further explored and developed to enable experienced nursing practitioners to play a greater part in teaching and research activities.

To conclude, there are many changes in prospect within nurse education and regulation as it emerges into the new millennium. The future for nursing in general, and district nursing in particular, is exciting and challenging.

REFERENCES

Bell R, Johnson K, Scott H 1997 Interprofessional education and curriculum development: a model for the future. In: Hennessy D (ed) Community health care development. Macmillan, London

Butterworth T, Faugier J (eds) 1992 Clinical supervision and mentorship in nursing. Chapman and Hall, London

Department of Health 1998 The new NHS – working together: securing a quality workforce for the NHS. DoH, London

Department of Health 1999a Making a difference: strengthening the nursing, midwifery and health visiting contribution to health and health care. DoH, London

Department of Health 1999b Review of the Nurses, Midwives and Health Visitors Act: government response to the recommendations. Health Service Circular 1999/030. DoH, London

Elkan R, Robinson J 1995 Project 2000: a review of published research. Journal of Advanced Nursing 22: 386–392

Hugman R 1995 Contested territory and community services: interprofessional boundaries in health and social care. In: Soothill K et al (eds) Interprofessional relations in health care. Edward Arnold, London

J M Consulting 1998 The regulation of nurses, midwives and health visitors: report of the review of the Nurses, Midwives and Health Visitors Act 1997. J M Consulting, Bristol

May N, Veitch L, McIntosh J, Alexander M 1997 Preparation for practice: evaluation of nurse and midwifery education in Scotland: 1992 programmes. NBS, Edinburgh

National Board for Nursing, Midwifery and Health Visiting for Scotland 1998 The network project. NBS, Edinburgh

Pateman B 1992 District nursing. In: Butterworth T, Faugier J (eds) Clinical supervision and mentorship in nursing. Chapman and Hall, London

SEHD 1999 Learning together: a strategy for education, training and lifelong learning for all staff in the NHS in Scotland. Stationery Office, Edinburgh

United Kingdom Central Council 1986 Project 2000: a new preparation for practice. UKCC, London

United Kingdom Central Council 1994 The Council's standards for education and practice following registration. UKCC, London

United Kingdom Central Council 1999a Fitness for practice. UKCC, London

United Kingdom Central Council 1999b The continuing professional development standard. UKCC, London

Warner M, Longly M, Gould E, Picek A 1998 Health care futures 2010. University of Glamorgan, Welsh Institute for Health and Social Care

Watson H 1999 The support of students in practice. Glasgow Caledonian University, Glasgow

White E, Riley E, Davies S, Twinn S 1993 A detailed study of the relationships between teaching, support, supervision and role-modelling for students in clinical areas within the context of Project 2000 courses. King's College London and University of Manchester, English National Board for Nursing, Midwifery and Health Visiting, London

White E, Riley E, Davies S, Twinn S 1994 A detailed study of the relationships between teaching, support, supervision and role-modelling for students in clinical areas within the context of Project 2000 courses. King's College London and University of Manchester, English National Board for Nursing, Midwifery and Health Visiting, London

FURTHER READING

Council of Deans and Heads of UK Faculties for Nursing, Midwifery and Health visiting 1998 Breaking the Boundaries: Educating Nurses, Midwives and Health visitors for the next millenium. A Position paper

English National Board for Nursing, Midwifery and Health Visiting 1998 Researching Professional Education: the role of the teacher/lecturer in practice. Research Report series No. 8

Walker E, Dewer B, Runciman P 1998 Developing professional practice: an evaluation of work-based learning in a community nursing degree. Queen Margaret University College, Edinburgh

10

Ethical and legal issues

Graham C. Rumbold

Key points

- Ethics and the law
- Respect for persons
- Consent
- Accountability
- Duty of care

Clearly, within one chapter it is not possible to discuss in depth the full range of ethical and legal issues which may confront a district nurse. Therefore, rather than run the risk of oversimplifying by covering everything, this chapter will focus on some of the key issues. The chapter begins with a discussion of the relationship between ethics and the law. It then explores, from both ethical and legal viewpoints, a range of issues subsumed within four themes: *respect for persons, consent, accountability* and *duty of care*. Suggestions for further reading in ethics and law relating to both those topics covered within the chapter and other pertinent topics are given at the end of the chapter.

THE RELATIONSHIP BETWEEN ETHICS AND THE LAW

Within the context of health care there are a number of issues which are of concern to both ethicists and lawyers. It would be true to say that all laws and legal decisions have an ethical dimension, but that there are some issues which are of concern to ethicists but in which there is little or no role for law. The two disciplines, ethics and law, while each being concerned with right and wrong, have distinctively different approaches.

> Ethics … is a reflective, or theoretical business. It aims in the first instance at understanding rather than decision … It steps back from the immediately practical and attempts to discover some underlying pattern or order in the immense variety of moral decisions and practices both of individuals and societies. (Baelz 1977)

Of course, this is not to say that ethics has no practical application. An understanding of ethical theories and frameworks enables us to formulate decisions about practical issues and to justify actions. Within the context of nursing it can provide a theoretical basis for making decisions at both the macro and micro levels. For example, at the macro level, should more resources be allocated to the elderly or to children, and at the micro level, which patients should be given priority? Different nurses may arrive at different decisions, each of which, if made on sound ethical reasoning, can be said to be *right*. On the other hand, there are questions to which definitive ethical answers can be determined (see, for example, the work of Immanuel Kant on truth telling).

Law, on the other hand, is often seen as being far more clearcut and prescriptive. Either one is allowed to do something or one is not. The law is as determined as ethics to establish what is right or wrong and in most societies is founded upon ethical principles.

RESPECT FOR PERSONS

The 18th-Century German philosopher Immanuel Kant wrote 'So act as to treat humanity, whether in thine own person or that of any other, in every case as and end withal, never as a means only' (Kant 1788). In other words, every person has an intrinsic value and to treat them as an object or means is to fail to treat them as a person. This notion of the value of persons, and the injunction that we should have respect for persons, can be seen to underpin much ethical teaching and 'For many modern thinkers it is close to the essence of ethics' (Cribb 1995). Respect for persons is clearly related to two of the central principles of traditional medical ethics: *beneficence – to do good*, i.e. to do what will benefit the patient, and *non-maleficence* – to do no harm.

Respect for persons also can be seen to be an essential component of professional and legal codes. The UKCC *Code of Conduct* (1992a), for example, states that the nurse must 'act always in such a manner as to promote and safeguard the interests and well-being of patients and clients'. Equally, respect for persons underpins much criminal and civil law. Examples in criminal law include the laws relating to murder, manslaughter and assault and battery, while in civil law examples include the laws relating to trespass, defamation and, essentially in health care, the principle of duty of care and the law of negligence.

The principle of respect for persons is a broad one and, as has already been noted, underpins much ethical and legal thinking. Here, three sub-principles to which it gives rise are discussed: respect for autonomy, respect for privacy and respect for property.

Respect for autonomy

Autonomy has been defined as 'the capacity to think, decide, and act on the basis of such thought and decision freely and independently and without let or hindrance' (Gillon 1986). Respecting the autonomy of another means allowing them to make decisions and to then act upon them. Within the context of health care this means allowing patients to make decisions about their health behaviours, lifestyle and treatment. However, it is important to recognize that in order to exercise autonomy an individual requires:

> possession of: the physical wherewithal to carry out one's chosen tasks (the environmental circumstances must also be suitable); a degree of knowledge sufficient to pursue an end; an understanding of the routes open towards that end, the pitfalls, and the ways in which the knowledge can be employed in order to achieve that end; and the possession of an ability (sometimes referred to as the possession of rationality) to select ends appropriate for that person. (Seedhouse 1988)

Vignette 10.1   George's story

George is 75 years old. He has suffered from emphysema for more than 10 years and he also has a long-standing venous ulcer on his right leg. Eighteen months ago he suffered a cerebral vascular accident (CVA), which has left him severely incapacitated. He has regained limited use of his left leg but has no use in his left arm. As a consequence he is unable to wash, dress or feed himself. The district nurse visits twice weekly to dress his ulcer and supervise his medication. A home carer visits daily to help him wash, dress and walk to his sitting room and to empty his commode. His main carer is his 50-year-old daughter, Joan, who is married with two teenage children. Joan visits daily to prepare his meals. She also does his shopping and laundry. Because George refuses to go to bed until 11.00pm, either Joan or her husband has to visit in the evening to undress him and help him in to bed.

Joan is becoming noticeably exhausted and complains to the district nurse that she doesn't feel she can cope much longer. Her family are feeling neglected and she and her husband can never go away or even have a 'good night out'. Joan wants her father to be admitted to either the hospital or a residential home, at least for respite care, though preferably on a permanent basis. Now that her children are older, she would like to return to work. George, however, flatly refuses. He says he's fine where he is and does not intend to leave his home until he is 'carried out in a box'. When the district nurse points out to him that Joan is finding caring for him too much of a strain and that she has a right to enjoy life with her own family, George states adamantly that she's fussing about nothing and that it is her duty to care for him. In his view she is being selfish and he has every right to live in his own home as long as he wants to.

The district nurse, perhaps more than her hospital counterparts, interacts not just with the patient but also with their family and informal carers. They too have the right to act autonomously and this can often lead to conflict and difficult decisions for the nurse. While the district nurse's first and overriding responsibility is the patient, she does also owe an element of responsibility to the patient's carers. It is important to recognize that the right to exercise autonomy, as with all other rights, is not absolute. No individual has the right to exercise their autonomy if in so doing they impinge upon or restrict the right or ability of others to exercise autonomy. Consider vignette 10.1.

What are the issues here? First, George is asserting his right to have his autonomy respected. However, the question is whether he has a valid claim. Clearly, in exercising his autonomy, he is impinging upon Joan's right to exercise her autonomy, her duty towards her family and the rights of her family. Furthermore, he does not possess all the faculties required to exercise autonomy; in particular, he does not possess 'the physical wherewithal to carry out his selected task' – the selected task being to remain in his own home. Second, Joan is asserting her and her family's right to autonomy. She and they appear to possess all the faculties required for the exercising of autonomy. The only constraint

placed upon them is George's demand on their time. On balance, then, George's claim cannot be upheld.

How, then, can the district nurse resolve the problem? She owes a duty of care to George. She cannot force a decision and has no legal weapon to force his move. One possibility is to increase the provision of care – to provide a home carer twice daily and to increase the number of nursing visits. George could be told that he either goes to bed at a time when help can be provided by the home carer or nurse or spends the night in his sitting room. The choice is then his. The nurse can only reason with George. The issue could be forced by Joan either withdrawing her help completely or by drastically reducing it, in which case George would become solely dependent upon the statutory services and have to adjust his lifestyle accordingly. While this might be said to be limiting his autonomy, it is justified because, as has already been noted, he does not possess the necessary faculties to exercise autonomy.

Respect for privacy

The right to privacy within the context of health care implies that patients have the right to three things. First, they have the right for their treatment to be carried out in private. Second, they have the right to have all information about their diagnosis, care and treatment held in confidence. Third, they have the same basic right as do all to *be private*; that is, to have time and space to themselves and to have time alone with their significant others.

The first of these seldom raises any problems for the district nurse, given that the majority of care is carried out in the patient's own home and therefore it is usually easy to ensure privacy. Similarly, the third is less of an issue in the community than it is in a hospital. It is the second that is of prime concern.

The UKCC *Code of Conduct* (1992a) states that each nurse must 'protect all confidential information concerning patients and clients obtained in the course of professional practice and make disclosures only with consent, where required by the order of a court or where you can justify disclosure in the wider public interest' (clause 10). Furthermore, in 1987 in order to make this clause more explicit, the UKCC published a document on 'Confidentiality'. This document concludes with an important set of principles, the second of which states 'That practitioners recognize the fundamental right of their patients/clients to have information about them held in secure and private storage'. This poses a problem for the district nurse. While some patient's records may be held in the health centre or other premises owned either by the trust or GP practice, it is customary for nursing notes to be kept in the patients' own homes. These notes may, in some circumstances, be accessed by those who have no authority to do so – a neighbour or other casual visitor. This is more likely to occur when the patient has little or no control over their environment or the actions of others within their home; for example, patients, who are immobile or confused. In such circumstances the nurse would be advised either to ensure that the notes are kept in as secure a place as possible in the patient's home or to remove them from the home altogether.

Because district nurses undertake the majority of care in patients' own homes, they are often privy to far more information about the patient, their family and their lifestyle than are nurses in a hospital. Much of this information has little or no relevance to their care and treatment but can nevertheless be considered 'confidential'. The information is acquired by the nurse as a result of her privileged position and therefore must be treated with respect for the patient's and their family's right to privacy.

As Clarke (1999) points out, should a district nurse be guilty of breaching confidentiality: (i) she may be subject to disciplinary action by the UKCC; (ii) her employer may take disciplinary action to ascertain whether she has been guilty of a breach of contract; (iii) the patient may sue her. A patient may try to sue a nurse for unlawful breach of confidence, although to be successful, the patient would have to prove that it the information were untrue, the disclosure was actuated by malice or if it were true, that they suffered harm as a result. In the latter case, the nurse may have breached her duty of care and therefore be negligent. Or the patient may sue the nurse under the Human Rights Act (due to come in to force this year) for the right to privacy and/or respect for family life.

Respect for property

The district nurse is, of course, a 'guest' in the patient's home. She is there by virtue of the patient's invitation and consent. The issues surrounding access to the patient's home are discussed in the next section; here we are concerned with respecting patients' property once access has been afforded. Obviously, nurses should not deliberately damage a patient's property, nor should they assume they have the right to handle anything without the patient's or their family's permission, even if they need to do so as part of the nursing care. Vignette 10.2 describes an event which took place several years ago and hopefully would not occur in quite the same way today. The principles raised are nevertheless still pertinent.

The actions of the senior nurse were not illegal but certainly unprofessional. They showed a distinct lack of respect for both the patient's property and, more importantly, for the patient himself and his family. It represented an infringement of privacy and resulted in a loss of dignity.

Vignette 10.2   Respect for property

Eric Jones was 60 years old and suffering from terminal cancer of the lung. He was a managing director of a large brewery and lived with his wife in a pleasant suburban neighbourhood. Because he was unable to get out of bed, the family had brought a bed into the dining room in order that Eric could remain part of family life and be able to have his meals together with the rest of the family. The room was expensively furnished and both Eric and his family were anxious that as far as possible a sense of normality be maintained. The student district nurse respected their feelings and made sure that all nursing equipment, such as drugs, catheter bags, washing bowl, etc. were kept out of sight. On the

student's day off, the senior nurse from the practice visited and expressed her disagreement with the way in which the room was organized. Without asking permission, she removed the silver and glass from the antique sideboard, covered the sideboard with paper towels and then arranged all the nursing equipment on it. When she had finished, she said, 'That's better. It looks more like a sick room now'. Eric and his family were greatly distressed by this and when the student returned the next day, made their feeling known, stating also that they never wanted 'that woman' in the house again. The student apologized on the behalf of his senior colleague and restored the room to its former state.

Obviously, district nurses frequently have to use items of patient's property in order to carry out their care. They need, for example, a work surface and storage space. It is essential that the nurse treat any such items with due care. Should the nurse damage a piece of furniture by not adequately protecting it, then she might well be sued by the patient or their family. Also, if the nurse fails to ensure that any equipment, or materials which she leaves in the house are not safely stored, resulting in a safety hazard, or that any equipment, such as a hoist, is not properly installed and as a consequence a member of the family suffers injury, she may well be sued by the family.

CONSENT

The UKCC (1996) states that all health professionals must obtain consent before giving any treatment or care. 'It is a basic rule of law that no one has the right to even touch another person without their consent' (Clarke 1999) and 'English law requires the nurse to obtain consent from the patient before treatment is given' (McHale 1995).

There is, then, both a legal and a professional requirement for nurses to obtain a patient's consent. Failure to do so may result in her being prosecuted in the criminal courts or the patient could sue in the civil courts for trespass to the person. This applies even if the patient has suffered no harm as a result and even where it has been done for their benefit. The likelihood of criminal prosecution for battery is minimal and it

is more likely that the patient would bring a claim in the civil courts. It is also worth noting that once a broad general consent has been given, a patient may still claim that they had been given inadequate information and sue for negligence (*Chatterson v Gerson* 1981).

The issue is not simply that consent has been given but that it is given on the basis of adequate information. The question is how much constitutes 'adequate' information. The answer to this question is by no means clear. The UKCC (1996) states that practitioners should share information freely, 'in an accessible way and in appropriate circumstances', and points out that 'it is not safe to assume that the patient or client has enough knowledge about even about basic treatment, for them to make an informed choice without an explanation' and 'it is essential that you give the patient or client adequate information so that he or she can make a meaningful decision'. Similarly, the Patient's Charter (1991) states that a patient has a right to 'be given a clear explanation of any treatment proposed, including any risks and any alternatives, before you decide whether you will agree to treatment'.

However, in the case of *Sidaway v Board of Governors of Bethlem Royal Hospital* (1985), Lord Templeman said: 'some information may confuse, other information may alarm a patient ... the doctor must decide in the light of his training and experience and in the light of his knowledge of the patient what should be said and how it should be said'. The law then allows the professional to withhold information from the patient if it is in their best interests. Such a decision must however be justified, and 'the nurse must make a very careful assessment of the degree of harm which may be caused to the patient by providing full information' (McHale 1995).

In obtaining consent two principles must be observed. First, consent must be freely given and patients should not be pressurized into consenting to care or treatment. Second, consent must not be obtained by deceit. All information given must be honest and factual. To obtain consent by lying about the effects of treatment invalidates the consent. Also, the nurse should provide the patient with the facts and not opinion. The essence of informed consent is that the patient makes their own independent decision.

Refusal to accept treatment

Any mentally competent adult can refuse treatment and the UKCC (1992a) advises that 'you must respect the patient's refusal just as much as their consent'. The key issue is what constitutes 'competent'. Earlier, it was noted that one of the faculties required to exercise autonomy is the possession of rationality. It is important, however, not to assume that if we consider the patient's decision to be irrational that they do not possess rationality. Frequently, health professionals only question a patient's rationality when they make a decision with which the professionals do not agree. A patient's decision to refuse treatment is often interpreted as a lack of rationality, while had the same patient consented to treatment his rationality would not have been questioned.

The law is not absolutely clear on this point. In the case of Re T (an adult) (refusal of medical treatment) 1992, 4A11 ER649, the court ruled that a young woman who refused a blood transfusion should be given it on the grounds that she was not in a fit state to make a valid decision. However, mental illness is not necessarily itself justification for deciding that a patient is incapable of making a valid decision. In Re C (an adult) (refusal of medical treatment) (Family Division, 1994, 1 A11 ER819), a patient at Broadmoor Hospital refused to undergo an amputation of a gangrenous foot. Although medical opinion was that amputation was the only way to avoid death, the court ruled in the patient's favour because the evidence showed that he understood the purpose and effect of the treatment and had made a coherent decision.

In the course of their work district nurses do meet patients who either refuse treatment or, more commonly, refuse the specific treatment the nurse recommends, preferring an alternative. The commonest examples are patients with venous ulcers. Frequently patients refuse to accept the treatment recommended by the nurse, e.g. four-layer bandages, because they cannot tolerate it, finding it uncomfortable. Or it may be they prefer an alternative because this means the nurse will have to visit more frequently. Their decision may not be considered entirely rational, in as much as the alternative treatment may not be as successful. However, there may be no just reason to doubt their mental competence. The nurse cannot enforce a particular treatment on a patient, nor can she, except under very exceptional circumstances, withdraw care. If despite full explanation and advice, the patient still refuses to accept the recommended treatment, the nurse has little option but to comply with patient's wishes, on no other grounds than that a less effective form of treatment is better than no treatment. To refuse to comply with the patient's wishes would be to not respect their autonomy.

Admission to property

'Normally, a community nurse will be a lawful visitor even when visiting a new family uninvited. But that does not mean that she has a right of entry to a client's house' (Clarke 1999). As a 'lawful visitor' the nurse is owed a duty of care. The occupier(s) have both a statutory and a common law duty to ensure the nurse's safety when on their premises. The Occupiers Liability Act 1957 states that occupiers have a 'duty to take such care as in all the circumstances of the case is reasonable to see that the visitor will be reasonably safe in using the premises for the purpose for which he is invited or permitted by the occupier to be there'. Thus, a district nurse would be justified in refusing to enter premises if she considered that conditions presented a threat to her safety. And her employer cannot require her to do so.

The nurse, though, may not enter a patient's premises without their consent. She only has the right of entry under common law in an emergency in order to save a life. If in any other circumstances she is unable to obtain entry, she would be advised to call the police who do have the right to force an entry legally. Nor should the nurse try to obtain entry via another route if unable to do so through the normal one. For example, if normally the occupier admits the nurse through the front door and the nurse is unable to obtain an answer when she rings the bell or knocks on the door, she cannot, unless having previously been told so by the patient, attempt to enter through the back door. Also, should at any time the occupier withdraw their consent, the district nurse has no right to remain on the property and if she does, she becomes a trespasser. The occupier has the right to use reasonable force to evict a trespasser; therefore the nurse, if asked or told by the occupier to leave, should do so.

ACCOUNTABILITY

Accountability is a term which occurs frequently in professional codes but which is seldom used in ethics, nor is it a term used within a legal context. This is not to say that it has no place in a discussion of the ethical and legal responsibilities of the nurse. Accountability means taking responsibility for one's decisions and actions and being held liable or accountable for the results of those decisions and actions. It can therefore be seen in ethical terms as exercising autonomy responsibility and in legal terms as a concept closely related to that of duty of care and negligence. The latter will be discussed within the final section of this chapter; here a number of issues related to the proper exercise of professional accountability will be explored:

- team working and delegation
- record keeping
- the scope of practice, with particular reference to nurse prescribing
- vicarious liability.

Team working and delegation

The district nurse frequently works as a member of a team. She is a member and, more often than not, a leader of a team of nurses. The nursing team may typically comprise a senior district nurse, other first-level nurses who may or may not possess a district nursing qualification, second-level nurses and health-care assistants or nursing auxiliaries. She is also a member of a multidisciplinary team, the primary health care team (PHCT), comprising doctors, health visitors, practice nurses as well as the district nursing team and possibly other health-care professionals. This complex working pattern raises a number of professional and legal issues for the district nurse, particularly as team leader.

As has already been noted, each individual is accountable for her own decisions and actions. Thus, when the district nurse delegates part or all of a patient's care to another member of the team, that person can be held accountable for their own actions and their results. However, this does not totally absolve the team leader from all responsibility. The team leader may still be held accountable for the care received by the patient. The UKCC in *The Scope of Professional Practice* (1992b) states:

The registered nurse, midwife or health visitor must, in serving the interests of patients and clients and the wider interests of society, avoid any inappropriate delegation to others which would compromise those interests.

It is therefore incumbent upon the team leader to ensure that any member of the team to whom she delegates care is competent to undertake that care. Failure to do so could mean that the team leader be held guilty of negligent delegation. It is also worth noting that this might also apply to care which the nurse delegates to a family member or other informal carer. 'For those tasks that are outside normal care that the family accept as their responsibility special training must be given or the nurse could be negligent in delegation' (Young 1995).

The law asserts that patients have the right to receive safe and adequate care, as indeed does ethics. Ethics would tend to place a higher standard than does the law and suggest that patients have the right to the best possible care. The law, however, is sometimes more pragmatic and asserts that care given should be that which is 'in accordance with a practice accepted as proper by a responsible body of medical men skilled in that particular art' *(Bolam v Friern Hospital Management Committee* 1957.) This ruling, which has become known as the *Bolam test*, applies across the professions and we shall return to it later in the discussion about negligence. Here it is noted as setting the standard of practice expected of a health professional.

The other crucial case that applies to undertaking delegated duties is that of *Wilsher v Essex Area Health Authority* 1987. In the case of Wilsher, the crucial ruling was that when care was carried out by a less qualified or less experienced person than the one who would normally be expected to undertake that care, they would be judged as if they were the postholder and not as a junior. In other words, if a junior nurse undertakes a task that would normally be undertaken by a more senior nurse, then applying Bolam, what would be reasonably expected of the more senior nurse would be the standard against which the performance would be judged. The same applies if a nurse undertakes a task which would normally be undertaken by a doctor. There are two implications of these rulings. First, it is incumbent upon the person delegating the care to ensure that the person to whom they delegate is competent to undertake it. Second, it is incumbent upon the person to whom the care is delegated to only undertake that care if they feel competent to do so, bearing in mind that they will be judged not on the basis of what can be expected of a person of their level of qualification but of their senior.

Record keeping

Record keeping is an integral part of nursing, midwifery and health visiting practice. It is a tool of professional practice and one which should help the care process. It is not separate from this process and it is not an optional extra to be filled in if circumstances allow. (UKCC 1998)

The importance of keeping accurate, up-to-date and comprehensive records cannot be overemphasized. First, because failure to do so may result in inappropriate or unsafe treatment being carried out, thus endangering the patient. Second, because records may be required as evidence in a court of law. Failure to maintain good records can lead to a breakdown in continuity of care a risk of medication or other treatment being duplicated or omitted and failure to note significant changes in the patient's condition, which could prove vital to others involved in their care.

There are certain basic principles which should be observed.

- Records should be made at the time of, or as soon as possible after, the events being reported.
- Records should be legible, using a pen. The use of pencils is not acceptable because of the risk of changes being made later.
- They should be clear and unambiguous (avoid phrases such as 'no change', no problems').
- Each entry should be dated and the time of entry included.
- Alterations should be made by scoring out, and initialled, much in the same way as making an alteration on a cheque. Never use tippex.
- They should be signed using full name and title, not just initials.
- Avoid abbreviations, other than those accepted as standard. Thus BP for blood pressure is acceptable but BWO for bowels well open is not – it could mean bladder washout!
- Finally, and by no means least, records should not contain any remarks about the patient or their carers which might cause offence, nor subjective comments about the patient which are unrelated to their care.

The UKCC also recommends that records should be written with the involvement of the patient or client and in terms they can understand. This is particularly important in the community where patients have more ready access to their records than do patients in hospital. It is in certain situations practice to keep two sets of records, those which are held in the patient's home and a further set held in the health centre or elsewhere.

The reason given is that there may be information which the nurse needs for her own use or to convey to colleagues which is pertinent to the patient's care, but which for various reasons she does not want the patient to access. Examples might be a patient whose condition is terminal but they have not been informed of this or a situation where the nurse suspects that the patient is being abused by their carer. The second is perhaps more justified than the first, provided that it is not totally subjective. However, two questions have to be asked. Does anyone have the right to record information about someone else without their knowledge? And whose information is it?

The Data Protection Act 1998 and the *Access to Medical Reports Act 1988 (Access to Personal Files and Medical Reports (NI) Order 1991)* enable patients to request access to all records held on them. There are some situations in which information may be withheld, but these seldom apply to records maintained by nursing staff. Furthermore, the UKCC (1998) makes clear its support for open access to records. It can also be argued that since the information is about the patient, it in essence belongs to them. To hide it from them is therefore an infringement of their rights.

The scope of practice

In 1992 the UKCC issued *The Scope of Professional Practice* in recognition of the fact that the scope of nursing practice was continually expanding in response to advances in health-care practice and research and changes in national and local policies. Two recent examples of national policy initiatives which have affected the role of the nurse are the reduction in junior doctors' hours and nurse prescribing. The former has greater implications for nurses working in hospital than for those in the community, while the latter represents a major development for all nurses in the community and for the district nurse in particular. Before discussing issues specifically related to prescribing, some general points will be discussed.

In undertaking any task which is encompassed within what is sometimes referred to as the extended role, the same principles apply as to the traditional role. That is, that a nurse should not undertake any task for which she has not been trained nor feels competent to perform, nor should she delegate it to others who are not competent to do so. Nor should the nurse undertake any task which she is not authorized by her employer to perform. This latter point can cause conflict within a PHCT. The district nurse is usually employed by the trust or health authority and not by the GP. Even if the nurse feels competent and the GP considers her to be so, she may not perform the task, except in an emergency situation, without the employer's authorization. Practice nurses, on the other hand, are employed by the GP and so the decision as to which tasks they might perform rests entirely with the GP and the nurse. GPs often find this difference in roles difficult to understand, given that both district nurse and practice nurse are qualified nurses, and may therefore at times put pressure on the district nurse to perform tasks which they are not authorized to do. It goes without saying that the district nurse should resist such pressure. One final, general point to be made is that when undertaking any 'extended role' task, the nurse should bear in mind the rulings in the Bolam and Wilshire cases referred to above.

Probably the most significant expansion of the district nurse's role in recent years has been the introduction of nurse prescribing. While the nurses' formulary is extremely limited and most of the items included within it are available over the counter, it does place additional responsibility on the nurse. On the one hand, as has often been remarked within district nursing, it has merely legalized what was fairly common practice and on the other hand, it has simplified the correct procedures, enabling nurses to obtain the necessary dressings or medicines for patients more quickly, thus benefiting patient care.

In many situations, for example the treatment of venous ulcers, district nurses have decided on the treatment and then requested the GP to write out the prescription, a practice which was acceptable to both nurse and GP, and within the law, but time consuming. Unfortunately, there were instances where the procedure was short-circuited and contravened the law. The author has in the past come across many instances where GPs signed blank prescription forms and allowed the nurse to complete them. In one instance the district nurse filled in blank prescription forms and had them made up by the pharmacist who then passed them to the GP for signature. Such 'arrangements' were clearly open to abuse and at least one district nurse was 'struck off' by the UKCC for using such an arrangement to obtain drugs for her own use.

The introduction of nurse prescribing, while making life easier, has at the same time increased the responsibility of the nurse. While all prescribing was undertaken by the GP, he shared accountability with the nurse. The nurse was accountable for her own actions when administering the treatment, but at least some accountability rested with the GP who prescribed it. Now that nurses can prescribe treatments, total accountability rests with them. This has two implications. First, it means that the nurse needs to ensure that she has the necessary knowledge in order to prescribe the most appropriate treatment. Failure to do could lead to a case for negligence. Second, it means that pressure is likely to be placed on nurses by manufacturers to prescribe their products. Witness the increase in advertising in nursing journals, particularly community nursing journals, by the manufacturers of those products contained within the nurses' formulary. This adds to the legal and professional dimensions an ethical one. Pharmaceutical companies, and doctors, have come under a lot of media criticism in the past for the, at best covert and at worst blatantly overt, bribes in the forms of gifts and weekend 'conferences' that have been associated with the introduction of new products. While nurses are not likely to be offered the same lavish treatment as doctors have been in the past, nevertheless they will have to ensure that their clinical decisions are not influenced by advertising or promotional campaigns.

Vicarious liability

So far, in this discussion of accountability it may have appeared that the nurse is liable to be sued for every mistake she makes. While the nurse is held individually accountable for her actions and may therefore be subject to disciplinary proceedings by either the UKCC or her employer, it is far less likely that she would be sued by a patient or their family, not least because there is little to be gained in suing someone for damages who has little money! What is more likely is that the patient or family would sue the nurse's employer. The doctrine of 'vicarious liability' means that employers are liable for any negligent acts committed by their employees. In order to establish that the employer is vicariously liable for the negligent act of an employee, the claimant has to prove three points:

- that the nurse was negligent
- that she was an employee
- that she was acting in the course of her employment.

Should the patient or family be successful in their action, the employer can then attempt to recoup their costs from the employee. However, this rarely happens, for the very same reason that complainants seldom sue nurses. The employer almost certainly will, if the case of negligence is proved, instigate disciplinary proceedings against the nurse concerned.

It is also worth nothing that it is the employer who can be held vicariously liable and not the manager or person in control. Thus the district nursing team leader cannot be held liable for the negligence of a team member, nor can the GP for the negligence of a district nurse employed by the trust or health authority. In the case of practice nurses, it is the GP who is the employer and can therefore be held vicariously liable for the practice nurse's negligence.

DUTY OF CARE

That nurses owe a duty of care to patients is an accepted notion professionally, ethically and legally. The UKCC Code of Conduct (1992a) spells out in some detail exactly what is expected of the nurse, midwife or health visitor in respect of the level of care to be afforded to patients/clients.

As a registered nurse, midwife or health visitor, you are personally accountable for your practice and, in the exercise of your professional accountability, must:

1. act always in such a manner as to promote and safeguard the interests and well-being of patients and clients 2. ensure that no action or omission on your part, or within your sphere of responsibility, is detrimental to the interests, condition or safety of patients and clients.

The ethical perspective

There are two fundamental principles which underpin health-care ethics – beneficence and non-maleficence. According to Frankena (1963), the principle of beneficence can be summed up as follows

1. One ought not to inflict evil or harm (what is bad); 2. One ought to prevent evil or harm; 3. One ought to remove evil; and 4. One ought to do or promise good. These four things are different, but they may appropriately be regarded as parts of the principle of beneficence.

'More simply, it is often seen as a moral injunction always to do good' (Rumbold 1999). In the context of health care, this means doing what will most benefit the patient or what is in their best interests. The principle of beneficence has its foundations in the Hippocratic Oath and clearly underpins professional codes of conduct, including the UKCC Code, as can clearly seen by the quote above. 'That any nurse, or health care professional, would want to act in any way other than for the benefit of the patient or client is not under debate' (Rumbold 1999). However, it does beg the question as to who decides what is in the patient's best interests. Space does not permit discussion of this question here but the reader is referred to the earlier discussion on respecting autonomy and to suggestions for further reading at the end of this chapter.

The second clause of the UKCC Code of Conduct arises out of the principle of non-maleficence, the idea that nurses have a duty not to harm patients or clients. The problem with taking the principle to its extreme is that a number of medical and nursing interventions do either in themselves inflict harm or carry a risk of harm. To give a patient a injection is to inflict some pain, yet the drug being injected is intended to benefit them. Clearly, in such a situation the harm caused by the procedure is outweighed by the beneficial results. Other situations may be

less clearcut. If the risk of harmful side effects of a treatment is high and those side effects are sufficiently harmful to outweigh the possible benefits, then it can be argued that there is a case for not giving the treatment. At a more basic level, the prime duty of the nurse is not to cause harm, by act or omission, when there is no benefit to be gained for the patient. The debate as to which principle – beneficence or non-maleficence – takes precedence is not clear and again the reader is referred to suggestions for further reading at the end of this chapter.

The legal perspective

Lord Atkin laid down the basis of the duty of care that we owe to others (Donoghue v Stevenson 1932). A person must take reasonable care to avoid acts or omissions that he can reasonably foresee would be likely to injure a person directly affected by those acts. This concept forms a cornerstone of the civil wrong of negligence where a breach of duty with resultant harm constitutes liability and later cases have only served to refine this. (Young 1995)

In order to successfully bring a case of negligence, the plaintiff has to prove three things:

1. that a duty of care is owed by the defendant to the plaintiff
2. that there has been a breach of that duty
3. that, as a result of that breach, the plaintiff has suffered harm.

That nurses owe a duty of care to their patients is beyond doubt. It is the second two points that are more difficult to prove.

First, the plaintiff has to be able to show that the nurse, by what she either did or omitted to do, has failed in her duty of care. In some cases this may be quite clearcut, for example if the nurse gave the wrong dose of a drug or failed to ensure the patient's safety by leaving an arthritic patient alone in the bath. In others, it may be less so, for example where a patient is referred by the hospital to a district nurse for the removal of sutures following an appendicectomy. The nurse removes the sutures correctly, assures herself that the wound is healing satisfactorily, gives the patient appropriate advice for continuing recovery from the surgery but omits to carry out a full assessment and thus is unaware that the patient is suffering from chest pain.

In assessing whether there is a case for negligence the test applied by the courts is the Bolam test. This test, to which reference has already been made, arose from the case in 1957 of *Bolam v Friern Hospital Management Committee*. In this case the judge advised the jury that:

Where you get a situation which involves the use of some specialist skill or competence, then the test as to whether there has been negligence or not is not the test of the man on the top of the Clapham omnibus, because he has not got that specialist skill. The test is the standard of the ordinary skilled man exercising and professing to have that specialist skill. A man need not possess the highest expert skill; it is well established law that it is sufficient if her exercises the ordinary skill of an ordinary competent man exercising that particular art.

This ruling has since been upheld in a number of cases, including ones heard in the House of Lords.

What this means in practice is that the courts will take advice from the ordinary district nurse, not the Chief Nursing Officer or a professor of nursing at a prestigious university. Thus, in the example above, where the patient is claiming that the district nurse is negligent because she failed to discover that he was suffering from chest pain, the court would seek advice from district nurses working in a similar capacity. The question asked of them would be, 'In such a situation would you expect a district nurse to carry out a full assessment a case such as this? If their answer is "yes", then there is a case to be answered. If their response is "no", then there is no case to be answered.

If the second point is proved – that there has been a breach in the duty of care – the plaintiff then has to show that they have suffered harm as a result. 'It does not matter, for the purposes of negligence law, how badly a nurse, midwife or health visitor practises if no injury is suffered' (Montgomery 1995). The harm has to be shown to be a direct result of the negligent action or omission. To return to the example above, suppose that in failing to assess the patient fully the district nurse was found to have failed in her duty of care and that shortly after her visit the patient suffered a myocardial infarction, it would still not necessarily be the case that she would be found negligent. The next question would be what would have happened if she had discovered that the patient was suffering from chest pain and whether any action she took could have prevented the infarction. Unless it could be proven beyond doubt that the nurse could have prevented the infarction, then the case would not be proven. Where there is doubt in cases of harm resulting from negligent actions, the courts tend towards leniency toward the defendant.

It is not, however, only actions or omissions that can give rise to a case of negligence. Negligence can also be applied to giving or failing to give information. If a nurse fails to give the patient sufficient information in order to make an informed choice and the patient makes their choice on the basis of the information given and as a result suffers harm, there may be a case for negligence (see Sidaway v Bethlem Royal Hospital 1985, referred to earlier). Equally if a district nurse gives incorrect advice to a patient or their carers and the patient suffers harm as a result, this too would be negligence.

If plaintiffs win their cases, they are entitled to damages. These are calculated on the basis of the nature of the injury or harm incurred, expenses, loss of earnings and cost of future care. The amounts awarded can vary considerably, although the courts have developed an approximate tariff in order to achieve consistency. However, as has already been mentioned, it is unlikely that it would be the nurse who would be sued and therefore liable for the damages. It is more likely that it would be employer who would have to foot the bill.

REFERENCES

Baelz P 1977 Ethics and belief. Sheldon Press, London.
Clarke A 1999 Community nurses and the law. Community Practitioners and Health Visitors Association, London

Cribb A 1995 The ethical dimension. In: Tingle J, Cribbe A (eds) 1995 Nursing law and ethics Oxford, Blackwell Science, ch 2

Frankena W K 1963 cited in Rumbold G 1999 Ethics in nursing practice, 3rd edn. Baillière Tindall, Edinburgh

Gillon R 1986 Philosophical medical ethics. John Wiley, Chichester

Kant I 1788 Critique of practical reason cited in Ross D 1969 Kant's Ethical Theory. Oxford University Press, Oxford

McHale J 1995 Consent and the adult patient – the legal perspective. In: Tingle J, Cribb A (eds) Nursing law and ethics. Blackwell Science, Oxford

Montgomery J 1995 Negligence – the legal perspective. In: Tingle A, Cribbe A (Eds) Nursing law and ethics. Blackward Science, Oxford

Rumbold G 1999 Ethics in nursing practice, 3rd edn. Baillière Tindall, Edinburgh

Seedhouse D 1988 Ethics: the heart of healthcare. John Wiley, Chichester

UKCC 1992a Code of conduct for the nurse, midwife and health visitor, 3rd edn. UKCC, London

UKCC 1992b Scope of professional practice. UKCC, London

UKCC 1996 Guidelines for professional practice. UKCC, London

UKCC 1998 Guidance for record, and record keeping. UKCC, London

Young A 1995 The legal dimension, In: Tingle J, Crubb A 1995, Nursing Law and Ethics. Blackwell Science, Oxford

FURTHER READING

Relationship between Ethics and Law

Rumbold G 1999 Ethics in nursing practice, 3rd edn. Baillière Tindall, Edinburgh, ch 16

Smith J P 1983 The relationship between rights and responsibilities in health care: a dilemma for nurses. Journal of Advanced Nursing 8: 437–440

Tingle J, Cribb A (eds) 1995 Nursing law and ethics. Blackwell Science, Oxford, ch 1, ch 2

Thompson I E, Melia K M, Boyd K M 1983 Nursing ethics. Churchill Livingstone, Edinburgh, ch 2

Respect for Persons

Campbell A V 1975 Moral dilemmas and medicine. Churchill Livingstone, Edinburgh

Ross D 1969 Kanto ethical theory. Oxford University Press, Oxford

Autonomy

Rumbold G 1999 Ethics in nursing practice, 3rd edn. Baillière Tindall, Edinburgh, ch 14, 15

Seedhouse D 1988 Ethics: the Heart of Healthcare. John Wiley, Chichester, ch 9

Seedhouse D, Cribb A (eds) 1988 Changing healthcare. John Wiley, Chichester

Consent

Clarke A 1999 Community nurses and the law. CPHVA, London

Freedman B 1975 A moral theory of informed consent. Hastings Centre Report 5 (4): 32–39

Rumbold G 1999 Ethics in nursing practice, 3rd edn. Baillière Tindall, Edinburgh Tingle J, Cribbe A 1995 Nursing law and ethics. Blackwell Science, Oxford, ch 6

Accountability

Fromer M J 1981 Ethical issues in health care. CV Mosby, St Louis, ch 1

Clarke A 1999 Community nurses and the law. CPHVA, London ch 1, ch 4

Thompson I E, Melia K M, Boyd K M 1988 Nursing ethics, 2nd edn. Churchill Livingstone, Edinburgh, ch 13

Duty of Care

Clarke A 1999 Community nurses and the law. CPHVA, London, ch 2

Rumbold G 1999 Ethics in nursing practice, 3rd edn. Baillière Tindàil, Edinburgh, ch 14

Tingle J, Cribbc A 1995 Nursing law and ethics. Blackwell Science, Oxford, ch 5

Other legal issues

Clarke A 1999 Community nurses and the law. CPHVA, London

Dimond B 1990 Legal aspects of nursing. Prentice Hall, Hemel Hempstead

Young A P L 1989 Legal problems in nursing practice, 2nd edn. Chapman and Hall, London

Young A P 1991 Law and professional conduct in nursing. Scutari Press, Harrow

Nursing and Health-Care Ethics

In addition to the texts cited above, the following provide a good discussion of the principles and issues of health care ethics.

Beauchamp T L, Childress J F 1989 Principles of biomedical ethics. Oxford University Press, Oxford

Benjamin M, Curtin K 1992 Ethics in nursing, 3rd edn. Oxford University Press, New York

Gillon R 1994 Principles of health care ethics. John Wiley, Chichester

Vargan A C 1980 The main issues in bioethics. Panlist Press, New York

District nursing within the management context

11

Management of care

Judith Canham

Key points

- Case load management
- Team nursing
- Primary nursing
- Hospital at home
- Care management (NHS and Community Care Act 1990)

INTRODUCTION

Existing strategies for managing care in district nursing appear to be service led and influenced by available resources and other factors external to the specialism. The purpose of this chapter is to enable an understanding of positive and negative influences on the management of care in order that district nurses may formulate for themselves effective systems for managing care that are patient centred and at the same time reflect the reality of primary health-care services.

Care management conjures up a number of different images for district nurses: a system of work organisation, a nursing strategy for providing care and a way of managing care packages within the NHS and Community Care Act (DoH 1990). This chapter begins by considering the strengths and weaknesses of caseload management in relation to the organisation of district nursing care. Second, there is an examination of specific care management issues using team nursing, primary nursing and hospital at home as examples of systems that have contributed to the development of managed care in district nursing. Third, in the review of care management (NHS and Community Care Act 1990) the intention is to stimulate debate through an analysis of social service and district nurse experience, before moving on to consider how future practice may be managed by utilising best evidence from both traditional and contemporary care management systems.

In all types of nursing, care management should need little explanation but briefly it is worthwhile suggesting that it is a strategy or system that provides an optimum way of ensuring that care needs are met appropriately and equitably and includes the way in which patients are referred and prioritised for assessment, the assessment process and the planning and evaluation of care.

Hidden agendas within any care management strategy may include cost effectiveness (the proper use of resources or working with limited resources), professional protectionism (the ways in which professions ensure that their micro and macro needs are met) and work-ease (the simplification or manipulation of strategies). At times these agendas may not be hidden, an example being the explicit requirement for value for money in care management. Whether agendas are covert or not, it is important that practitioners recognise exactly what the system of care management they utilise says about patients, health care, cost effectiveness, the profession and the ease or difficulty of implementing that strategy in real-life situations. This necessitates a critical evaluation of how all aspects sit together. For example, taking into consideration all explicit and implicit agendas, district nurses should be able to judge whether or not primary nursing is the best strategy for managing care in their particular practice.

Strategies of managed care may be tightened by introducing quality mechanisms that act for the patient group (Ross & Mackenzie 1996) and loosened by such factors as a lack of practitioner ownership (Hadley & Clough 1996). These concepts relate to the development of and rationale for the strategy of care management; if it was intended to improve the management of patient care and if it was planned and developed in conjunction with patient groups and practitioners. Above all, any strategy of care management requires a common intention and purpose that is easily understood, applicability in any situation and an assurance to all parties that the system will make a beneficial difference to care.

Providing the best system of care management is particularly relevant within the new NHS and the requirement for clinical governance (DoH 1997). Here there is little question that district nursing must be able to articulate how it manages care, justify why it manages care and present evidence of quality care with positive outcomes for both patient groups and primary care groups.

Until fairly recently, district nursing's methods of managing care were not dissimilar to those identified within social service departments prior to the implementation of the NHS and Community Care Act in 1993, where care was primarily organised around existing resources, as opposed to initiating or activating resources in relation to need (Lewis & Glennester 1996).

CASELOAD MANAGEMENT

Although not a true system of care management, conventional caseload management is as good a place as any to start describing the traditional modus operandi of district nursing. The district nursing caseload will have changed significantly since the implementation of the NHS and Community Care Act 1990, yet the principles of caseload management may retain old values and beliefs that act against the tenets of needs-led care.

At its simplest, caseload management is an organisational technique, undertaken by a district nurse with overall responsibility for an identified caseload, the aim being to ensure that each patient receives the appropriate care at the appropriate time and by the appropriate person. However, the district nursing caseload is no easy thing to define as it is not restricted by ward size or beds and, at its worst, is not limited by inadequate staffing resources or frequent seasonal caseload bulges (Dimond 1997). Additionally, the caseload is staffed by nurses with a variety of skills and qualifications and the range of care provided is exceptionally wide and often unpredictable.

This variability suggests that caseload management is a deceptively complex technique that should include responsibility for managing assessment and reassessments; delegation; caseload review, monitoring and evaluation; critical decision making; record keeping; staff development, staff support and team leadership. In reality, research and experience suggest that where traditional caseload management is the only operational strategy for managing patient care, the system will adhere to a simplistic, organisational model, due to a lack of professional consensus that articulates the philosophy and principles of care management for patient-led care.

The referral and admission processes

Until fairly recently, patients were formally referred to district nursing only by certain professionals, mainly hospitals and general practitioners, and this would theoretically ensure a degree of professional 'screening out' prior to district nurse assessment, with most referred cases being needy of some form of care. Despite a more open referral system, the district nurse caseload is still mainly dependent on professional referrals and 'screening out' continues. The frustrations of the referral system are epitomised within palliative care where early referrals could ensure a reduction in problems and create a secure and trusting nurse–patient–carer relationship and yet district nurses frequently cite late, crisis referrals despite the wealth of policy guidance (DoH 1994, DoH/SSI 1991, 1995).

Even though the system of referral to the caseload appears to be formalised, the reality is that the system is ad hoc and dependent on the skills, knowledge and understanding of the referrer (Worth 1998) (Vignette 11.1).

Caseload review

The lack of review of district nurses' caseloads was noted to be problematic by Badger et al

---

Vignette 11.1   District nurse

It's just ridiculous. Sometimes you get an excellent complete referral from a hospital and sometimes you may simply get a name and 'please assess' from a GP. What galls is that you are expected to visit on that minimal information and I think it could be downright dangerous. But when you try to phone the GP or hospital for more information you can't get through to the right person – 'Oh the primary nurse isn't here' – and you have to consider that some poor soul is waiting for you to visit so what can you do? You get there and find out that either there are so many problems they shouldn't even have been discharged or you spend an hour or so finding out that the referral was inappropriate and they really need an OT.

(1989) who identified that factors such as 'expectation of re-referral', 'the intensity of the relationship' and 'patient complaints' affected district nurse criteria for caseload review. District nurse caseloads grew until natural processes (cure or death) intervened; evaluation was largely notional and, if it took place, simply maintained the status quo of the caseload (Badger et al 1989).

The somewhat idiosyncratic individuality of district nurses' management of caseloads is also reflected by Griffiths & Luker (1994) and suggests that district nurses have yet to identify a corporate or professional philosophy for caseload management. Additionally, Griffiths & Luker note that there are a range of covert organisational rules (hidden agenda) that may act against needs-based care. For example, qualified district nurses may be reluctant to interfere or disagree with a colleague's plans for care, even when to do so would be in the patient's best interest. In district nursing, the majority of care is provided without direct supervision and this has implications for the accountability of the caseload manager in relation to ensuring acceptable standards of care, the overall quality of care provided and the degree of collaborative activity utilised to meet care goals.

Consumerism in caseload management

A relatively recent change to the way that district nurse caseloads were organised resulted

---

Vignette 11.2 Staff nurse – district nursing

It's not the patients or their carers, although they do sometimes say 'What time do you call this.' It's more to do with managers and being seen to have everything sorted out into immovable bands of time. They should know that district nursing doesn't work like that and that despite all good intentions you get stuck at someone's house and it would be unprofessional or unethical to leave so you are very late or have to leave your next patient until the afternoon. The system should be able to cope with that but no, it's 'you should have visited' or 'they'll complain'. I get the feeling that time banding has become a management stick and that they are so obsessed with it because it's one way in which they can say 'look, quality, quality' to *their* managers.

Vignette 11.3 G grade district nurse

I know that I could manage my caseload better if I could make better use of the district nursing team's skills but I'm not allowed to. To give you an example, in this trust only the G Grade can assess patients but sometimes it's the staff nurse or F Grade who would be most capable. X has recently completed the care of the dying course, has a BAC counselling diploma and does bereavement counselling outside work but she can't assess for palliative care. So I take her with me cause, to be honest, she's damn good at it.

Our auxiliary is excellent at taking blood, a natural, but venepuncture has to be by a first-level nurse. Now our staff nurses are run off their feet and the auxiliary hasn't got enough work. Recently I've been asked for my ear syringing certificate. Well I haven't got one and I'm going to carry on regardless. I've got so much experience but the trust wants a certificate. This makes a mockery of Scope.

I think that as caseload manager the trust should do what they said at interview and in the job description – make me accountable and responsible but all they do is make me feel frustrated that I can't manage the caseload properly.

---

from the Patient's Charter (DoH 1992) and in particular the recommendation for time-banded visits. Meeting the standard expectations of patients is not straightforward and before Charter publication, Ong (1991) was discussing the difficulties of structuring the working day of district nurses to suit patient need in that many patients are deemed to be of equal priority; equally sick and equally needy. In some cases, meeting Patient's Charter standards (DoH 1992) has become a matter of juggling the caseload rather than managing the caseload to professional standards (Vignette 11.2).

Concepts such as empowerment and partnership in relation to the provision of skilled nursing care in the community are essentially professional and not service management issues. As the majority of patients on the district nurse caseload are severely disabled, acutely ill or dying, the translation of concepts into nursing policy needs to be carefully considered in light of individual patient/carer needs for nursing care. It is likely that district nurses are somewhat better than health service managers at rapidly moving away from a market-led consumerism, critically questioning the health service conceptualisation of empowerment and identifying that partnership in primary health-care situations means more than shared responsibility for care. If nothing else, the Patient's Charter (DoH 1992) and other repeated calls for patient participation (Hodder & Gallagher 1998) ensure that district nurses remain acutely aware of the patients' role

in caseload management and the need to move quickly in the direction of a needs-based service.

Bureaucracy and caseload management

As district nurses attempt to manage patient needs and rights in a professional manner and be accountable for their decisions, one of the major problems they face is that caseload managers are themselves dependent on the way that district nursing is managed, organised and resourced by others. The district nursing workforce significantly outnumber other workforces in the community (NHSME 1992); the service employs both qualified and unqualified staff and utilises a vast amount of community NHS trust and general practice resources (DHSS 1989). To contain financial outlay and exercise control over this disparate workforce, district nursing has traditionally been a strictly managed service where staff non-conformity is unwelcome. Often the 'rules' of practice overwhelm professional decisions and may not be in the best interests of patient care management (Vignette 11.3).

On a more mundane level, trying to contact district nursing services is often difficult as in many cases administrative support for district nursing remains at the level of an ineffective answerphone (Ong 1991) and somewhat obscure 'contact times'. It is rare to find dedicated administrative support which is surprising considering district nursing's theoretical 24-hour service and the high-tech care that is now provided. The frustrations of trying to manage care within the existing bureaucratic management structures of the NHS are not unique to district nursing and not new to nursing. It is evident that district nursing is not autonomous as it may appear because its decisions rely partly on medicine and partly on NHS management. However, this lack of absolute autonomy should not adversely affect quality care, as long as district nurses are aware that accountability includes all their actions related to caseload management, despite or notwithstanding bureaucracy in the system. Accountability implies that district nurses should have full control of their caseload management or care management, but this will only be possible if there is evidence that relevant strategies are credible in terms of care and that this is seen to be feasible to NHS management.

Delegation by numbers

Until relatively recently the service was top-heavy with qualified district nurses. The work was often equally spread out among a usually large team and although there was delegation of certain aspects of work, by and large caseload management was based on an artificial concept of equality (Smith et al 1993) and had more to do with numeration of cases than care management (Vignette 11.4).

The rationale for maintaining such inappropriate practices could relate to the traditional, work ethic of nursing (Melia 1987), task orientation stemming from a medical model approach (Jolley & Brykczynska 1993) or may have more to do with the quantification of nursing outcomes (Hodder & Gallagher 1998). There is a well-founded fear that within a quantified quality system, a reduced number of district nursing visits implies that the need for services is decreasing, rather than suggesting that the quality and depth of care are increasing. As the patient mix and care mix within the district nurse caseload have fundamentally changed over the last decade (Barrett & Hudson 1997, Groves 1997), district nurses should reclarify, at a local level, patient need in relation to skill mix in the context of quality professional care. The issue of caseload management and audit is also of relevance to district nursing's ability to make a decision about its future role; what it could do and what is not feasible for future practice.

To summarise this section, the traditional district nurse caseload was prescreened, assessments were simply to enquire how often, evaluations were often ineffective (Badger et al 1989, Luker & Kenrick 1992) and the service's proper use of its available human resources was questionable. Although the situation has changed considerably, the old system of caseload management is noteworthy in that it identifies those areas of work that may benefit from a considered and coherent strategy of care management.

TEAM NURSING

In district nursing, although one person is ultimately responsible for a caseload, care management is often based on a team approach. In team nursing patients may belong to an amalgamated caseload, managed by one (usually senior) district nurse and semi-managed by other qualified

---

Vignette 11.4   F Grade district nurse

I'm not sure what their rationale is for delegating care. It seems to be, 'Well, we've all got 10 patients so that's okay, isn't it'. What doesn't count is that you've got two assessments and three complex cases while someone else has got dressings and eye drops. I've tried to get them to look at patient dependency and caseload weighting but they're not interested – I don't know why. Things can get really bad if you've only got five or six patients as someone will inevitably add some extra patients to your list. Usually these are patients you don't know and so it takes a lot longer. I think I'm seen as a whinger or a skiver when I complain, as they say, 'Well, I've got the same as you'. If you can't get through your list it's seen as your fault – like you're inefficient. It wasn't like this in my last (DN) practice as the work was organised on skills, dependency, priorities and travelling time.

district nurses, a system similar to the traditional ways of managing a hospital ward. Other qualified and unqualified district nurses will provide support to the entire team and patient care will be delegated to all members of the team by the senior district nurse. Patient allocation may be randomised or geographically organised and this can cause problems in relation to continuity of care and in defining responsibility for individual patients or families. A further problem of team nursing is that although, through good delegation, skills may be used appropriately within the team, members of the team may be frustrated by a lack of overall responsibility for patients. Qualified district nurses working within this system may not use their leadership or management skills on a regular basis and may find that they are utilised as another pair of hands.

The potential benefits of team nursing include scope for engendering good working relationships that can help to support staff, especially those who are new to practice or undertaking care in difficult circumstances. Team care management could also encourage the emergence of team performance review to promote both staff development and the quality of patient care. Additionally district nurses practising team nursing may be able to transfer the experientially learnt skills of collaboration to other multidisciplinary teams. On a more basic level, team nursing enables the successful management of the 'problematic weekend' which other systems fail to address to any degree of satisfaction, though team nursing across a 24-hour day does seem to be a rather remote prospect.

Contrary to beliefs that district nursing has fully embraced primary nursing, anecdote suggests that team nursing is still the preferred way of managing care and this may be beneficial to the future of care management in district nursing, especially if lines of responsibility and accountability are clearly identified.

PRIMARY NURSING

Within this popular system of managing care, the primary nurse, as case holder, has 24-hour responsibility for planned care, for ensuring that the patient has been appropriately assessed and that the care has been appropriately planned (Manthey 1988). Both primary and associate nurses are responsible for the implementation of care and this means that in their absence, primary nurses are not responsible for the inadequate implementation or inappropriate delegation of care that has been properly planned.

Overall primary nursing appears to answer many of the problems associated with district nursing's lack of evident care management. At first glance, a recognised system of patient allocation within a broad clinical management system appeals and more so as district nursing may feel that it has been implementing a similar strategy (patient allocation in team nursing) for many years and so can easily adapt to primary nursing. Whether or not this is the case, primary nursing is an attractive concept as the importance of the nurse–patient relationship is stressed and it allows community staff nurses responsibilities similar to those which they have been used to in the acute sector. Additionally, primary nursing begins to answer some generic nurse management problems of responsibility and accountability that district nursing has not adequately answered. However, the individual professional responsibility for decision making associated with primary nursing (Manthey 1988) also raises concerns related to the isolated and largely unsupervised nature of district nursing work.

In many cases primary nursing in district nursing has allowed a reduction of qualified district nurses as the district nurse heads an increasingly large caseload that may be made up of a number of 'old' caseloads. Within this large caseload, smaller caseloads are delegated to the primary nurse who is more often than not an unqualified district nurse. Although theoretically caseload management and overall responsibility and accountability will still rest with the qualified district nurse, there is increasing anecdotal evidence that district nursing practice is insidiously moving toward a system where primary nurses (usually community staff nurses) have largely unsupervised responsibility for a caseload. This would be good news for nurse management, who would have a cheaper workforce and higher levels of devolved responsibility, and for some staff nurses who, as primary nurses, would relish the wider spectrum of care, greater professional autonomy and responsibility. It may not be such good news for the qualified district nurse with overall responsibility for an increasingly unwieldy caseload or for the mandatory district nurse qualification or, and most importantly, for the assurance of high-quality care (Vignettes 11.5 and 11.6).

One of the major concerns arising from the experiences of primary nursing in district nursing is that there is little evidence of evaluation and most studies have been carried out in the acute sector where the appropriateness of qualifications and direct supervision relates to a different practice in a different context. If district

nurses are to consider implementing a system of primary nursing, they should examine its potential benefits and question its applicability to district nursing practice (Boxes 11.1, 11.2 and 11.3).

Without doubt, primary nursing is the first organised system for managing district nursing care provision to all patients, though issues related to this system of singular professional

---

Box 11.1   Potential benefits of primary nursing

- Fosters individualised patient care
- Ensures a wider spread of tasks
- Increases individual autonomy and accountability
- Makes use of all nurses within district nursing

Box 11.2   Questions about primary nursing

- Is there a primary nurse or associate nurse on duty at all times?
- What are the qualifications required of the primary and associate nurse in district nursing?
- Do available resources (physical and human) act for or against increased responsibility and accountability?
- Is there a strategy (i.e. clinical supervision) in place to support primary nursing?
- Is the primary nurse able to be accountable through appropriate education and empowerment?
- Do district nursing hours allow for person-to-person (e.g. primary nurse to associate nurse) communication?
- Can primary nursing exist without a 24-hour continuous service?
- Can primary nursing be practised at weekends?
- Primary nursing – best for whom?

Box 11.3   Potential problems of primary nursing in district nursing

- Assessment and evaluation may be based on the primary nurse's previous (acute sector) care experiences
- Overinvolvement in long-term care situations
- Limit to the number of patients the primary nurse can safely be responsible for
- Caseloads are likely to be unequal in terms of patient dependency
- Does not encourage teamwork and cooperative practice
- Implications for accountability of the team leader/caseload holder, where primary nursing is largely unsupervised

---

Vignette 11.5   District nurse student

I was a primary nurse in the community for 2 years before coming on this course and I have always had my own caseload, admitting and discharging patients and only referring to a qualified district nurse if I felt out of my depth. I thought I was good at it. What I realise now is how little I knew.

I had most of the clinical skills, better than a lot of older nurses, but I didn't have the interpersonal skills or in-depth knowledge of the community. What is most worrying is that when you were talking about assessments taking 2 hours or more I thought you were talking some theoretical rubbish, as I could do an assessment in 20 minutes. I now know what I missed, what I didn't consider, my short comings and my tendency to be fast and slick, the quicker the better. Having observed and been involved in proper assessments carried out by qualified district nurses with experience and a wider range of skills than I could ever dream of, I realise that I was only skimming the surface.

Vignette 11.6   Community staff nurse

Well, you know they say that there's always a qualified district nurse on (duty) but that isn't always an active district nurse and could be a manager. I've been the most qualified, well, most experienced member of the team on at weekends and because we're all primary nurses we all do our own thing, admissions and so on. You don't ask for help from the manager on call and, well, you don't really ask for help from a qualified district nurse in another centre, cause you are a qualified nurse and should be able to cope.

responsibility should question not only who can manage care but also if care management should be an individual or a team responsibility.

HOSPITAL AT HOME

Although not systems of care management, hospital at home (HAH) schemes are relevant to care management in that the focus is on either preventing admission or enabling early discharge from hospital, the difference being that HAH patients are in need of health care. HAH had its origins in a 1961 French initiative 'hospitalisation a domicile' and by the 1970s UK projects were under way. The longest surviving and best known example of HAH is the Peterborough HAH scheme started in 1978 (King's Fund 1989). The push for HAH services was initiated by a number of factors including spiralling hospital costs and long waiting lists, the real and anticipated change in elder demography and the health risks of hospital admission (King's Fund 1989). Additionally, though perhaps of lesser importance, was the change in public expectations, particularly around choice and empowerment.

Of interest to district nursing is that the impetus for HAH arose within the acute sector (the gist of hospital at home) presuming that nursing at home care should be organised by experts in that speciality (i.e. orthopaedics). The early management of HAH was generally that of an outreach style of nursing service and this caused problems for district nurses (Dimond 1997) who were responsible for the care of ill patients at home and yet that care may have been instigated and managed by others. Outreach workers did not work in the community and were likely to have had limited knowledge about influencing community factors.

Although the management of present HAH schemes varies (Ross & Elliott 1995), many are now linked to district nursing. For instance, after referral to HAH a district nurse may be required to assess the patient before liaising with or referring on to the HAH scheme manager. HAH care is usually provided by a team of skilled and unskilled staff and bank nurses and, depending on the organisation of the scheme, district nurses may or may not continue to be involved with care. The district nurse may remain as care manager for the duration of the patient's stay on the HAH scheme.

Cooperative working practice within an incomplete integration of HAH and district nursing ensures that both services protect care provision to their patient group (although it should be noted that frequently the district nursing service supports patients on HAH schemes) and their own professional integrity. Full integration may be problematic in terms of prioritising patient needs, increasing workloads and losing dedicated budgets. This is particularly important to district nursing as patients receiving district nurse care are less likely to be considered care priorities (Shickle 1998) when competing against hospital waiting lists, blocked beds and consultant demand (King's Fund 1989). The issues that affect district nursing's involvement with HAH are similar to those that may affect its involvement with care management and district nurses may find it useful to consider how able or willing they are to manage a complete system of nursing care provision in the community.

Of specific interest to care management is that HAH schemes rely on concrete eligibility criteria (King's Fund 1989), otherwise the schemes would be chaotic and introduce unwanted risk to patients. An example of eligibility criteria is the confirmation of possible readmission to hospital should that be necessary (King's Fund 1989). The eligibility criteria used in HAH schemes may legitimately be compared with those used in care management for a considered evaluation of the ability of care management to provide safe optimum care in *all* situations.

The changing role of the district nurse

HAH schemes in the UK were designed to meet identified need and, interestingly, it was other professionals who moved quickly to fill subsequently identified gaps in community nursing provision, e.g. diabetic and cancer specialist nurses (Haste & MacDonald 1992). Although there were some questions asked about the lack of district nurse involvement in the specialist nurse services in the community (Murray & Canham 1989), district nurses appeared generally unmoved by these encroachments on their role (Haste & MacDonald 1992). Although the suggestion is that district nurses lacked initiative, it was NHS management that organised the introduction of the new specialist services outside the remit of district nursing and there was little or no consultation with practising district nurses before implementation.

The introduction of specialist nurses made some small change to the district nursing role but it was not until the Griffiths Report (Griffiths 1988), *Caring for people* (DHSS 1989) and eventually the NHS and Community Act 1990 that the first real threat was posed to district nursing's raison d'etre, its monopoly over care in the community. Other factors around this time were a direct result of general practitioner and primary care influence on district nursing and included the traditional assumptions of who does what (in district nursing) (NHSME 1992) and the influence of general practitioners as potential employers (Lewis & Glennester 1996). In short there was every reason to suggest that district nursing would have to change and that change would be imposed rather than arise as a result of professional consensus.

More recently, there has been evidence of much innovative practice (Ross & Elliott 1995) and district nurses have been involved with telephone triage, rapid response teams, community hospitals and nurse-led clinics (Dimond 1997, Smith et al 1993). However, despite the sheer number of innovative schemes, the district nurse has generally been utilised to provide a service and overall, these schemes have not been directed to improving or developing district nursing services. The significance of district nursing's unquestioning acceptance of change to its role in the context of overly directive management systems cannot be overstated in relation to the future of care management.

The whole scenario leading up to the implementation of the NHS and Community Care Act in April 1993 suggests that the management of care within district nursing had not been a process planned by district nursing to meet the needs of its client group. District nursing had deferred to others and, although useful to the NHS, it had not established any independent effectiveness in relation to how its management of care would meet the needs of patient groups, government or primary care.

CARE MANAGEMENT

Introduction

Although the ideology of community care is rarely disputed (Hadley & Clough 1996; Lewis & Glennester 1996), it has come to suggest something less than idealistic in that it is not care but a shift of containment based on economic resource management and a relocation of responsibilities. The relevance of the concept and policies of community care to care management is fundamental in that care management arose directly from the NHS and Community Care Act 1990.

Putting the NHS restructuring part of the NHS and Community Care Act 1990 firmly to one side, the community care element was partly a move to change an ineffective system into an efficiently managed system. Without doubt, there were problems within the existing social, mental health and physical health services, the system was inflexible, with an overall lack of accountability, and was paternalistic and professionally led (Audit Commission 1986, Ross & Tissier 1997) but also without doubt, community care is now no better off than it was preimplementation in 1993 and is in certain aspects worse (Hadley & Clough 1996). The overall impression is that before the NHS and Community Care Act 1990, care was provided on idealistic principles that may not always have been met, whereas now it is driven by economic principles that must be met (Lewis & Glennester 1996). Although some of the underlying principles of community care may be consistent with the philosophies of district nursing (i.e. patient and carer participation), not all aspects sit comfortably with individualised and interactive care based on need and an examination of the major points indicates that a degree of caution should be applied before welcoming care management as a beneficial development to district nursing practice.

Care management is a process and not a job, its intention being 'to make proper assessment and good care management the cornerstone of high-quality services' (NHS and Community Care Act 1990). The assessment and planning of care-managed services is focused on the individual client and/or carers with usually one Social Service department (SSD) team or individual being responsible for care management (Sines 1995). The essence of care management is similar to that of individualised patient care in that it is the process of 'tailoring services to individual needs' (DoH/SSI 1991) but it is explicit that care provision is by a range of services (Sines 1995).

The process of care management

Originally, care management had five main elements (DHSS 1989) though this has been extended to seven core tasks (see Box 11.4).

The immediate impression of these seven core tasks is that although there are some similarities with the management of care in district nursing, the care management process appears to be more clearly delineated. In fact, aside from the core

tasks and the necessity for some protocol to be in place, there was no direct government guidance as to how care management should be implemented and as a result, a variety of models have been adopted by SSDs (Bergen 1997).

The care management process appears to be more of a business strategy than a system for providing optimum care and this largely relates to the conception and inception of the NHS and Community Care Act 1990. The main focus of this was a review of public funds and, in particular, supplementary benefits for residential care which were to be curtailed by properly assessed and managed care. In other words, the previously unrestricted Social Security monies for private rest homes and nursing homes were to be strictly controlled. The focus on finance within the core tasks is thus to be expected. Local authorities were charged with the statutory responsibility for assessment that might lead to residential care. The assessment was to be needs led and result in packages of care similar to those studied earlier by the Personal Social Service Research Unit (PSSRU) (Challis & Davies 1986). Interestingly, as far back as 1979, district nurses were involved in schemes in Oxfordshire for the frail elderly and a number of similar collaborative schemes were shown to reduce admission to Part III (local authority accommodation (Baker et al 1987).)

Box 11.4 The seven core tasks of care management (DoH/SSI 1991)

1. Publishing information
   This may include plans for care management that are jointly agreed by the social and health services. Information may state the areas of responsibility and how much services cost service providers and users. This information should be made accessible to service users.

2. Determining appropriate level of assessment (see p. 195)

3. Assessing needs (see p. 195)

4. Care planning
   The care plan is likely to involve a number of other providers from the statutory services and voluntary and private sectors. Care planning is a resource-conscious exercise and the costed care plan will be authorised by (usually) a senior SSD manager before

implementation. The care plan should be agreed by users and providers.

5. Implementing the care plan
   Here the responsibility is to ensure that the care plan is implemented rather than to implement it. Implementation will include negotiating resources and the senior SSD manager ensuring that the necessary finances are secured.

6. Monitoring services
   The progress of care plan implementation is monitored by the care manager on an ongoing basis. Where necessary, the care plan is fine-tuned or reorganised.

7. Reviewing
   This is a formal process usually undertaken by the care manager at 6-monthly intervals.

In brief, the thinking behind the NHS and Community Care Act 1990, and specifically care management, centred on the premise that the care of the frail elderly could be successfully managed at home, with less cost to the state purse. However, it is accepted (Hadley & Clough 1996) that the planning and preparation for the NHS and Community Care Act 1990 by the Conservative government of the day was both underresearched and ill conceived. Although the care-managed projects in Kent, Gateshead and Darlington showed comparative cost effectiveness (Lewis & Glennester 1996), these studies focused on people who were on the verge of being admitted to long-term care and thus likely to benefit from packages of care provided in a community setting. The difference is now that care management is asked to consider extraordinary cases in ordinary circumstances and without the benefit of controlled evaluation (Hadley & Clough 1996). For instance, the early PSSRU projects utilised local informal carer support, but this has been problematic outside projects where issues of carer safety and education need serious professional consideration in terms of accountability, responsibility and possible litigation.

Whereas the concept of care management was almost entirely new to SSDs in 1989–90, individualised patient care was not new to district nursing. Likewise, the concept of the care manager as responsible for assessment and service coordination, tailoring help to meet individual needs, was seen as akin to elements of caseload management, primary nursing and HAH schemes. However, what was new and potentially difficult for district nurses to take on board was the budgeting responsibility and the additional focus on client enablement (though the conceptualisation of enablement as empowerment was later found to be erroneous) but this must be viewed in the context of how district nurse caseloads were managed before the NHS and Community Care Act 1990.

More specific district nurse concerns related to the issues of differentiating between health and social care and the fear for the well-being of the 'non-health' patient. The 1990 NHS and Community Care Act's lack of definition of either health care or social care caused rifts between SSDs and NHS trusts and, in at least one case, legal action (Tadd & Tadd 1998). SSDs and NHS Trusts had to quickly establish definitions of health and social care and although there may still be inevitable overlap, considering the interdependence of health and social issues (Ross & Mackenzie 1996), most eventualities are addressed within community care plans and eligibility criteria.

However, the social–health divide continues to cause some problems in the practice setting and in relation to referral from hospitals. Whereas clear cut medical-nursing referrals from hospital to community cause little concern, when the problem is social and health, the patient is likely to be assessed prior to discharge by a hospital-based social worker and the involvement of the district nurse in these assessments varies (Hadley & Clough 1996). Misunderstanding health problems, understating their importance and the potential impact of a seemingly minor health problem on the individual are some of the continuing concerns that district nurses raise about the social service assessment of health. Similarly, SSDs have concerns about the ability of others to assess the social aspects of care (Lewis & Glennester 1996).

The care manager

The role of the care manager within the NHS and Community Care Act 1990 is to assess, identify and deploy the services that are required for an individual client (Sines 1995). The NHS & Community Care Act did not specify who the care manager should be or what skills they should possess and within SSDs there seems to be no consensus (Lewis & Glennester 1996) though in most cases it is a person with acknowledged assessment skills, such as a social worker or home care organiser. Although the NHS and Community Care Act 1990 suggested that district nurses could, where appropriate, be care managers, individual SSDs have developed policies that may actively disbar district nurses from care management roles. However, there are a number of district nurses either working in SSDs as care managers and/or assisting the care management process (Dunderdale et al 1998, Ross & Elliott

1995) or working within the district nursing services and accepting care management responsibility with the (cautious) blessing of SSDs (Ross & Elliott 1995). Some local authorities (e.g. Rochdale) have determined that the care manager should be either 'the Practitioner who knows that client, user or carer best or the Practitioner with the most appropriate skills' (Rochdale Joint Care Planning Team 1994).

Enablers and brokers

SSDs within local authorities were to be enablers of community care and not primarily providers. This was supported by the government's insistence that 85% of the Special Transitional Grant (the monies to implement care management) went to independent bodies (i.e. private or voluntary care agencies). (This is viewed as a political move by the Conservative government of the day, particularly reflecting Margaret Thatcher's antipathy to local authorities (Lewis & Glennester 1996).) Additionally, the Audit Commission (1992) suggested that the care manager should be a purchaser and not a provider in order to reduce the potential conflicts of interest, in particular professional affiliations with care provision. Lewis & Glennester (1996) note that the intention implies that providers have a vested interest that could affect the objective assessment of need. Although the separation of assessor and provider is cited as one good reason why district nursing should not accept the care management role, Hadley & Clough (1996) argue that this separation is false and that in this kind of personal service, the work should be 'continuous and interactive'.

Although true to the spirit of social work, the concept of enablement caused much SSD concern, especially as enablement within the NHS and Community Care Act 1990 suggested a different translation of the concept: enablement as procurement and not as empowerment (Hadley & Clough 1996). Initially, traditional or innovative social work practice did try to address enablement as empowerment. However, as implementation of the Act took hold, the concept of enablement moved more toward brokerage

where care managers procure care for clients (Dimond 1997, Ross & Mackenzie 1996) and this may rightly be viewed as appropriate to the market mentality of the time.

The purchaser–provider dichotomy facing care managers in SSDs is immense (Hadley & Clough 1996, Lewis & Glennester 1996) and a similar dilemma will confront district nurses who either work in SSDs or who intend to be care managers within the district nursing services. The question is not simply how an individual district nurse can purchase, enable or broker care but whether district nursing per se wants to separate itself from the provision of care (Bergen 1992). It was noted earlier that district nursing was working toward care partnerships and the direct conflict between the concept of partnership and the conceptualisation of enablement as procurement (Lewis & Glennester 1996) is one that merits serious debate. Interestingly, there are increasing calls for district nursing to be involved in purchasing processes (Smith et al 1993) but this is largely seen as something district nurses can do well because they are also providers of care. (This particular issue centres on the purchaser requiring objective information about need and the provider subjectively and objectively knowing that need.)

Eligibility criteria

As the actual care management protocols and definitions of the care manager are partly local decisions, so eligibility criteria for care management are partly based on policy and then finalised by SSDs, usually in consultation with health authorities and NHS Trusts. The Audit Commission (1992) demanded that criteria for care management acceptance be clearly laid out and, controversially, that as resources were limited and could not outstrip need, eligibility criteria must screen out rather than screen in; 'a concept at odds with needs-based assessment' (Lewis & Glennester 1996). Additionally, eligibility criteria are set at various levels according to the client group; for instance, people who are HIV positive receive mainly DoH monies and this will be reflected within the eligibility criteria.

Continuing care (DoH 1995) has also had an effect on eligibility as the Department of Health stipulated NHS responsibilities for providing health care to specific target groups.

Working within Audit Commission and Department of Health guidance, SSDs will have established eligibility criteria for care management, often known as the care management target group. An example of a person fitting the criteria of a care management target group might be an elderly person with Parkinson's disease who is becoming increasingly dependent on an informal carer (Rochdale Joint Care Planning Team 1994). Each SSD will have similar eligibility criteria for care management and district nurses should contact their local SSD for relevant detail.

Assessment

Although the NHS and Community Care Act 1990 contains a right to assessment, it does not confer the right to have those assessed needs met. Additionally, the right to assessment is also very clearly focused on people who may need care management services (Lewis & Glennester 1996) and thus assessment for care management is not a universal right.

Whereas the theoretical relationship between individual need and a tailored care package is not questioned, there does appear to be some doubt about the ability of SSDs to develop that relationship (Nolan & Caldock 1996). For example, the gap between identified needs and available provision had led to SSDs devising ways to ensure that the documentation will not lead to litigation (Lewis & Glennester 1996); DoH advice is that assessment documentation should only include 'what is the least that is necessary to know' (DoH/SSI 1991). Generally, it is accepted that in care management there is a recognised difference between defined needs and eligible needs (Lewis & Glennester 1996) but although the assessment of need within care management may be considered to be anachronistic, it is the only way in which people with intense social-health need can gain access to costed services.

Care management assessment is considered to be a one-event procedure (even if carried

out over time) and is not a continuous process, as in district nursing. Most SSDs have three or four levels of assessment from which the screening 'assessment' is excluded.

Screening

At duty officer level, decisions are made through the referral documents as to what level of assessment should be implemented. There is a level of anticipation here which district nursing should recognise as being problematic; in other words, how is it possible to know without assessing that the person does not need assessment? However, within SSDs the screening process is to determine who would most likely not need to progress to Level II, care-managed assessment; this could include simple referrals for aids for living or a request for meals on wheels.

Simple assessment

This type of assessment is usually categorised as Level I and is not a care-managed assessment. It would most likely include the two examples given above or be a precursor to the core assessment.

Core assessment

This is normally considered a Level II assessment and is the basis of the care-managed assessment in which the needs of the client are identified and at least part of the core assessment form completed. The core assessment will elicit (most of) the information necessary to propose a care plan. It is explicit that the assessment for care management should be a participative process (Ross & Mackenzie 1996) though this may not always be realised in practice.

Complex assessment

This type of assessment is generally categorised as Level III and invariably involves other agencies, although the logistics of bringing all relevant agencies together for one assessment event is often unrealistic. At this level, a district nurse may be asked to participate in the complex assessment or may undertake a separate specialist assessment of a client if a health needs deficit is suspected. As in the specialist assessment, the district nurse needs to be able to make decisions about the appropriateness or ability of the district nursing service to provide care.

Specialist assessment

This assessment may be considered to be Level IV or may fall into the Level III category. It is the type of assessment with which district nurses are most frequently involved and may take place in the patient's home or in a secondary care setting. The assessment is either to contribute to the care plan and to gain access to appropriate resources or to confirm the client's inability to be care managed within his own home. As its name suggests, it requires the specialist, expert opinion of the district nurse, yet all too often anecdote suggests that this level of assessment is delegated (by district nurses) to an unqualified district nurse. Specialist assessments may be problematic to SSDs if district nurses (or other specialist services) are reluctant or show a lack of urgency toward the process and in these cases, specialist nursing assessments will by necessity be taken on board by the SSD (Lewis & Glennester 1996).

The specialist assessment document will only request specific information relating to the specialism as other more general details and information relating to other agencies will have been undertaken previously or simultaneously. The assessment form may be only one page, depending on the SSD, and this should be considered in relation to the previous levels of assessment and not that health needs are considered to be of lesser importance. District nurses may find it useful to obtain care-managed specialist assessment information from their local SSD before they are asked to be involved in the process.

Budget holding

Although the initial thoughts stemming from Challis & Davies (1986) were that budgets should be held by care managers, in reality this has not occurred (Lewis & Glennester 1996) and in the main budgets are held at senior SSD level (Bergen 1992). This senior SSD manager is able to commission or purchase services more efficiently than a single budget holder would be able to do (Ross & Tissier 1997) and although the care manager has the budget responsibility to purchase provision on behalf of clients, authorisation comes from the senior SSD manager. (This is similar to the way in which continuing care (DoH 1995) budgets are managed in district nursing.)

There are two inherent problems in this system: first for the practitioner, in that professional assessment may be at odds with budget constraints, and second for the organisation, in that non-budget holding practitioners may be overly liberal in their assessment of needs, thereby defeating the purpose of the exercise.

As financial assessment and budgeting is a major issue within care management, local authorities, through SSDs, may be reluctant to allow district nurses (as care managers) to have direct access to LA/SSD funds though there are examples of district nurses, either working in SSDs or working collaboratively with SSDs, having access to the care management budget (Bergen 1992, Dunderdale et al 1998, Ross & Elliott 1995).

Documentation

One of the outcomes of the NHS and Community Care Act 1990 was that SSDs had their documentation in good working order by April 1993 as the provider workforce was to be largely unqualified and needed clear, explicit documents (Hadley & Clough 1996). However, the negative aspect is that paperwork relating to budgeting and financial assessment has grown out of all proportion and has increased the bureaucracy of SSDs, to the dissatisfaction of social workers (Hadley & Clough 1996). Even given district nursing's propensity to ever increase the quantity of its documentation, the sheer weight of SSD documentation is awesome and should be considered as a serious constraint to a provider service (Dunderdale et al 1998). The documentation in care management does appear to have more to do with a paperwork exercise than assessment, in that although it is complex it is relatively limited in relation to the philosophy of professional assessment. As noted earlier, this does need to be considered in relation to the aims of the NHS and Community Care Act 1990.

Quality

The 85% Special Transitional Grant rule resulted in the increase of unqualified workforces in the private community care sector. These workforces are also low paid and it is hardly surprising when their ability to provide more than simple care tasks is questioned. To district nurses without a care management role or district nurses largely divorced from the working of SSDs, this is a contentious issue as district nurses can see gaps in social care that they know they previously would have met. Quality issues such as policy implementation, training and education appear to be met piecemeal within the voluntary and private agencies and the ability of SSDs to ensure quality within such agencies is problematic (Dimond 1997, Hadley & Clough 1996). Hadley & Clough suggest that most private and voluntary agencies have little preparation and lack the appropriate management experience to take on the task of care provider.

Collaboration and cooperation

One of the reasons put forward for the NHS and Community Care Act 1990 was that service provision was fragmented and concerns have been raised for many years about the lack of cooperative working practices (DHSS 1989, Dalley 1990). Unfortunately the Act may have resulted in movement from indirect cooperation and agreement of services to competition and confrontation (Hadley & Clough 1996), especially in the continuing social – health divide debate agitated by separate budgets for SSDs and NHS trusts.

At the practitioner level, reasons for a lack of collaboration are categorised by Dalley (1990) as competing professional ideologies and tribal and cultural differences. These differences are rarely explicated to the other groups and remain a matter for internally expressed discontent directed toward the outsiders. Each group has the same but different problems with themselves and each other and it is pointless to suggest that any one group should change to accommodate another or that all groups should homogenise. What is more realistic is that all groups should understand their differences and concentrate on removing tribalism, without threatening role erosion.

Roles and responsibilities in social work and district nursing have been subject to over a decade of change and concerns have been expressed regarding role boundaries. In 1992 Bergen noted that community nurses and social workers needed preparation, training, support and supervision if they were to work together successfully and although this has not occurred to any great degree, it appears that workers from these two agencies have begun to devise their own ways of cooperating. Increased collaboration at the grass roots level (Lewis & Glennester 1996) is usually through informal and formal meetings and although this is helpful, district nurses (and social workers) should seriously consider working through differences and similarities together (see Box 11.5) if they are to enable true collaboration in practice.

Box 11.5   Collaborative practice: issues for discussion

- How are the organisations managed?
- What are the geographical limitations of practices?
- What are the procedures of the organisations?
- How are standards set and monitored?
- What are the roles and responsibilities of staff?
- What is the working environment like?
- What are the channels of communication?
- How does communication work in out-of-hours emergencies?
- What is the work ethic?
- What are the attitudes toward patients/clients/other workers/the organisation?
- How are practice concepts expressed?
- Is there a unique practice language?
- Are there any shared values?
- What are the areas for possible conflict?
- Is there a possibility for joint education?
- Can students cross boundaries to learn about other practices?
- Is there the potential for joint documentation?
- What are the lines of accountability?
- Is there the possibility of shadowing?

Collaboration is not simply an ideological concept but a practical concern to avoid duplication, repetition and the inappropriate use of services. Collaboration in this sense means working together in joint or shared enterprises and not sleeping with the enemy. It is about true professionalism and a real concern for the patient or client.

Change in social work role

Change to the social work role as a result of care management policy appears widespread and if UK society were to require increasing expert social work intervention, it may well find this shelved to make room for care management. As social workers become more focused on the legal principles of care management, other community health workers are doing what social workers did, particularly in relation to active case work (Hadley & Clough 1996).

One of the casualties of care management has been early preventive work, with most SSDs acting only on crisis intervention (Hadley & Clough 1996). This shift in role emphasis has left social workers in the position where they have few active cases as they act primarily as assessors before providing a care plan for implementation by others. There appears to be a general consensus that care-managed cases only remain active in the planning and evaluation phases (Lewis & Glennester 1996) and that care management has become a 'hit and run' activity. Even within the care management process, Hadley & Clough (1996) note that the need for a qualified social worker is being questioned as the financial focus of assessment negates the need for social work skills. The nature of professional roles in care management may in time return to that envisaged by Challis & Davies (1986) but in the interim district nurses may be wise to heed the experiences of their social work colleagues.

Implications of care management for district nursing

If district nurses were to take on the care management role within the remit of the NHS and Community Care Act 1990 or adopt a care management strategy based on the principles of the Act, district nursing could also lose its traditional identity (Bergen 1992). District nursing continues to appeal as it 'goes back to the patient' (Mackenzie 1992) and permits the district nurse to provide high-quality and specialist care within a series of intense, temporary or long-term relationships (McMurray 1993) where loss and grief are experienced by all parties when the partnership ends by death or recovery (Ong 1991). The district nurse uses high-level interpersonal skills to develop and maintain these relationships for the purpose of delivering quality care. Within a structured care management system, qualified district nurses are likely to lose that nurse–patient intimacy and there should be no illusions that less experienced carers will be providing more direct care.

Of specific interest is that the highly organised and widely used systems of caseload management and care management are not synonymous with the management of care for patients. Case or care is not insignificant in that cases are impersonal but easy to organise, while care is personal,

---

Vignette 11.7   District nurse practice educator

It's funny but you tend to forget that you are setting up a syringe driver or redressing a nasty burn or taking blood as these things are on automatic pilot. What you think about very carefully is what you are saying and the impact you will have on this person or this family. You are looking for clues as to why they are so tense or if they are not telling you how they really feel. You spend more time counselling than doing health education. When you come out of the house it can be a surprise to realise how much you have actually done and certainly the psychomotor skills are not as important to me as interpersonal skills. Without them you would never get anywhere. I remember a very shocked student asking me why I was so lax in one house. It was because I had taken weeks to get my foot in the door and pushing too much on them too quickly might have made the door close on me forever. The patient was dying and lived with her son who was on heroin and dealing. The conditions were pretty awful but she wanted to die there and the son wanted to care for her. I had to adjust my care to them and yes, it was less than perfect, but she died well and the son did care for her. I couldn't have let them do that if I was less experienced. My decision was based on professional judgement and I knew and was comfortable that I was accountable for my actions.

fragile and dependent on human interactions. Although district nursing is a complex combination of clinical and interpersonal skills, lay and quality audit assumptions are that skilled nursing care relates primarily to psychomotor skills, possibly as these are relatively easy to define, capture and quantify. In reality, functional district nursing skills may be secondary to the main objective of promoting an appropriate environment for providing care, through the development of partnerships (Vignette 11.7), and the real needs of patients and carers may be overshadowed by a preoccupation with a purely functional approach.

The management of care in district nursing

The apparent maintenance role of the district nurse was dramatically changed by the implementation of the NHS and Community Care Act in 1993 and Barrett & Hudson (1997) note that although district nurses' patients are generally less dependent as a direct result of losing highly dependent social – health care patients, the caseload requires more skilled nursing input. Alongside care management and the reshaping of the NHS, district nursing has also been affected by other modernising health strategies such as minimal access surgery. This situation suggests that the present (and future) situation will contradict previous claims made by the Audit Commission's Value for Money Unit (NHSME 1992) on the required skill mix in district nursing and that, as noted previously, district nurses need to reclarify patient need and district nurse interventions (Vignette 11.8).

The infinite nature of the district nurse caseload (Hadley & Clough 1996) is of relevance to district nursing's ability to take on additional cares, services and the care management role, especially in the light of SSDs difficulties, even when waiting lists are commonplace. District nursing does not normally operate a waiting list system and the caseload is thus infinite. This, when combined with iller patients, has implications for district nursing's ability to radically develop the range of cares. District nurses' work within the NHS and Community Care Act 1990 has been additional to existing responsibilities for care (Cain et al 1995,

Ross & Tissier 1997) and although this willingness is admirable, it may be less than desirable within a focused professional service.

Although the suggestion is that district nursing is too willing to accept others' strategies and too amenable to unplanned change, this inherent flexibility may be an advantage if district nurses are able to do so while still maintaining the integrity of their main work (Bergen 1992). A clear articulation of the nature of district nursing will assist practitioners to determine for themselves how care should best be managed within the existing and future health services. A coherent, credible and feasible strategy for care management in district nursing should utilise the best and reject the evidently problematic aspects of traditional and contemporary models. However, no strategy will work unless district nurses possess the skills, knowledge and attributes (see Box 11.6) to develop and maintain a care management system.

Vignette 11.8   G Grade district nurse

Control has been taken away from the DN and collectively they are expected to do things that individually they would not. This means filling in for social workers and physios when they have staff shortages. We never ask anyone else to do our work. We need to be more focused on health.

Box 11.6   Knowledge, skills and attributes for care management

- Specialist clinical skills to know what care is necessary and the internal and external issues that may help or hinder care provision.
- Leadership skills that enable the team to work constructively, playing the same tune; includes communication, staff development and support.
- Management skills: budgeting, planning, organising, information sharing and gathering. The willingness to be involved in decision making and risk taking.
- Teaching, educative and facilitative skills to foster an appetite for lifelong learning and to demonstrate how appropriate education can improve nurse–patient partnerships.
- Interpersonal skills to listen, communicate and relate within the DN team and in the broader teams and to demonstrate by example how nurse–patient partnerships work.

Conclusion

It is clear that the first 6 years of care management have not been trouble free and that the system is flawed by a number of factors including the lack of appeal to professional values and the dictatorial manner of its implementation. The lack of relevant research related to primary nursing questions its applicability in the professional practice of district nursing, while caseload management throws up visions of case versus care and quantity versus quality. Nevertheless, all these systems have something to say about the nature of care management in district nursing, even if that evolves through a consideration of the problematic.

There can be no doubt that the community will continue to need skilled district nursing care and to ensure that care is provided equitably, professionally and sensitively, there is a need for care management strategies that appeal to practitioners, managers and patients. It would go against the grain for this chapter to suggest to district nurses how they should manage their care; specialist practitioners should not rely on others to set the future parameters of care. District nurses should be able to determine for themselves a suitable strategy for care management that is cost effective, accessible, feasible and able to be evaluated in both quantitative and qualitative terms but, above all, that has practitioner ownership so that district nurses can feel passionate about its potential success.

REFERENCES

Audit Commission 1986 Making a reality of community care. HMSO, London
Audit Commission 1992 Community care: managing the cascade of change. HMSO, London
Badger F, Cameron E, Evers H 1989 District nurses' patients – issues of case load management. Journal of Advanced Nursing 14: 518–527
Baker G, Bevan J M, McDonnell L, Wall B 1987 Community nursing: research and recent developments. Croom Helm, London
Barrett G, Hudson M 1997 Changes in district nursing workload. Journal of Community Nursing 11 (3): 4,6,8
Bergen A 1992 Case management in community care: concepts, practices and implications for nursing. Journal of Advanced Nursing 17: 1106–1113
Bergen A 1997 The role of community nurses as care managers. British Journal of Community Health Nursing 2 (10): 466–474
Cain P, Hyde V, Howkins E 1995 Community nursing: dimensions and dilemmas. Edward Arnold, London
Challis D, Davies B 1986 A more comprehensive approach to the care of the elderly: the community care approach. Personal Social Services Research Unit, University of Kent
Dalley G 1990 Collaboration. In: Hughes J (ed) Community health care: enhancing the quality of community nursing. King's Fund Centre, London
Department of Health 1990 NHS and Community Care Act, DoH, London
Department of Health 1992 The patient's charter. DoH, Leeds
Department of Health 1994 Hospital discharge workbook: a manual on hospital discharge practice. DoH, Leeds
Department of Health 1995 NHS responsibilities for meeting continuing health care needs. DoH, Leeds
Department of Health 1997 The new NHS: modern, dependable. HMSO, London

Department of Health and Social Security 1989 Caring for people: community care in the next decade and beyond. HMSO, London
Department of Health: Social Services Inspectorate 1991 Care management and assessment – a practitioner's guide. DoH, Leeds
Department of Health: Social Services Inspectorate 1995 Report of the National Inspection of Social Services Department. Arrangements for the discharge of older people from hospital to residential or nursing home care. DoH, Leeds
Dimond B 1997 Legal aspects of care in the community. Macmillan, Basingstoke
Dunderdale N, Pink H, Caan W 1998 Aiming for the goal with a foot in both camps. Journal of Community Nursing 12 (5): 10, 12
Griffiths R 1988 Community care: agenda for action. HMSO, London
Griffiths J M, Luker K 1994 Intraprofessional teamwork in district nursing: in whose interest? Journal of Advanced Nursing 20: 1038–1045
Groves E 1997 Adult care. In: Skidmore D (ed) Community care: initial training and beyond. Edward Arnold, London
Hadley R, Clough R 1996 Care in chaos: frustration and challenge in community care. Cassell, London
Haste F H, MacDonald L D 1992 The role of the specialist in community nursing: perceptions of specialist and district nurses. International Journal of Nursing Studies 29 (1): 27–47
Hodder P, Gallagher A 1998 Standard-setting. In: Chadwick R, Levitt M (eds) Ethical issues in community care. Edward Arnold, London
Jolley M, Brykczynska G 1993 Nursing: its hidden agendas. Edward Arnold, London
King's Fund 1989 Hospital at home: the coming revolution. King's Fund Centre Communication Unit, London

Lewis J, Glennester H 1996 Implementing the new community care. Open University Press, Buckingham

Luker K, Kenrick M 1992 An exploratory study of the sources of influence on the clinical decisions of community nurses. Journal of Advanced Nursing 17: 457–466

Mackenzie A 1992 Learning from experience in the community: an ethnographic study of district nurse students. Journal of Advanced Nursing 17: 682–691

McMurray A 1993 Community health nursing: primary health care in practice. Churchill Livingstone, Melbourne

Manthey M 1988 The practice of primary nursing. Blackwell Science, Boston

Melia K 1987 Learning and working: the occupational socialisation of nurses. Tavistock, London

Murray C, Canham J 1989 The community specialist. Journal of District Nursing 8(6): 10–12

NHSME: Value for Money Unit 1992 Skill mix in the district nursing service. HMSO, London

Nolan M, Caldock K 1996 Assessment: identifying the barriers to good practice. Health and Social Care in the Community 4 (2): 77–85

Ong B N 1991 Researching needs in district nursing. Journal of Advanced Nursing 16: 638–647

Rochdale Joint Care Planning Team 1994 Level 4: inter-agency care management assessment of complex needs for implementation by all agencies. Unpublished policy document, Rochdale MBC Social Services Department, Town Hall, Rochdale

Ross F, Elliott M (eds) 1995 Innovations in primary health care nursing. Community and District Nursing Association UK, Edinburgh

Ross F, Mackenzie A 1996 Nursing in primary health care: policy into practice. Routledge, London

Ross F, Tissier J 1997 The care management interface with general practice. Health and Social Care in the Community 5(3): 153–161

Shickle D 1988 Rationing of health care: why do acute hospital services have higher priority? In: Chadwick R, Levitt M (eds) Ethical issues in community care. Edward Arnold, London

Sines D (ed) 1995 Community health care nursing. Blackwell Science, Oxford

Smith P, Mackintosh M, Towers B 1993 Implications of the new NHS contracting system for the district nursing service in one health authority: a pilot study. Journal of Interprofessional Care 7(2): 115–124

Tadd W, Tadd V 1998 Concepts of community. In: Chadwick R, Levitt M (eds) Ethical issues in community care. Edward Arnold, London

Worth A 1998 Ethical issues in the discharge of patients from hospital to community care. In: Chadwick R, Levitt M (eds) Ethical issues in community care. Edward Arnold, London

12

Management of change

Sue Plummer

Key points

- Why change?
- Culture – what it is, why it is and its importance in change
- The change process
- Attitudes, pressures and behaviour in times of change
- Common elements in securing agreement to change
- The personal impact of change
- Change as a source of stress

INTRODUCTION

Change is not made without inconvenience, even from worse to better.

This quote, taken from the writings of Richard Hooker (1554?–1600) and cited by Johnson in the preface to the *Dictionary of the English Language* (1775), neatly sums up the essence of change: that it always carries a cost, even when the outcome is improvement.

The world in which we live is continuously in change; change in relationships between our organisations and others, in the character and culture of organisations. Change between members of our organisations and in work patterns. Change in the dominant norms and values governing society, in the make-up of 'haves' and 'have nots'. These changes impact on us at a personal level and affect our working lives. We have to learn to be both proactive and reactive in responding to these changes which make demands on our time and skills and often involve taking on new roles and responsibilities.

As recipients, initiators and managers of change, district nurses must learn to take an optimistic view of it and look at the opportunities offered. They must look for ways to increase the gains and reduce the real or perceived losses. To do this, district nurses must understand the change process and the factors that influence their own attitude and behaviour towards it, and that of others.

The ways in which people change are best explained by reference to social cognitive theory as developed by Bandura (1986). The assumptions of the theory are that: people make conscious choices about their behaviours; the information they use to make their choice comes from their environment; their choices are based on the things that are important to them, the perception they have of their ability to behave in certain ways and the consequences they think will flow from the choice they make. The more desirable the outcome, the more likely it is that people will engage in the behaviour they believe will lead to it. The more confident a person is that he can assume a new behaviour, the more likely he is to try it. Despite this, even when the benefits of change seem clear and appear to outweigh potential costs and the behaviours required seem achievable, there will be people who react negatively to it and who will resist it.

Understanding why these differences in attitudes and behaviour occur is the first step in planning to manage a change programme and achieve the goal of changing a questioning or seemingly obstructive attitude into a commitment to change. This chapter looks at some of the factors that affect people's perception of change and their consequent behaviour.

When planning any work programme, it is often helpful to break the whole picture down into its component parts. The change effort should be approached in the same way. There are key questions that have to be asked and answered at each stage of the process by those involved. To neglect these questions is to risk limiting the chance of successful implementation of the change. This chapter considers what these questions are and the approaches that may be used to get answers to them.

Beckhard & Harris (1987) describe resistance as 'a normal part of the change process'. Rather than viewing this as an unduly pessimistic statement which becomes a self-fulfilling prophecy, it should be used as the catalyst to thinking and discussion of the potential barriers and sources of resistance. By being prepared, the effects of these 'hitches' can be planned for and managed more effectively. Some tried and tested approaches to the successful management of resistant behaviour are therefore outlined.

Change can be exciting, a time of high energy and anticipation of improvements to come. For some, however, it can bring worry about security of employment, doubts over competence in the envisaged new environment, fear of the true 'costs' of the change. It also requires an increase in the capacity to accept disruption. District nurses have to manage this on a personal level and in their dealings with patients and their families. The stress that results from change, at whatever level, can be significant and can have a detrimental effect on health. It is important that district nurses are equipped to not only recognise the warning signs of 'overload', in themselves and others, but also to suggest ways of dealing with the more negative elements of some change efforts. We will look briefly at some of the coping mechanisms that can be employed to reduce or dilute the stress that sometimes accompanies change.

WHY CHANGE?

When we try to bring about change in our societies, we are treated first with indifference, then with ridicule, then with abuse and then with oppression. And finally, the greatest challenge is thrown at us: we are treated with respect. This is the most dangerous stage.

This quote, which expands a well-known statement by Mahatma Gandhi, is taken from a speech made by Ariyaratne (1983) at an international community leadership summit. Ariyaratne is one of the world's most successful community organisers and his words remind us that it is easier to begin initiatives than to realise enduring change. The stage at which change leaders are treated with respect is the most dangerous because it is then that they, and others, can believe that the work is finished. In fact, this is usually just the starting point.

The drivers of change are multifaceted. Many lie outside our immediate sphere of influence. Those political, economic, social and technological developments that we often welcome for the improvements they bring also engender feelings of concern over the real or perceived 'costs' to ourselves and others. The technological advances, for example, that have led to enormous improvements in many areas of our lives have often resulted in reductions in the size and/or location of the workforce, with consequent economic and social costs for many in society. We live in an age where premature death from previously common conditions has become a thing of the past. The corollary of this is that we now have an increasing number of dependent people to be cared for and the associated economic and social costs to be considered and catered for.

Some of the drivers for change are 'internal' to a team or organisation. Again, these may include the size and skills required of the workforce, the style of leadership needed, the direction in which the organisation is moving and the culture it exemplifies, changes in roles and responsibilities within the team. District nursing has experienced, and will continue to experience, examples of many of these changes. The shift in emphasis to a primary care-centred service, the increasing focus on keeping people in their own homes and the early discharge of patients from hospital care have led to changes in the complexity and size of workload managed by district nurses and in the skills and knowledge they need to perform their role effectively.

Self-managed teams are one example of a response to the challenges imposed by these changes. The shift to self-management demands a change in culture and working practice, with many of the functions traditionally carried out by nurse managers being assumed by the nursing team.

Similarly, the new direction for the health service is one of partnership working, with collaboration replacing competition. Health service staff have to 'unlearn' the behaviours and attitudes associated with the market-oriented culture built around the Thatcher-led policies geared to 'rolling back the state' (Ranade 1994). Trying to teach old dogs new tricks is not always easy, even when they want to learn, and it is made more difficult when the learning curve is steep and the deadline short.

The agenda for us all is about multiple challenges, stretching aspirations and ambiguous issues. The dilemma in this turbulent environment is how to maintain the stability needed to allow everyday work to continue and at the same time adapt to outside forces, stimulate innovation, change assumptions and often change the culture of the organisation itself.

The one certainty about change is its inevitability. It is therefore important to understand it and to learn to manage it, and help others to manage it, effectively. Fundamental to understanding the change process is an awareness of why the change is necessary. The next section looks at the questions that should be addressed by those proposing the change. Unfortunately, they are often ignored, sometimes because people simply don't know what the questions are, sometimes because they don't want to know the answers.

Should we be doing this?

The endpoint of any change process should be improvement of the current position. However, people and organisations sometimes get so caught up with initiatives that they don't link them to a goal; some don't even have a goal. The golden rule is: if the change doesn't offer benefit, think carefully about the need to do it. There are plenty of things that will add value that can be pursued without wasting time and effort on initiatives of dubious value.

When deciding whether a change is 'right', one should question its organisational, ethical, social and economic desirability and cultural feasibility and address these issues from the perspective not only of those proposing the change but of those who will be affected by it. The example of the 1998 changes in the organisation of the health service can be used to demonstrate this.

The key themes underpinning the Labour government's policies on the health service are cooperation and partnership working. This would seem to fit with the service and collectivist ethos of the National Health Service. However, since 1989 the NHS has been configured to meet the demands of a market-oriented system based around contracting. Staffing of the system, the processes put in place, the cultures fostered in organisations all focused on what was needed to service this environment.

This organisational set-up no longer fits with the new order. The new messages demand a radical shift away from the market culture and its associated behaviours to a more inclusive, collaborative environment. Discussion and joint working are now the name of the game, with clinical involvement in all appropriate decision making. The old bureaucracies are to be broken down in an effort to remove what are perceived as unnecessary layers of administration between clinicians and patients. The new working arrangements have a direct impact on a large number of people who were recruited because their skills and aptitudes were those wanted in the purchaser/provider environment. Many may make the journey into the new world, some may choose not to try. For others, the decision may be made for them, their culture and style simply having no place in the new picture. So, while the change may be desirable from an organisational and economic perspective and may be culturally feasible, the social costs are likely to be high.

Another example, which will be familiar to district nurses, is the introduction of nurse prescribing (Chapter 8). If this change is tested against the above framework it comes out rather well. Prescribing systems are already well established in the UK to support prescribing by medical and dental colleagues. The changes needed to allow for the administration of nurse prescribing are relatively small. Organisationally, once training programmes have been drawn up and approved and the necessary funding

arrangements agreed, the roll-out of the scheme should be unhampered by problems. The staff are in place, the universities are geared up to providing the training needed for nurse prescribing, the validating and regulatory bodies are in situ and prescribing monitoring systems well established.

Although there were initially concerns in some quarters about the potential impact of nurse prescribing on the overall prescribing budget, the evidence so far has not borne this out. Most prescribing appears to be substitute prescribing and has not therefore incurred significant increased costs. This may of course change if or when the range of prescribable items is expanded, but at the moment the change is economically sound.

In terms of costs and benefits to patients, the costs are very low but the gains high. Although very limited to date, work does suggest that patients are positive and encouraging about the change. They welcome, for example, the lack of delay in issuing a prescription for dressings that is part of the process when the nurse has to ask the GP to prescribe a given item.

Culturally the change fits well with the teamwork models that the new NHS is expected to demonstrate, where best and most appropriate use is made of people's skills and experience. Patients, nurses and their medical colleagues recognise that in many instances the change has merely legitimised age-old practice, where the nurse told the doctor what was needed for a patient and why and the prescription was issued by the doctor on the basis of his confidence in the nurse's ability to make the correct judgement.

Not all changes will be so clearcut. In many cases, there is an equal balance in each area in terms of costs and benefits. A decision then has to be made about which issue is the most important, how much of a risk can be taken in implementing the change and accepting the consequences or, alternatively, risking the consequence of *not* changing. Cultural feasibility may in some instances be the deciding factor. The dominant culture of a family, group or organisation can help, hinder or completely block any change effort and therefore it is important that district nurses appreciate and understand its significance.

We have all been in situations where we have not given enough, if any, consideration to the cultural framework within which other people operate. We have all embarked on proposed change programmes for the right reasons and with the best of intentions but, in an effort to get results, rushed ahead with the implementation plan before doing the groundwork. A very necessary part of this groundwork is understanding the 'norms' and values of those one is working with and accepting that they may be very different from one's own. Barriers often go up when trying to initiate change because the questions being asked by those proposing the change are not understood by those targeted by it. Work with people from ethnic minority groups has shown, for example, that questions posed by health-care professionals are often not understood by the target 'audience'. This is not because of language difficulties but because the question simply does not make sense in cultural terms.

Because culture is such an important element in all change programmes, it is worth devoting time to looking at this vague term and somewhat ambiguous phenomenon.

CULTURE – WHAT IT IS, WHY IT IS AND ITS IMPORTANCE IN CHANGE

Culture is an organisation's body language. It has been described as 'the way we get things done around here' (Bower 1966). More formally, culture is the set of artefacts, beliefs, values, norms and ground rules that define and significantly influence how the organisation operates (Box 12.1). For organisation, read family, team, group. It can be affected by powerful individuals within the structure and is sometimes used as a means of control. The culture of any organisation pervades everything that happens within it, affecting the 'dominant logic' of the surroundings. This in turn influences leadership styles, orientation, the decision-making models operating within the organisation or group, how success is measured and how members treat each other.

Interest in the culture of organisations peaked in the 1980s when a link was suggested between culture and success (Peters & Waterman 1982).

Box 12.1 The four elements that constitute the culture of an organisation (Trice & Beyer 1984)

- *Company practices*
  Annual awards scheme, social gatherings

- *Communications*
  How members of the 'tribe' communicate and express themselves. It may be through stories, sagas or symbols and slogans. Witness the logos adopted by NHS trusts.

- *Physical cultural factors*
  Senior staff dining rooms, for example, or the starched aprons and silver buckles once so loved by nurses.

- *Common language*
  The modes of internal communication and the language used. Health-care professionals often 'protect' their difference by using professional 'jargon'.

Cultures which promote innovation, teamwork and commitment were seen as the secret of the success enjoyed by many companies. Some of this work has since been discredited but there is no doubting the significance of culture on the behaviour of an organisation. Equally, there is no doubt that culture is difficult to understand and one should never underestimate the Herculean effort needed to change it.

Handy (1985) describes four cultures: power culture, role culture, task culture and person culture.

Power culture

This is often drawn as a web, with a central source of power and rays of influence spreading from this point. There are few rules or procedures and little bureaucracy in this culture where control is exercised by a central elite. This central group will do everything personally if they can. If those at the centre of the web are 'weak' in any way, the whole team/organisation will be weakened.

In the power culture, size is important. The web can break if too many activities are linked; it therefore usually thrives where there is a small number of people. This environment is rich in personality and is an exciting place to be if you are in the elite group and share the beliefs of the spider at the centre of the web, less comfortable if this is not the case.

The power culture is able to respond immediately and intuitively to opportunities and crises because of the short lines of communication and centralisation of power. People who are power-oriented, politically minded risk-takers who rate security as of little importance thrive in this environment. Some clubs and primary health-care teams display a power culture.

Role culture

The structure of this organisation will be pyramidal, composed of boxes filled with job titles. These 'job boxes' will be joined together purely to get the work done. The emphasis is on functional strength and there are processes for everything. These processes are coordinated at the top by a narrow band of senior managers.

The role culture is seen where working practices are governed by the need to ensure that a given set of tasks is carried out on time: ensuring that scheduled payments are made on the correct dates, for example. Job descriptions are tightly defined and there is little room, or need, for creativity or individuality. Role occupants, not individualists, are required.

Some people like this culture because they know exactly what is expected of them, what they have to do, how they have to do it and when. There are no 'gaps' or room for ambiguity.

This culture is typically slow to perceive the need to change, sometimes with unfortunate results.

Task culture

A net depicts the task culture. It is job, or project, oriented and is often seen in a matrix organisation. The emphasis is on getting the job done, making best use of the skills and resources available. Influence is based on the level of expertise. It is a team-based culture where there are no hard boundary lines and working practices reflect respect for each team member's different contributions. People are encouraged to take the lead because their skills fit with the demands of the goal to be achieved rather than because of status or position within the team or organisation.

This environment demands commitment. It wants people who are self-confident, forward looking, constantly working on new challenges. It is a questioning culture, which chafes at routine. The team demonstrates extensive cross boundary working both inside and outside the organisation.

This is the type of culture that most of us probably feel we should strive to achieve and think that we would like to work in. It looks attractive. The emphasis on 'allowing' people to use their skills most appropriately and to fulfil their potential is very important in terms of job satisfaction and personal and professional development. The task culture is not all roses, though.

The team or organisation that displays a task culture can be a very uncomfortable place because of the constant drive to question, to challenge, to improve, to change. People working in this environment need to have the confidence and stamina to keep up with the pace and scale of change, both of which can be quite punishing.

Person culture

This can be drawn as a cluster of unconnected stars. It is rare and is focused on the individual. The desire of the individual takes precedence over the organisation's objectives. The organisation is in effect the resource for the person's talents.

This is a difficult culture. People in it may be influenced or persuaded but cannot be managed. It can be epitomised by the scientist who devotes his working life to the pursuit of one line of scientific enquiry, which may ultimately lead to glory. In the meantime, the employing organisation provides all the resources needed to support this work in the knowledge that it may never gain a reward for its input but if it does, it will be worth waiting for. The person culture may be full of stars but will be devoid of team players.

Each of these cultures meets a different need and will be attractive to different types of people. The things that motivate people in each of these environments will look very different, as will the leadership styles and decision-making models.

There have been attempts in the past to try to create a 'common' culture in organisations with diverse interests. Some very large organisations are known to only want people who can fit comfortably with the culture developed for their organisation. Most teams and organisations, however, require a mix of development and maintenance roles if they are to be effective. The challenge lies in fostering a blend of cultures and an understanding of the need for, and desirability of, retaining essential differences. Change programmes must preserve these differences, unless they are completely at odds with the strategic direction in which the organisation or team has to move.

In a nurse/patient change plan the district nurse must recognise that the factors which will motivate the patient to change his behaviour, or accept a change in treatment, may be very different from those that would encourage her to change. Similarly, the way in which the district nurse 'packages' the change will need to be different to suit the culture of different patients and families. Before they will consider change, they have to believe that the benefits will outweigh the costs and the benefit has to be real from the *patient's* perspective and fit with *their* belief system and culture, not that of the health-care professional.

To embark on any change without thinking about the cultural significance of what you are asking of those involved is to neglect an important part of the planning stage. If a cultural 'fit' cannot be achieved, the change has little chance of success and certainly no chance of endurance.

THE CHANGE PROCESS

'If you don't know where you're going, you might end up somewhere else.' Stengel, management theorist and one-time manager of the New York Yankees, makes a simple but often neglected point. Similarly, if you don't know where you are starting from it is difficult to plan the journey.

The change process always involves three states: the present, the future and the bit in between. This seems obvious, but at least one of these stages is often ignored when planning and implementing change. Thinking about these three states helps to define and clarify the work that needs to be done to manage the change, whether trying to effect change in a patient's behaviour, encourage acceptance of a different pattern of care or for those who are embarking on organisational change. The change process is illustrated by vignette 12.1.

The guiding principle and starting point in all change effort should be the identification and definition of the reason for change and the desired end result. The questions to ask, and answer, are:

Vignette 12.1   Record keeping for cancer patients

Why change?

The complexity of care often needed by a patient with cancer demands that communication between the various people involved in the management and provision of care is good. An effective channel of communication needs to be built between the patient and all those who are involved, in whatever capacity, in activity aimed at ensuring provision of integrated advice, care and support.

Different record-keeping arrangements can reduce access to pieces of information by members of different organisations and by the patient and his carers. A patient-held record provides a 'one-stop' source of information and, importantly, places responsibility for control of this record with the patient.

Defining the desired future state

All patients with a diagnosis of cancer whose care is provided outside as well as inside the hospital setting should hold their own records. These records will detail their specific and agreed needs, including details of chemotherapy regimes, radiotherapy, medication and personal notes.

The present state

The patient's hospital records stay inside the hospital records department. Only the information given on the discharge letter is conveyed to the GP and community staff. There is often little liaison with other professionals or organisations who may be involved in the patient's care, including the patient and his carers.

Vignette 12.1 Cont'd

The information collected by members of the primary health-care team who care for the patient at home is recorded on a separate document which is kept in the patient's home and is available for the family and patient to see. The degree to which this is accessed by the patient and his carers, and the level of responsibility they feel for it, is variable. In most cases, it still feels very much like the 'nurse's notes'.

Getting from here to there

A group was convened composed of community and hospital-based nurses, GPs, secondary care colleagues and Marie Curie nurses. The groups' remit and authority to make decisions had been agreed with those bodies whose support was crucial to implementation.

This group discussed the advantages and possible concerns about introducing a patient-held record. They used examples of patient-held records from other areas as a basis for discussion and development of the idea.

The representatives agreed a core of information that needed to form part of the record that would accompany the patient on his journey through the system.

It was felt important to agree with the patient who should have access to this record.

Local 'champions' from each of the organisations represented were identified. These were seen as people who would be enthusiastic and influential in taking this change forward.

A timetable for implementation, evaluation and monitoring was agreed by the group.

Plans were agreed on how patient acceptance and satisfaction with the self-held record would be measured.

The routes of communicating the proposal for change, the reasons why, the how and the timetable were drafted by the group. It was agreed that the outline proposal would be circulated to those who would be affected by the change (including relevant patient groups) for comment.

Following the agreed consultation period, the patient-held record was introduced.

- Where do we need to be – *and why?*
- Where are we now?
- What do we need to do to get from here to there?
- Part of the planning process is about painting very robust pictures of these three states.

Change models

Change models can be used to help guide this exercise. The choice of model depends on the reason for the change. Some look at very specific elements of the change programme. Most take a wider view. All emphasise the fact that it is impossible to change one part of the system without affecting others. A good rule when choosing a model is – keep it simple.

One model which is often used is the seven Ss (Fig 12.1). The seven elements can be viewed as change levers. If pressure is exerted on any one lever, it has an impact on the others. The implication is that change has to be carefully orchestrated so that a balance is maintained between all seven.

Beckhard & Harris (1987) (Fig. 12.2) describe a practical model for planning and implementing change which is particularly helpful in moving between the three stages and in helping to plan for each of them. In looking at the need to change, one examines the source of demand for change and the potency of that source. There are occasions when an organisation, team or individual has no choice over whether or not to change. The choice lies in *how* the change will be managed. It is also important to understand the magnitude of the planned change.

- Is it adaptive or transformational?
- What is its scope and pace? Is it evolutionary or revolutionary?

If it is a slow change there is likely to be time to plan and consult. In fast-paced change, external threats may force an authoritative style of leadership. These factors will clearly influence how those on the receiving end feel about the change, and the management of it, and must be built into the pictures.

The following three steps are important when initiating the change process.

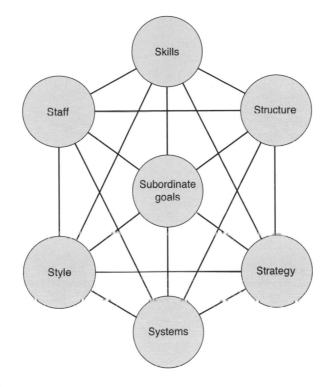

Figure 12.1 The seven Ss.

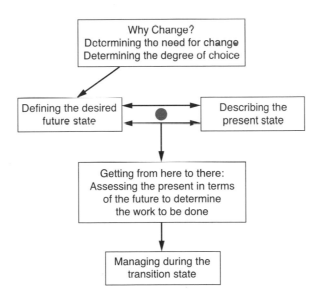

Figure 12.2 Model for planning and implementing change (Beckhard & Harris 1987).

Step 1

The vision of the future state is the first to be developed. It should be approached unhampered by history or the problems of the present. These can stifle creativity in goal setting by raising concerns of perceived impracticability, creating a 'no can do' mindset instead of promoting a 'why not?' attitude. There needs to be a very clear definition of what the future needs to deliver and why; what the leadership's vision of the endpoint is. It is also impor-tant to have a 'midpoint' picture that represents what you want/need the picture to look like at a given time on the way to reaching the final destination. This is particularly important for changes which are likely to take longer and which involve a number of parts of the 'system'. The goals for reaching the midpoint should be detailed in order to motivate those involved to invest time and energy in the change effort.

The description of both the endpoint and the interim have to be detailed to be of value (Vignette 12.2).

Spelling out the behaviour required of those involved in the change helps people to visualise their place in it so they can start to see what will be expected of them. Uncertainty can be reduced because the 'mystery' of the change has been removed. Importantly, by going through this process, those planning the change can be guided away from attacking symptoms to addressing the root cause of the need for change. It also allows people to decide whether they want to be part of this change or need to opt out. It can identify training and education issues that may be tackled at an early stage and used to help to facilitate the change. Importantly, the exercise allows people involved in, and affected by, the change to participate in planning for it – a key issue in gaining commitment.

Step 2

The next step, developing a detailed picture of the present, is a vital part in the management of change. This picture should be built up taking into account the desired future state and will include elements of the 'hard' and and 'soft' parts of the system, i.e. IT, structure, culture, communication, people issues.

This has to be a very honest picture and may include the perspectives of different groups from within the family or team. One then has to ask how this fits with the picture of the future.

Approaches to building the picture of the present depend on the reason for, and size of, the change. In organisational change, the management team may commission a major study of the organisation to provide it. Another way, and one which is more relevant to district nurses, is to bring together a team of people who are informed about the current state by virtue of their day-to-day interaction with the relevant groups/individuals. The team then develops an accurate and detailed assessment of the present state based on their knowledge of the circumstances and characters involved (Box 12.2). This 'team' can include all those perceived to be key players. It should not be seen only as the territory of health-care professionals.

Vignette 12.2   Example of developing the end vision for an organisational change

In a move to self-managed teams, for example, the picture should include a comprehensive definition of what the responsibilities of the team will be, what the structure will look like, the reward system, personnel policies, where the authority to make decisions – and which decisions – lies, individual responsibilities, performance review systems, relationships within the team, with other colleagues and with external agencies and expected performance outcomes. The actual elements included and the description will vary from team to team, but all should address each of the relevant issues and be very clear about what is expected. Only with this degree of clarity can one be sure that the goal the team is working towards is the same one. The single greatest threat to successful change is the lack of attention to defining the desired endpoint.

> **Box 12.2** Developing the picture of the present state in a family-centred change programme
>
> - What facilities are available in the patient's home?
> - Who in the family makes all the decisions?
> - Where does the power lie?
> - What levels of support are available and what are they?
> - Are the family aware of the diagnosis/prognosis?
> - Is the patient aware of the diagnosis/prognosis?
> - What is the communication style in the family?

Without this detailed picture, it is impossible to determine what needs to be changed, and when, and what can remain as it is. Part of the exercise therefore involves prioritisation. There are usually a host of things that need to look different at the end of the change process. The district nurse should be clear about those that need to be addressed first, *and why*. This will help to identify potential 'show stoppers' – those things that have to be tackled in order to allow other things to happen. A brief description of what the issues are is often helpful and should specify *who, what and how*. The nurse can use this description to work with others, including the patient and his carers, to agree on what needs to happen to help reduce the likelihood, or effects, of these problems.

An assessment of the readiness and capability for change can be made at this time as this will inevitably influence the change programme. Readiness has to do with willingness, motives and aims. Capability involves power, influence, authority and often the possession of information, and skills required to carry out the necessary tasks and responsibilities.

The readiness of people and organisations to change depends on attitudes towards the change. Are families, for example, ready for the major disruption in their lives that may be caused by taking on more responsibility for the care of a relative? If one is asking a patient to take responsibility for some aspect of his own care, an insulin-dependent diabetic for example, he may be very capable of doing so in terms of information and skills but may not be motivated to do so. He may see himself in the sick role and managing this aspect of care dilutes the effect.

Similarly, families may be very capable of managing areas of care for relatives but may be unwilling to do so because of loss of personal freedom or fear of loss of support from the statutory agencies if they agree to the proposed change. This can work in reverse and individuals may be very willing to take on new responsibilities but do not have the skills required to do so. The change effort therefore has to focus on equipping them with the necessary skills and information to allow this change to happen *safely*.

Change strategies have to find a way of increasing either the readiness or the capability of the key players in the situation.

Step 3

Before embarking on a new journey, particularly a long and complicated one, it is sensible to plan the route you will take. The change programme should be approached in the same way. Having painted the first two pictures, the next stage helps to develop the map for change. This will determine the type of changes required, identify where these changes need to happen, when and the domino effect of change on the various parts of the system. The plan will determine where to intervene and identify any perceived problems together with plans to manage them. If different structures are needed in the transition stage they will be described. Managing during the transition state requires one to think of strategies geared to gaining commitment to the change. These may involve education and training, role modelling, changing reward systems, sometimes forced collaboration and often resistance management.

ATTITUDES, PRESSURES AND BEHAVIOUR IN TIMES OF CHANGE

We are all interested in change but there are many things which hold us back. During any change, whether as an individual or at organisational level, people go through a series of stages, including resistance, confusion, integration and finally commitment. As we have already seen, change is not a simple process and the transition from one stage to the next is seldom a clean one.

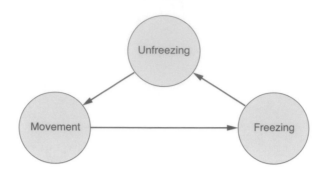

Figure 12.3 Milestones in the change process (Lewin 1951).

Lewin (1951) describes a three-step model showing the three distinct milestones in the process and the behaviours associated with each of the stages. (Fig 12.3) In Lewin's model one has to demonstrate, or sometimes invent, dissatisfaction with the present in order to encourage people to 'unlearn' current behaviours and attitudes. This unfreezing process allows them to move to something better. This process must take into account the threats the change presents to people and the need to motivate those affected to attain the natural state of equilibrium by accepting change. New responses are developed based on new information and people then enter the freezing stage where stability is achieved and a new balance created.

To achieve commitment, people have to move successfully through each of the three steps. Some people will, for many reasons, find the 'unfreezing' process difficult; others will get stuck at one point and take time to move on. Some will never complete the journey.

For those implementing the change, it is wise to accept the fact that all change will be resisted. The difference comes in the degree and source of resistance encountered. Resistance cannot be overcome. It has to be managed. To manage it, one has to understand the root cause of it. This is important as some causes of resistance are easier to deal with than others.

Resistance to change

When people are confronted by change, their attitudes to it will be affected by several things,

including their personality and the conflicts generated by the nature of the change and its manner of implementation. These factors will interact in a complicated way and will determine individual feelings and behaviour.

In *Making it happen* (1988) Harvey-Jones says that the brake on change is fear: fear of the unknown and fear of the future. In change situations people have to give up the familiar for the unfamiliar, the certain for the uncertain. Change often threatens our sense of security and predictability, it takes away the 'comfort blanket' and leaves people feeling exposed. In these circumstances people's perceptions of what the future will be like for them are all-important in determining their attitudes to the change. As well as giving people reasons why they should change, it is important to define the risk of not changing. When people understand the full picture their perception of the change may alter.

Resistance often stems from a perception that the change threatens an individual's core skills and competence. Some people build their power around the knowledge and information they hold. A change may result in loss of this power base and associated loss of status. This threat often results in the fiercest source of resistance. In families, one sees this when illness forces a reversal of roles, with the parent being 'reduced' to the place of the child. This is particularly difficult – for the parent and children – when the parent figure has been quite powerful.

The dominant feelings and attitudes often displayed in these situations, i.e. fear, anxiety and

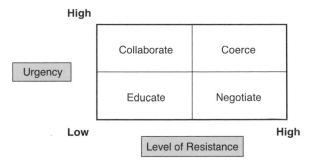

Figure 12.4   Urgency of change versus level of resistance.

anger, are all at the opposite end of the spectrum to those required to enter any new situation, where a degree of courage and self-confidence is essential. Lack of information, or misinformation, often makes this situation worse and if there are historical factors that lead individuals to be distrustful about what is planned, the barriers to the change are likely to be high and will take significant effort to overcome.

Similarly, if people cannot see the benefits of the change, or perceive the costs to outweigh the gains, they will be more reluctant to go along with it. The trigger for change is sometimes referred to as the 'burning platform'. Sometimes it is necessary to 'invent' this platform, to create a 'felt need' for change. District nurses often have a powerful 'ally' when trying to build this platform with patients – trust. If people trust those who are proposing the change, they are more likely to believe that their interests will be looked after as a result of the change. This trust will be built on a series of consistent interactions, which have demonstrated to the patient that the nurse will work to help achieve the best outcomes for him. In poor relationships, distrust of the initiator of the change will lead to increased resistance to the change itself. It is important not to abuse this trust but to use it constructively to encourage open discussion about the proposed change and its implications and so reduce resistance to it.

These situations need careful handling if the nurse, and others, are to move through Lewin's model and come out at the other end committed to the change.

Box 12.3   Dealing with resistance

- Obtain support from *all* key players.
- Avoid surprises.
- Ensure participation.
- The change must not increase the burden – real or perceived – on people.
- Recognise the feelings of those involved.
- Incorporate values and ideals of those involved.
- Offer new, worthwhile experiences.
- Avoid threats to autonomy and security.
- Be adaptable.
- Recognise the need to bring in 'new blood' to help implement the change.
- Learn to 'let go'.
- Keep it simple.
- Take small steps.
- Get the timing right.
- Be explicit about the choices – including the choice to opt out.
- Be explicit about the implications of the choices.

Handling resistance

There are some general guidelines for dealing with resistance which are helpful in any change situation (Box 12.3).

The issue of letting go is often a particularly tough one. There are occasions when the person or people who thought of the change are not the best ones to implement it. They have to recognise this and bring others in who may then get all the kudos.

If these pointers are followed, the barriers that go up may be considerably lower and easier to get over than those erected if shortcuts are taken. Ignoring any of them may result in a much longer and more difficult change journey

Table 12.1 The situational model

Approach	Commonly used when	Advantages	Drawbacks
Education and communication	There is a lack of information or inaccurate information and analysis	Once persuaded, people will often help with implementation of the change	Time consuming if lots of people are involved
Participation and involvement	The initiators do not have all the information they need to design the change. Where others have considerable power to resist	People who participate will be committed to the change	Time consuming. Participants may design an inappropriate change
Facilitation and support	People are resisting because of adjustment problems	No other approach works as well with adjustment problems	Time consuming, expensive and may still fail
Negotiation and agreement	Someone or some group will lose out in a change. Where that group has considerable power to resist	Sometimes it is a relatively easy way to avoid major resistance	Can be too expensive in cases where it may alert others to negotiate for compliance
Manipulation and cooption	Other tactics will not work or are too expensive	Can be a quick and inexpensive solution to resistance problems	Can lead to future problems if people feel manipulated
Explicit and implicit coercion	Speed is essential and the change initiators possess considerable power	It is speedy and can overcome any kind of resistance	Can be risky if it leaves people mad at the initiators

than necessary. The strategies employed will depend on the urgency of the change and the forces driving it. There are several models that are useful in helping to identify these factors.

Models for managing resistance

• **Urgency of change versus level of resistance** In cases where the levels of urgency and resistance are high, coercion may be a necessary tactic to employ. It is usually seen where there is no choice over whether to change or not and where the change is urgent and important. Coercion can backfire if the resistors are a powerful group (Fig. 12.4).

Education can be employed where the levels of urgency and resistance are low. There are many ways of using this tactic and the choice will depend on the circumstances of the change and the audience.

• **Situational model** This model can be used to 'mix and match' a number of approaches that can be used to target interventions at the likely source(s) of resistance (Table 12.1).

• **Force field analysis** (Lewin 1951) (Fig. 12.5) How resistance is handled depends on where the resistance comes from and the power of the resistors. In any change which affects a number of people there will be a range of attitudes and some will be more positive than others. It is

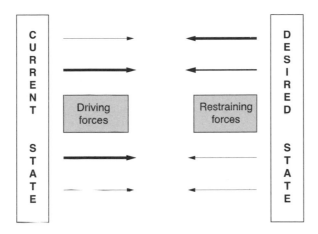

Figure 12.5   Force field analysis.

important to know where support and resistance are coming from and how strong they are.

The force field analysis is a useful tool in identifying and assessing these factors. It can also be used to map the motivation of people to change and the helpfulness, or otherwise, of change processes.

The analysis looks at the driving forces behind the change effort and at what are termed 'restraining forces'. For a successful change effort, the driving forces have to be stronger than the restraining forces.

The strength of the force is indicated by the thickness of the line: the thicker the line, the stronger the force. A thicker arrow can also be used to signify the power of the stakeholders in either camp to influence or control the change.

COMMON ELEMENTS IN SECURING AGREEMENT TO CHANGE

Many of the models employed in managing resistance to change include the same tactics. The first two examples given here reflect this 'common core'. This is not surprising since they are built on experience of the strategies that have been found to be most effective. Because of their importance it is perhaps worth saying a little more about them.

> **Box 12.4**   Key questions for understanding the change process
>
> - Why is there a need to change at all?
> - What is the long-term objective of the change?
> - What are the short-term goals?
> - What has to change?
> - How?
> - When is the change to take place?
> - Who is to be involved?
> - How will those involved be affected?
> - What will the situation be after the change?
> - What are the potential benefits?
> - What do we have to do to accomplish these objectives?
> - How should the information be communicated?

Education, understanding and communication

When as many of those involved in a change understand as much as possible about it and its consequences, their resistance is likely to be reduced. In a nurse – patient relationship, it is up to the nurse to develop this understanding. To do this, the district nurse must know what is to be understood.

Box 12.4 gives questions that need to be answered as fully as possible.

Whatever the scale of the change, the questions will always be the same. The difference comes in how the answers are handled. Communicating information, for example, may be most effectively done in a nurse – patient change on a face-to-face basis, with written back-up if appropriate. In an organisation or team, newsletters, news releases or posters may be used. Formal training courses or group discussions are other media that can be employed. The more complex the change, the greater the variety of methods that may be needed.

The important factor in transmitting the information is that it is understood. It must therefore be factual, accurate and accessible. It must be given in a form or language that is comprehensible to the recipient. It must answer the right question, i.e. not only what is to happen but how, why, when and to whom. Finally there must be a way to confirm that real understanding has been achieved. This may mean that the nurse has to give the patient time to think about what has been proposed, check if the initial purpose of the change is understood and be prepared to go back to it as the patient raises more questions or concerns over the course of time. This is the most effective way of hitting all the above targets for communication, particularly in a trusting relationship where patients will feel comfortable about telling the district nurse their greatest hopes, or fears, of the change.

Participation and involvement

There is some evidence to suggest that participation leads to commitment to, and not merely compliance with, a change.

These are strategies which do take time; there are also certain prerequisites that have to be fulfilled (Box 12.5).

Box 12.5 Prerequisites for participation and involvement

- The recipients want to participate and be involved.
- The person 'in charge' feels confident in that role.
- There is no 'hidden' agenda, i.e. the decision has not already been taken regarding a course of action.
- There must be a willingness to give credit and recognition openly to all contributions of value.
- Those involved must be willing and feel able to express their opinions and suggestions.

Participation is easier than involvement, which requires you to give something of yourself. Involvement, to use the Americanism, is about 'walking the walk and talking the talk'. It's about practising what you preach. Both participation and involvement demand a climate of trust, credibility, tolerance and time.

Facilitation and support

These factors provide the 'safety net' for innovation. They are about building confidence and might include training in new skills or simply listening and providing emotional support. These methods are probably most useful when anxiety and fear are at the heart of resistance. Nurses are usually accomplished in these skills and adept at recognising when they need to be employed.

The important questions to answer when they are used are:

- What is the appropriate level of support?
- What goes in its place when it is taken away?

This last question is often a particularly difficult one in changes affecting patients and their families and it may be that a range of options are considered, and tried, in order to reach a satisfactory solution.

Negotiation and agreement

This is a good way to inform through a formalised process, perhaps less helpful on a 1:1 basis, although even there it does have a place. There are examples of nurse – patient contracts based on these principles that are used to agree courses of action or care.

The emphasis of negotiation in times of change should be on 'integrative bargaining'. This involves the process of mutual problem solving. Its aim is to achieve a win – win situation.

Manipulation and cooption

Manipulation in this case means the selective use of information and often the conscious structuring of events. A common form of manipulation is cooption where an individual or group is given a desirable role in the design or implementation of the change. Coopting is different from participation; in the former the initiators don't want the advice of those coopted, merely their endorsement of the change objectives.

Compulsion and coercion

Many change processes have an element of compulsion. In situations where speed is vital and where changes will not be popular however they are dressed up, coercion may be the only option. It does bring risks with it. It can backfire; it can also work against the environment needed to support change, where one needs to encourage a climate where people feel free to think creatively, to come up with new initiatives. Authority tends to restrict the development of the discretion needed to allow people to think and act in a different way and so discourages the generation of ideas.

It is important that change strategies are consistent. Efforts that are not clearly planned get bogged down in unanticipated problems. On the other hand, prolonged implementation of change runs the risk of becoming stalled. Identifying the likely sources of resistance, and by so doing allowing planning of the most effective ways of managing them, can help to balance these tensions and ease the implementation of the change.

The chances of success are enhanced if those initiating the change begin by looking at the 'playing field' (Box 12.6).

When considering individual resistance, think about why it is happening. Use the generic guidelines to identify where the source of discomfort might be. Think about the unfreezing process that people have to go through or be helped to get through. Is this happening? If not,

---

Box 12.6 'The playing field' - What needs to be considered before implementing change

- What are the drivers for change?
- Where might resistance lie – at both an individual and organisational level? How powerful is the resistance likely to be?
- What power do the chief players hold?
- Whose cooperation is essential?

---

why not? How can people be helped through the unfreezing process? What strategies can be employed to facilitate the process?

At an organisational level, the culture of the organisation will be the guiding factor in resistant behaviour. Consider the recipe that makes up the organisation's value system and use that knowledge and understanding to help manage the situation. Think about the power of the systems within the organisation. The urgency of the change may dominate your choice of management and may reduce the power of some of the resistors.

How you handle resistance will depend on the reason for and urgency of the change and the type and degree of resistance. If we accept that resistance is a feature of change and that it cannot be overcome, it is helpful to develop skills that will allow effective management of resistant behaviour.

Moving through the change process, managing resistance to it, keeping people on board is demanding and stressful. For those responsible for managing and implementing change or those on the receiving end of it, dealing with stress in themselves and others is a crucial part of the change programme. In order to manage stress, we need to understand what it is, what it does to us, where it comes from, what affects it and what coping mechanisms can be employed to manage it effectively.

THE PERSONAL IMPACT OF CHANGE

Stress is widely accepted as a common feature of modern life. The word is now part of our everyday vocabulary and, as such, often suffers from a lack of definitional clarity. Because its effects on people have been studied from the perspectives of a wide range of disciplines, the concept has been variously defined in the literature. Cummings & Cooper (1979) offer the following definition:

A stress is any force that puts a psychological or physical factor beyond its range of stability, producing a strain within the individual. Knowledge that a stress is likely to occur constitutes a threat to the individual. A threat can cause a strain because of what it signifies to the person.

This definition highlights the importance of understanding the individual perception of stress. The negative impact of psychological factors, for example, depends on one's perception of what is stressful and on one's personal capacity to deal with some stressors better than others. What determines our experience of stress is usually not the event itself but the way we think and our perception of the degree of control we have over the situation.

We all need a degree of pressure to stimulate us into action and a certain amount of stress is healthy. This 'positive stress' allows us to stay alert and it stops life from being boring. When we are subjected to stress, a series of hormonal reactions take place which are designed to protect the body, causing it to prepare for physical action – the 'flight or fight' response. The heart rate and muscle tension increase and blood sugar is released to fuel the exercising muscles. We have all experienced these reactions, waiting for an examination to begin, preparing to speak in public, before an interview. In these situations stress can be stimulating; it gives the 'buzz' which can help to enhance performance.

However, when the pressure or stress is prolonged or excessive, the individual feels unable to cope and performance and health can deteriorate. If, for example, the 'flight or fight' response is constantly triggered but the individual does not engage in any physical activity, the body will be activating the hormonal response unnecessarily. This is particularly pertinent today when many stressors don't require a physical response.

The level and type of stress that can be experienced by people before ill effects are felt varies according to the individual and across different situations. These 'negative' effects are often referred to as 'distress' and the distress cycle refers to the behavioural, physiological, emotional and cognitive changes experienced by people experiencing stress overload. These changes include changes in eating and drinking habits; people typically feel restless and are unable to concentrate. They complain of palpitations and may also suffer from sleep problems, which exacerbate their feelings of being unable

to cope or concentrate. Any combination of these effects leads to decreased well-being, decreased functioning, decreased productivity and decreased enjoyment of life. This becomes a vicious circle that some people are unable to break out of without help.

Feeling stressed is not reserved for those who feel they have too much to do. Boredom and lack of intellectual or physical stimulation can equally be the source of stress. People entering retirement, the unemployed, patients whose illness incapacitates them, all may experience the same symptoms of stress as those felt by people with very busy lives. The challenge is to achieve the balance that provides the optimum level of stress – the type and degree of stress that facilitates effective performance, that provides the 'stretch' that we all need, without going into overload. It is at this optimum point that people are at their best, where their performance is most effective. The danger is that this is also the point at which people feel able – and willing – to take on more, which can tip the balance the wrong way.

CHANGE AS A SOURCE OF STRESS

The number of potential sources of stress are infinite and touch on personal and work life.

For patients and families, the stress of coping with the effects of illness often throws them into stress overload. They feel that they have no control over the course or outcome of the situation that has been forced on them. There may be financial worries that result from their changed circumstances or changes in family role. In some cases there is the added burden for carers of having to stay well. Who will care for their partner if they become ill?

At work, there is research to suggest that stress is caused primarily by the fundamentals of change of control and a high workload. Common sources of stress among health-care professionals have been identified as understaffing, high levels of demand and the threat of change. The changing face of the organisations in which we work, the changing nature of the work itself and the demands for a more flexible workforce have placed greater emphasis on multi-skilling, creating insecurity for many health-care professionals.

Changes in role, role ambiguity, role conflict all create stress and can occur in work and personal life. In self-managed teams, for example, the appointment of a team leader or coordinator typically sparks conflict if not well managed. The lack of definition of the role and responsibilities associated with this post can result in confusion and anger. One of the essential tasks in making the shift to self-management is to clarify the responsibilities associated with this role and to involve members of the team in this definition. It is important that everyone has the same understanding of what is expected of this person, where the boundary lines lie and the skills and behaviours that will be required of the post holder.

In families, illness can result in role change and ambiguity about the position taken by some of those caring for the patient. Patients often face a number of major changes at once. They may, for example, suddenly find themselves excluded from the workforce as a result of illness. If this is permanent, their role within the family is changed. The way they perceive themselves and are perceived by others changes. There is an infinite number of other variables that can be added to this picture, the stressful effects of which are additive (Box 12.7). The end result is often conflict and anger caused by resentment of the imposed change and the perceived or real lack of control over it.

Certain people may also be at risk because of their personality. Theory and research support the notion that a major factor underpinning stress is the lack of control, power and influence possessed by those affected by the change.

Box 12.7   The problems that exacerbate stress

- Lack awareness or insight into the change.
- Are not motivated to change.
- Do not possess the skills and/or knowledge needed to respond to the new situation.
- Lack the resources needed to implement and manage the change.
- Have inadequate support.

Cooper & Smith (1985) found, for example, that as one moves down the organisational (and social) hierarchies, the amount of stress symptoms and stress-related illness rises. One of the keys to successful management of stress is therefore the same as one of the essential elements of a successful change programme, i.e. the involvement and participation.

The district nurse, as change agent, will often have to cope with stressors in her own life as well as being called on to help others affected by change. It is therefore important that she is able to effectively manage stress.

Research has found that there are a number of things that can be done to increase one's ability to cope more effectively with periods of stress and so reduce the risk of suffering from stress-related illness (Taylor & Cooper 1988). The adoption of a 'healthy' lifestyle is one. This is about the maintenance of physical, mental and social health. Nurses need to put into practice many of the messages that they encourage patients to take on board. This means paying attention to their diet, taking the recommended level of exercise and, importantly, allowing time for relaxation. It is also important to look carefully at one's usual response to events perceived as stressful and to group responses under four headings.

- *Initial reaction.* There is often a tendency to panic, to make hasty decisions or to try to do everything at once. It is more helpful if the individual learns to stand back, stay calm and respond to the incident step by step.
- *Dealing with feelings.* It is important to express one's feelings and show emotions. If change generates anger or conflict, these feelings have to be addressed. Similarly, being 'upset' has to be recognised as a reasonable response to some events. Happily, the culture of not getting 'involved' with patients and their families has now changed and expressing sorrow at the death of a patient, for example, is no longer frowned on. Nevertheless, district nurses do sometimes have to suppress emotions and if this is prolonged or when the district nurse has no social network where she can freely express her

feelings, the effects build up and the associated stress can be overwhelming. The need to provide a support system for district nurses dealing with terminally ill patients is recognised and has been addressed by clinical supervision which has been introduced into many primary care trusts. We all need to be able to 'offload' our feelings now and again. The creation of a safe and supportive environment is an important aspect of personal and work life.

• *Developing relationships.* This is particularly important in times of change when district nurses need to explain or discuss the changes and the planned action with everyone involved in the effort or affected by it. They need to discuss the programme with those in a position to help and must know when to seek help and/or advice.

• *Confronting underlying issues.* People involved in change may reach a point where they have to confront the issues underlying particularly stressful incidents. Burying one's head in the sand will not help.

District nurses, because of the nature of their work, will be in contact with people who are under pressure and strain. If they are to be of assistance to these people, they must recognise that they are stressed and then provide practical help or advice on ways of managing this pressure. One of the essential features of this management is to identify the root cause of the stress rather than simply helping people to cope with the symptoms.

In general, such interventions seek to keep people informed while providing a supportive climate in which individuals are encouraged to participate.

The basic rules are:

• let people know what's going on
• listen to them
• involve them
• encourage behaviour that is goal directed.

Staying in control

Marcus Aurelius, the philosopher and Roman emperor, wrote in his *Meditations* that 'Our life is

---

> **Box 12.8**   Five rules for positive thinking (Makin & Lindley 1991)
>
> • Accept achievement.
> • Deal in specifics, not generalities.
> • Realistically address the chances of your worst fears happening.
> • Imagine the worst-case scenario.
> • Do your best, then resign yourself to whatever happens.

what our thoughts make it'. Positive thinking is a way of making life more positive (Box 12.8). It is as easy to think negatively as positively. Henry Ford summed this up when he said 'Whether you think you can or you cannot, you are absolutely right'.

It is important to boost your ego and to encourage others to look at their successes now and again. This is important for patients and families who often get so caught up with the perceived downward spiral of illness that they miss the good things that happen and the improvements, however slight, that occur.

Learn to relax. Relax *before* a potentially stressful event. Take just a moment or two to unwind, take a few deep breaths and than tackle the business in hand. Relax *during* stressful events. You want to stay in control, so don't wait to unwind until after it's all over. Relax *after* stressful events. Remember that the effects of stress are additive. Several relatively minor stressors can contribute to a major impact.

There are many excellent publications on relaxation and relaxing techniques and it is not appropriate to go into the detail of the various tactics here. There are, however, one or two 'tips' that we would all do well to follow.

1. Taking a break is one. Work done many years ago demonstrated that a physical worker was more productive when he took time to rest, even for only a short period. Mental fatigue is just as debilitating as physical activity and we should all learn to take time to 'shut down' for a few minutes. Even a 'micro break' of 60 seconds or so is useful to just call a halt. Micro breaks are also useful when you feel you may be responding to a challenge or perceived threat more out of emotion than reason.

2. Develop a release mechanism. Find out what works best for you, it may be cooking, listening to music, walking, sport. Build it into your regular routine.

By becoming aware of these approaches the district nurse is better placed to advise patients and others on some of the tactics they may employ to help deal with stress, whatever the cause.

CONCLUSION

The start of the chapter raised the dilemma of facilitating and managing change and development and at the same time carrying on the day-to-day work. To effectively accomplish this demanding task, nurses must have a clear vision of where they need to be as a result of the change, the milestones on the way, detailed maps of the journey route, a clear understanding of the capacity of those involved to make the change and the ability to get the best out of everyone involved. Their management of this complex agenda involves the ability to deal with ambiguity, skills in managing conflict, reducing resistant behaviour and a real concern for people and their potential.

The chapter has provided district nurses with some of the techniques and tools to equip them to be effective in meeting these challenges. The change process and its management have purposely not been approached from a purely nursing angle. District nurses are increasingly being asked to think more widely, to contribute to discussions on issues that span a spectrum of services and circumstances, where nurses and nursing may be only a minor player. It is therefore important for district nurses to gain a broad understanding of the change management process and of its developmental and interdependent nature as a necessary condition for success in any change effort.

A 'blueprint' for change management has not been suggested, nor would it be appropriate to do so. The uniqueness of every change effort, in terms of the drivers for change, the culture of those involved, the strength and source of resistance and support and the stress associated with

> **Box 12.9** Five fundamental issues to achieving lasting change (Judson 1990)
>
> - Understanding
> - Commitment
> - Resources
> - Measuring and monitoring
> - A climate of accountability

the change, must be recognised and addressed in ways which are most appropriate to these local circumstances.

District nurses should have recognised many examples of the use of skills and techniques that are integral to their everyday practice (Box 12.9).

These are all elements of good nursing practice, underpinned by effective communication.

One of the key messages to take from the chapter is the need to continually ask 'why?' when proposing change. If you can't give satisfactory answers, how can you expect to take people on the change journey with you? What may make good sense to you may be less comprehensible to a bewildered and cautious patient or carer. Similarly, what may appear like a gain to you may be perceived as a loss by others.

Change presents many challenges, including making best use of the instability, tension and conflict within families, groups and organisations, which we all find difficult to cope with at times. These factors are intimately linked with creativity and innovation and can therefore be put to good use; we just have to get the environment right to let it happen.

To move from the status quo it is also necessary to stop worrying about the 'what if?' and turn the environment from one of planning to one of learning. There is a need to be proactive *and* reactive in response to change, creating the conditions for learning and acting simultaneously. This is a tall order but nursing is used to facing, and meeting, exacting agendas.

These are exciting times for the health service and for nursing. Changes in the planning and provision of services, in terms of both format and location, will demand significant adaptations.

The increasing emphasis on public involvement in these discussions will require a change in attitudes and expectations of health-care professionals and the public. By developing a sound understanding of the change process, nurses can realise, and help others to realise, the benefits of change, whether at a personal, team or organisational level.

Remember:

...change is always a threat when it is forced upon us, but it becomes an opportunity when we are involved. (Kanter 1983)

REFERENCES

Ariyaratne A T 1983 Speech at international community leadership summit, Winrock, Arkansas, March

Bandura A 1986 Social boundaries of thoughts and action: a social cognitive theory. Peters Hall, Englewood Cliffs, New York

Beckhard R, Harris R 1987 Organisational transitions: managing complex change. Addison Wesley, Reading, Mass

Bower M 1966 The will to manage. McGraw Hill, New York

Cooper C L, Smith M J (eds) 1985 Job stress and the blue collar worker. John Wiley, Chichester

Cummings T, Cooper C L 1979 A cybernetic framework for the study of occupational stress. Human Relations 32: 395–419

Handy C 1985 Understanding organisations. Penguin Books, London

Harvey-Jones J 1988 Making it happen. Collins, Glasgow

Judson A 1990 Making strategy happen. Transforming plans into reality. Blackwell, London

Kanter R 1983 The change masters. Unwin, London

Lewin K 1951 Field theory in social science. Harper and Row, New York

Makin P E, Lindley P A 1991 Positive stress management. A practical guide for those who work under pressure. Kogan Page, London

Peters T J, Waterman R H 1982 In search of excellence. Harper and Row, New York

Ranade W 1994 A future for the NHS. Health care in the 1990s. Longman, London

Taylor H, Cooper C L 1988 Organisational change: threat or challenge? The role of individual differences in the management of stress. Journal of Organisational Change Management (1):

Trice H M, Beyer J M 1984 Studying organisational cultures through rites and rituals. Academy of Management Review 9: 654

FURTHER READING

Bate P 1994 Strategies for cultural change. Butterworth–Heinemann, Oxford

Covey S R 1989 The seven habits of highly effective people. Simon and Schuster, New York

De Bono E 1990 Six thinking hats. Penguin, London

Handy C 1994 The empty raincoat. Hutchinson, London

Pfeiffer J 1991 Theories and models in applied behavioural science, vol 3. Pfeiffer, San Diego

13

Quality and clinical effectiveness

Heather Marr

Key points

- Grasping the concepts and making them real
- The patient's perspective
- The district nurse's perspective
- Audit and clinical effectiveness
- Service excellence in district nursing

INTRODUCTION

District nurses are major providers of care in the community, fulfilling a diverse and varied role while delivering care in a vast number of settings over which they have little control. They are often required to make decisions in isolation, not only with their patients but also patients' families, friends and significant others. In addition, they deliver care within many resource constraints as part of a nursing team and as part of a multidisciplinary team. They are frequently the 'known and trusted face', providing advice not always seen to be directly related to nursing care but which does impact on the well-being of the patient and family.

The public's expectations of health care have changed considerably over the past few years and will continue to do so as the principles of the White Papers (DoH 1997, Scottish Office 1997) are put into practice. With the changing roles, relationships and approaches to care and caseloads, the need to develop appropriate and cost effective care is of paramount importance in order to assure a consistently high standard of care and meet optimal outcomes while reducing complications and preventing adverse events.

Vignette 13.1 Changing culture

A group of district nurses clearly highlighted in discussion that there has been a major culture change for them in their *wards without walls*. The group highlighted the change of skill mix within the team that had taken place with fewer trained district nurses and a more cost-effective team with the district nurse as team leader. They described the dramatic change in their caseloads which now included so much more teaching and support to family carers and the growing collaborative work and relationship with social work colleagues.

It was important for them to discuss 'getting rid of the old red tape of bureaucracy' and the clinical freedom they

had found after giving up the 'nurse as doctor's handmaiden' role. Many of them now had a degree and had achieved this alongside their work as community nurses. They talked of how this 'piece of paper had changed things for them'. While bringing greater credibility from other members of the health and social care teams it had given the district nurses greater confidence. 'We are now in a better position to question and challenge.'

Reflecting on the past few years, they remarked how 'the internal market has divided us as colleagues and did little for the patients ... we are looking forward to a more collaborative future'.

Accountability will increase along with multidisciplinary and interagency collaboration, while the standards of the care and service delivered to patients will have to include those aspects deemed most important by patients and therefore systems and approaches designed will have to be more patient centred.

Many aspects of the district nursing role are intangible and unquantifiable, making the measuring of effectiveness difficult, yet there is the need to make quality explicit and demonstrate the positive difference district nursing can make to patients.

Vignette 13.1 captures many of the key issues and challenges currently facing district nurses.

GRASPING THE CONCEPTS AND MAKING THEM REAL

We struggle constantly to make sense of new terms ... buzzwords which we read in the literature or which are presented to us by colleagues, educators and managers. Quality assurance, quality improvement, quality control, total quality management (TQM), continuous quality improvement (CQI), audit, review, standards, monitoring, clinical effectiveness, evidence-based practice, clinical governance, service excellence. Back in 1993, prior to the latest proliferation of terms, Norman & Redfern put it rather well.

What is immediately striking on entering the quality arena is the lack of consistency in the way in which

common terms are used in the voluminous literature. Ninety-six terms for the review of care can be derived by combining either *medical, health, clinical* or *professional* with *care, activity, standards* or *quality* and with either *assessment, evaluation, assurance, audit, monitoring* or *review* ... This confusion in terminology may be partly the result of the rapid expansion of interest in quality and quality assurance in health care, as a result of which a number of terms have become current before their meaning is clear.

We should learn not to make this same mistake again with the inception of clinical governance and any associated jargon.

Definitions of quality, service quality and learning from the industrial model

In the literature, *product* quality and *service* quality have been extensively explored. (Oakland 1993, Zeithaml et al 1990). It could be said that the product of district nursing is the care package designed for and delivered to each patient while the service aspects take account of how the care is delivered, the interpersonal aspects, communication and feedback. When reading the literature on quality, it is useful to remember that *product* quality and *service* quality differ in a number of ways and these are presented in Box 13.1.

Worldwide, much has been read and even more written on quality, most of which has been based on the foundation work of three of the leading authorities on quality in the USA: Deming (1986, Walton 1989), Crosby (1980, 1989) and

---

Box 13.1 Features of service quality

Intangibility. A product can be seen, touched and measured during its development and subsequent use, while the delivery of a service has many intangible aspects and, because of the high human input, can be felt but not touched, making measurement and management more complex and difficult.

Simultaneous production and consumption. A product is developed and then subsequently delivered to the customer. Rework can be done prior to the customer receiving it. In service delivery, the service is delivered by the producer(s) while at the same time it is being taken up and used by the consumer. It is altered within this relationship to meet the needs and this also makes it heterogeneous.

Heterogeneity. A product is homogeneous and therefore has a sameness about it and is produced to specification, while a service is heterogeneous, with a high people input in the delivery.

Juran (1988). The 14 points in Deming's management agenda (1986) clearly place the responsibility for quality within the sphere of management and give a high value to people and ongoing training. Juran (1988) emphasises the importance of the customer and the need for improving quality by a project-based approach, embracing quality planning, quality control and quality improvement. Crosby has developed 14 steps which provide a systematic approach to total quality management, the emphasis being on early commitment at the top of the organisation and total involvement through teamwork. Although originating over 35 years ago from the work of Deming and the rebuilding of Japanese industry, many of the key concepts are as relevant today.

Some definitions of quality worth considering at this point from the above work include *fitness for purpose intended* and *conformance to requirements*. The definition given in the International Standard ISO 9000 is 'the totality of features and characteristics of a product or service that bear on its ability to satisfy stated or implied needs' (B SI 1994).

Over the last 15 years in the USA and more recently in Britain, there has been a move to include consumer-oriented definitions of quality within the service industry and these have been applied to health-care service delivery. Literature

on delivering service quality is extensive and the most quoted literature is the work undertaken by Zeithaml et al (1990) on the perception–expectation (P–E) gap; the gap between what customers expect and what they actually receive. This work is expanded upon in the final section of this chapter.

Within health-care delivery, our own British experiences over the last 10 years have taken us through a maze of changes and learning experiences, not only as professionals and managers designing and delivering care but also as members of the public, patients and clients. In health care, quality has become such an overused, abused and misunderstood term that it seems to have lost its meaning. Quality can be seen as relative or absolute, simply meeting a stated requirement or an idealistic but unachievable state. It can be value laden, as meaning something good, 'a degree of excellence' or it can be valueless, 'what makes a thing what it is'. Such varied definitions make striving to achieve quality difficult.

Some of the key foundation work on quality in health care can be found in the writings of Maxwell (1984), Donabedian (1966, 1970, 1980, 1982, 1985, 1992) and Øvretveit (1992).

Maxwell (1984) defined quality in six dimensions: effectiveness, efficiency, equity, accessibility, acceptability, appropriateness to need. Many organisations have subsequently used this framework when defining, monitoring and improving service delivery. In striving to achieve quality in these dimensions, the trade-offs need careful consideration.

Take the example of closing a local community hospital located in a rural area and referring the local community to the nearest district general hospital 20 miles away for care and treatment that cannot be delivered from the local health centre. This can be considered under each of Maxwell's six dimensions as shown in Box 13.2.

As Professor Emeritus at the University of Michigan, Avedis Donabedian has written extensively on the quality of medical care since the 1960s. He proposed that the quality of medical care could be defined and evaluated within the well-known structure-process-outcome framework, explored the technical and interpersonal aspects of

---

Box 13.2 Maxwell's dimensions (Maxwell 1984)

Taking each dimension in turn, how might this be affected by the decision? Is it likely to increase or decrease? Why? Who is in the best position to judge this?

Dimension	Increase/decrease) (why	best position to judge
Efficiency		
Effectiveness		
Equity		
Accessibility		
Acceptability		
Appropriateness to need		

Who is likely to make the final decision to close the hospital?
On what grounds do you think the decision might be made?
Would you make a similar decision?

---

care along with the impact of amenities and examined the professional roles and responsibilities of practitioners. Some of his writings, which form the foundations of later work on quality in health care, are expanded upon in this chapter.

At a seminar on quality in health care in 1992, Donabedian distributed a paper outlining his comparison of models for quality assurance, shown in Box 13.3.

John Øvretveit (1992) defined quality as 'fully meeting the needs of those who need the service most, at the lowest cost to the organisation, within limits and directives set by higher authorities and purchasers'. His definition recognises that a quality health service is one that satisfies a number of sometimes conflicting requirements and interest groups and involves three dimensions: client, professional and management quality (Box 13.5).

Box 13.3 Models for quality assurance (reproduced from Donabedian 1992 with permission)

Two models for quality assurance from two distinguishable 'families', the health-care model and the industrial model, are compared within the following framework:

- the nature of quality
- the scope of quality
- the nature of 'the quality problem'
- the strategies of quality assurance and improvement
- the methods of quality monitoring.

Industrial Model	Health-care Model
The nature of quality	
Quality is whatever consumers desire, endorse, buy	Quality is what is good for consumers, as defined jointly by themselves and their health-care advisors, subject to societal guidelines
The customer–seller interaction is less prominent as a component of quality	The patient–practitioner relationship is very complex and its management is an integral part of quality
The consumer is a coproducer of quality by competence of use	The consumer (patient) is even more intimately and decisively a definer and coproducer of quality
Low cost is a component of quality. The added cost of added quality can often be counterbalanced by efficiency of production and more sales (quality is free)	Low cost is less emphasised as a component of quality. The added cost of added quality is not so easily counterbalanced by efficiencies in production or higher sales and it is added to by longevity (quality costs money)
Optimality and equity are less important issues	Optimality and equity are important issues of policy and implementation
The scope of quality	
Emphasis on 'total quality' to include:	Emphasis primarily on the performance of professional
1. lowering of cost as well as meeting consumer requirements	personnel and primarily in technical care but with expansions to include the patient–practitioner interaction,
2. all steps in the process of designing, producing, selling and servicing	the patients' contribution to care, and social issue of access and equity

---

Box 13.3 Cont'd

3. everyone in an organisation, at all levels, in all units

When applied to health care there is a danger of paying less attention to clinical care and more attention to supportive activities, with preponderant emphasis on cost saving	The danger is preponderant attention to the technical performance of physicians, with less attention to other professionals and no attention to others
Can be criticised as 'marginal' or 'peripheral'	Can be criticised as 'partial', 'less than total'
The nature of the 'quality problem' Most problems of quality arise from defects in the design of systems, products and processes of production. They arise less often from failures of production workers to perform their duties	The contributions of structural characteristics are recognised, but the competence of health-care professionals is a major structural characteristic and variability in their performance an important problem
The strategies of quality assurance and improvement Emphasis on changing structural characteristics, but includes worker retraining or reassignment	Emphasis on influencing professional performance more directly by education, retraining, supervision, encouragement or censure
Management maintains ultimate responsibility but empowers production workers to monitor their own work by delegation of responsibility, education and training in methods of monitoring and offering financial and non-financial rewards for improvements in quality	What the industrial model advocates is already an established tradition in the self-monitoring and self-governance of physicians. But the two models would be even more similar if: (1) similar privileges were extended to other professionals and non-professionals; (2) physicians and others received more training in methods of quality assurance; and (3) the role of management in quality assurance was strengthened
The organisation is altered to become less hierarchical, more participatory	The aim is continuous improvement of performance
The methods of quality monitoring There is monitoring of production, using process and outcome measures, compared to relevant standards This takes two forms: (1) concurrent monitoring, during the production process, by workers and supervisors, aiming for speedy detection of significant deviations and their correction (2) terminal monitoring of samples of finished product, aiming to prevent sale of defective lots and learning how to prevent defects in the future	There are corresponding forms of monitoring process and outcome, using analogous standards, except that services given cannot be recalled. However, services planned can be countermanded; care can be monitored while it is being given; and care can be assessed after it is completed, so as to learn from past success and failure and make appropriate adjustments
Monitoring is seen as a continuous cycle of activities meant to verify performance; determine the reasons for unsatisfactory performance; take appropriate action; and check the effect of such an action	Monitoring is seen in similar terms; as a cyclical activity, with an analogous succession of steps
The aim is continuous improvement of performance	The aim is continuous improvement of performance
A rather specific set of methods is advanced for problem identification; consensus development; description of performance; determination of causation, etc. Statistical control methods are highly developed and widely used	Similar methods are available, especially in the armamentarium of descriptive and analytic epidemiology, but clinical case review is the dominant method and statistical-control methods have not been widely used
Some conclusions Despite differences in vocabulary, there are remarkable similarities between the two models and many of the differences that remain are justifiable. The industrial model, rather than being a negation of the health model, is a 'professionalisation of industrial production'.	The main dangers of applying the industrial model to health care are: • adoption of an oversimplified definition of quality • deflection of attention from clinical effectiveness to the efficiency of supportive activities.

Box 13.3 Cont'd

The main lessons we can learn from the industrial model are:

- a new appreciation of the fundamental soundness of our traditions
- the need for even greater attention to consumer requirements, values and expectations
- the need for greater attention to the design of systems and processes as a means to quality assurance
- the need to extend the self-monitoring, self-governing tradition of physicians to others in the organisation

- the need for a greater role for management in assuring the quality of clinical care
- the need to develop appropriate applications of statistical control methods to health-care monitoring
- the need for greater education and training in quality monitoring and assurance for all concerned.

Bibliographic note:
This lecture outline is based on a more complete treatment in a paper entitled 'Continuity and change in the quest for quality' scheduled to appear in *Clinical Performance and Quality Health Care*, Vol 1, Number 1, January 1993.

Box 13.4 Perspectives on quality

Questions for the district nurse
Are you delivering a quality service?
Yes?
How do you know this?
Where is the evidence which would support your answer?

Consider the following responses.

A manager: Yes I am, 90% of my district nurses are trained district nurses so yes, I must be.

A district nursing sister: Yes, I am up to date in all of my practice. My caseload is very large but I always make it through the day and my patients don't have any complaints.

Question for patients
Are you receiving a quality service?

Patient: Certainly the nurses are all good though some seem better than others. They are very busy and overstretched, but I know they do their best, often in very difficult circumstances.

Think of a recent encounter that you had with a patient while delivering care.

- Was the care you delivered good-quality care?
- What aspects did the care actually consist of?
- Was there technical care involved?
- Was the interaction/interpersonal relationship aspect of good quality?
- What are you using to judge this against?

Box 13.5 Perspectives of quality (Øvretveit 1992)

Client quality
What clients and carers want from the service (individual and population)

Professional quality
Whether the service meets needs as defined by professional providers and referrers and whether it correctly carries out techniques and procedures which are believed to be necessary to meet client needs

Management quality
The most efficient and productive use of resources, within limits and directives set by higher authorities/purchasers. This refers to designing the service and implementing it without waste, duplication and mistakes

Øvretveit (1992) stresses the importance of integrating the perspectives of these three major interest groups when specifying the quality of a particular service.

Joss & Kogan (1995), however, in developing quality further highlight how complicated this actually is.

One of the major concerns would be how to define quality, given the different perceptions and requirements of different groups of staff and the wide range of stakeholders in the NHS – government, regional and district purchasers, trust boards, doctors, paramedics, nurses, patients, clients and their carers. This is illustrated in Box 13.4.

Issues of quality are complex and the processes of improvement are neither easy to implement or to put in writing. However, it is clear that any approach adopted involves defining or specifying current best practice and subsequently

---

Box 13.6   Clinical governance

Clinical governance is the vital ingredient which will enable us to achieve a Health Service in which the quality of health care is paramount ... Clinical governance will not replace professional self-regulation and individual clinical judgement, concepts that lie at the heart of health care in this country. But it will add an extra dimension that will provide the public with guarantees about standards of care. (Sam Galbraith MP, Minister for Health (Scotland), June 1998)

Key principles
- Responsibility for quality of care is a trust's explicit statutory duty with the trust chief executive being accountable for the quality of care in the same way as

he/she is currently responsible for proper use of resources
- The delivery of consistently high standards
- Quality of patient care is given the highest priority at every level
- The planning and delivery of services take full account of the perspective of patients
- Systems are in place which ensure that care delivered meets relevant standards and unacceptable practice is detected and addressed
- Good practice is identified and disseminated
- Lifelong learning
- Evidence-based practice is in daily use
- Openness
- Cooperation and partnership

---

ensuring that this is implemented consistently within budgetary limits.

This section has explored a number of definitions, dimensions and frameworks for quality, service quality in general and health-care quality in particular. Defining, monitoring and improving the quality of district nursing will be addressed in more detail later in the chapter, referring when necessary to these frameworks, definitions and concepts.

The final definition to be introduced at this point is of the term 'clinical governance' (Box 13.6), described as a framework for designing and delivering care for a new health service. Two definitions of clinical governance which may be helpful are:

1. corporate accountability for clinical performance (Scottish Office 1998a)
2. a framework which helps all clinicians – including nurses – to continuously improve quality and safeguard standards of care (RCN 1998).

Cook (1999), in attempting to demystify clinical effectiveness for community practitioners, introduces clinical governance as 'probably the worst term for one of the best things to have happened to clinical practice in years'. She goes on to say that those practising in the community should see clinical governance as good news for their patients and clients as its principal aim is to raise

the standard of service to patients. Furthermore, it is important to practitioners as 'its aims are inseparable from those enshrined in professional ethics and the Code of Professional Conduct'. Since most practitioners have at times expressed concerns about quality of care they should welcome the systematic appraisal of practice across different disciplines working in primary care against agreed standards, with the additional commitment to share good practices and change and improve as necessary.

The key principles of clinical governance and its implications for patients, district nurses and trusts will be addressed within each relevant section.

THE PATIENT'S PERSPECTIVE

The last 10 years have seen a major move from the 'nurse knows best' and 'trust the caring professions' mentality to a questioning and challenging of information from patients (Box 13.7). The publishing of the Patient's Charter (DoH 1992) demanded that clear standards be shared with the public so that they know the level of service to expect and how to complain if necessary.

It has to be asked how prepared both professionals and the public were for the Patient's Charter and its consequences and again, there is a lesson to be learned as the key principles of clinical governance in involving patients and the public are implemented in practice. The

---

Box 13.7   Client quality (Øvretveit 1992)

As previously stated, Øvretveit (1992), in defining and measuring quality, reinforces the importance of clients' perceptions of the service at both individual and population levels and breaks this down further into:

- what a client wants from the service; that is, what they would like to receive and what it should ideally provide but this is rarely a demand
- what a client realistically expects from the service; that is, what they think it would provide
- what the client thinks they need, which may be different from what they want.

He states that a client's perceived experience of the service will be different at different times and this in turn will be different from their global and enduring perception or image of the service. All of this makes defining quality very complex and difficult … and that is before other perspectives have even been considered!

---

public now have easy access to information and guidelines and can arrive for their appointment at the health centre with guidelines applicable to their condition which have been downloaded from the Internet.

Generally speaking, there are patient/client groups who use their voice, for example women requiring maternity care, while other client groups are known to have little voice, for example the older person, people with learning disabilities and people with mental health problems. Although some changes have taken place, with advocacy systems being set up and greater 'watchdog' and public involvement, being heard may still be a struggle and facilitating the interests of patient and family remains in many cases within the control of the professional. For example, professionals decide how much patients should be told about their illness and professionals invite patient representation on to their groups.

Williamson (1992) puts forward a theoretical framework for understanding consumerism in health care and its relation to professionalism. She presents an insight into acting in the 'patient's best interests', consumer groups, ideologies and standards and gives examples of existing good practice. An optimistic conclusion is reached with increasing compatibility of interest between professionals and consumers. Williamson (1992) states that formulating new

standards that respect patients' wishes is a matter of urgency and cites some examples of progress in the area of information sharing and involvement, including a dermatology ward in the Queen's Medical Centre, Nottingham, where patients write their own care plans regarding the application of ointments and dressings. This is seen to assist understanding of and compliance with treatment. She goes on to say that health-care professionals call these innovations 'patient education' and self-care. However, she would prefer to see them as restorative and treating patients as people.

Within the White Papers (DoH 1997, Scottish Office 1997) which lay out the renewal of the health service, clinical governance is put forward as the vital ingredient which will enable the achievement of a health service in which the quality of health care is paramount. Quality of patient care is to be given the highest priority at every level and the planning and delivery of services should take full account of the perspective of patients. What is important to patients will be paramount. For a number of years now, involving patients and the public has taken place in a variety of ways. Service reviews have sought patients' views, patient satisfaction surveys have been undertaken and responded to, comments and feedback have been encouraged, as have the work of pressure groups and watchdog organisations such as health councils, to name but a few. While for some, involvement and consultation have been meaningful, for others there has been a degree of tokenism.

In national guideline development in Scotland there is patient representation and it is acknowledged that 'patients also have an important role in promoting guideline implementation … and they should have access to information on the recommendations of published guidelines' (SIGN 1999). SIGN has also established a Patient Information and Participation Subcommittee to take forward relevant issues and there are opportunities for discussion at national open meetings which is part of the consultation process during guideline development.

At a recent conference entitled Clinical Governance: Sharing Power and Opportunity, one service user gave some sound advice to the professionals in the audience. 'We need to learn your language, the jargon ... and that takes time; we need to learn how to make a meaningful contribution to the discussions and how these meetings work.' In response to a question on how to get patients involved in groups, the simple answer was 'pay them'.

A number of clear messages came over during the presentation and the discussion brought home again the power and control of the professional and the very different worlds patients and professionals inhabit, albeit that one can be a district nurse today and a patient tomorrow!

In her study which examined patients' views of the care given by district nurses, Davy (1998) stated that district nurses needed to take account of their legal and professional duty to care (UKCC 1996) and ensure that the care given is of a sufficiently high standard to justify the trust of patients, their families and society in general (RCN 1990). The principal finding was that 'good nurse/patient relationships are a necessary foundation for helping to create an atmosphere of trust and security in which effective physical and psychosocial care can take place' (see Box 13.8). The interpersonal process has been identified by several authors as being a necessary part of caring (Astedt-Kurki & Laitila-Haggman 1992, Clarke Wheeler 1992, Ford 1990, Fosbinder 1994).

Many of the aspects of good practice which Davy (1998) identified are reflected in the elements of good service quality identified in the SERVQUAL model. These are outlined in Box 13.22.

The one-to-one relationship of district nurse and patient enables each patient to be treated as a unique individual in her own setting and provides an opportunity for each patient to be treated as a person and feel valued and important.

Making the patient (customer) central to the design and delivery of care reflects one of the key elements of clinical governance and a key component of a continuous improvement approach to quality. Its achievement demands that the culture, systems and approaches of an organisation facilitate this centrality. This means listening to patients, valuing what they say, seeing things from their perspective, treating them as people and seeing them as individuals. Reflect on a traditional patient journey through the system, from entry point to possible exit, and consider any duplication, gaps and care that may be given, much of which seems more professionally led rather than patient focused. This journey is highlighted in Box 13.9.

Box 13.8 Key findings (Davy 1998)

District nurses need to take an interest in the people they nurse as individuals rather than merely as patients and also to extend that interest towards their carers and families.

Trust and security between patient and nurse seemed to arise from the proficient use of interpersonal skills and by exhibiting reliability and flexibility. This was demonstrated by district nurses visiting as planned and by being available when problems arose.

Expert knowledge also appeared to help create an atmosphere of trust and security.

Working with patients and not 'taking over' was also deemed important. This again requires knowing patients as people.

There is an overwhelming need to reiterate the importance of nurses integrating patients' views of their care into their endeavour to meet the needs of patients in the process of caring.

Box 13.9 A traditional patient journey

Visits GP – history taken
Investigations commenced
May be referred to nurse – history taken
Letter sent to hospital consultant re further investigations
Waits for appointment
Visits hospital for outpatient appointment; history taken, repetition of some investigations
May revisit hospital for other investigations
Waits for results
Visits hospital/GP for results
Admitted to hospital
Personal details documented
Medical history taken
Nursing history taken
Paramedical history taken
Treatment given
Discharged following treatment
Appointment with GP
Discharged – may be referred to nurse

> **Box 13.10** Professional quality (Øvretveit 1992)
>
> Whether the service meets needs as defined by professional providers and referrers, and whether it correctly carries out techniques and procedures which are believed to be necessary to meet client needs.

> **Box 13.11** Definition of quality (reproduced from Donabedian 1989 with permission)
>
> - The goodness of technical care judged by its effectiveness
> - The goodness of the interpersonal relationship judged partly by its contribution to effectiveness
> - The goodness of the amenities

THE DISTRICT NURSE'S PERSPECTIVE

As accountable health-care practitioners district nurses are required to give some assurance that their activities make a significant impact on the quality of health-care delivery, whether in health gain or palliative care. Sines (1997) states that in the new world of community health practice, nurses will be required to develop and change, drawing on the very best of their past experience and becoming increasingly reliant upon the production of research evidence to inform their future practice. Griffiths & Luker (1997) assure us that although at this time district nursing is underresearched as a subject in its own right, it can import evidence to underpin practice from neighbouring disciplines and this is already the case in the management of such clinical conditions as venous leg ulceration, pressure sores, urinary incontinence and terminal cancer, to name but a few. As professionals, district nurses need to be clear about their philosophy, values and professional standards.

Ultimately, the clinical judgement of clinicians should not be underestimated. The White Papers (DoH 1997, Scottish Office 1997) indicate that the framework implemented for clinical governance will not replace professional self-regulation and individual clinical judgement, concepts that lie at the heart of health care in this country. But it will add an extra dimension that will provide the public with guarantees about standards of care. Professional quality is defined in Box 13.10.

Demands are being made for nursing practice to be evidence-based, as necessary for the district nurse as any other. Evidence-based practice will be considered later in the chapter. In considering evidence-based practice, techniques and treatments come easily to mind but what about critical thinking, decision-making processes,

diagnosis of the problem, what about the evidence on which your communication is based?

In one of his definitions of quality Donabedian (1989) draws out the importance of the interpersonal relationship as a separate element alongside the technical aspects of care as shown in Box 13.11.

The client–practitioner relationship was originally outlined by Donabedian in 1972. In Box 13.12 you will find some attributes of a good patient–practitioner relationship. This relationship is an important component of quality as its attributes are desirable in themselves. Furthermore, patients often see the quality of this relationship as evidence of good technical care. The interpersonal relationship can certainly contribute to effectiveness in technical care through greater patient cooperation and compliance. Although Donabedian endeavoured in 1972 to put forward some attributes to enable the evaluation of the interpersonal relationship, even today professionals state that this is an area largely unexplored which is at times described as 'touchy–feely', therefore immeasurable and intangible. This is illustrated in vignette 13.2.

When defining and giving consideration to evidence-based practice, district nurses, as a group of professionals, should make efforts to ensure that 'evidence' is not limited to the technical aspects of care but extends into these other aspects which are deemed important by our patients.

Implementing evidence-based practice will require an effective continuing professional development programme for district nurses. One strategy to assist in its implementation is to set up clinical supervision in nursing. Structures to support clinical supervision have been around for some time in other professions and are gradually being introduced into nursing. In *A vision for the future* (DoH 1993) it was recommended

Box 13.12   Some attributes of a good patient – practitioner relationship (reproduced from Donabedian 1972 with permission)

- Congruence between therapist and client expectations and orientations
- Adaptation and flexibility: the ability of the therapist to adapt her approach to the expectations of the client and also to the demands of the clinical situation
- Mutuality: gains for both therapist and client
- Stability: a stable relationship between client and therapist
- Maintenance of maximum possible client autonomy, freedom of action and movement
- Maintenance of family and community communication ties
- Maximum possible degree of egalitarianism in the client–therapist relationship
- Maximum possible degree of active client participation through:

1. sharing knowledge concerning the health situation
2. shared decision making
3. participation in carrying out therapy
- Maintenance of empathy and rapport without undue emotional involvement of the therapist
- Maintenance of a supportive relationship without encouragement of undue dependency
- Confining the therapist's and the client's influence and action within the boundaries of their legitimate social functions
- Avoidance of exploitation of the client and of the therapist economically, socially, sexually or any other way
- Maintenance of the client's and therapist's dignity and individuality
- Maintenance of privacy
- Maintenance of confidentiality

Vignette 13.2   Lasting impressions

Among the many examples of good practice discussed with a group of district nurses, their work caring for the dying and bereaved left a lasting impression. Their interpersonal skills as well as their technical knowledge base and commitment to caring for the whole family were obvious as they recounted particular personal experiences. As well as carer, advisor and teacher, they had become a trusted family friend.

that clinical supervision should become 'integral throughout the lifetime of practice, thus enabling practitioners to accept personal responsibility for and be accountable for care and to keep that care under constant review'. Clinical supervision has been defined as 'a formal process of professional support and learning which enables individual practitioners to develop knowledge and competence, assume responsibility for their own practice and enhance consumer protection and safety of care in complex clinical situations' (DoH 1993). Butterworth & Woods (1998) state that there is an obvious relationship between the good practice of clinical supervision and the responsibilities necessary for effective clinical governance and suggest that it should be part of the systems of clinical governance. In addition the recent introduction of the clinical governance

framework places greater value on and provides direction for staff development to ensure that staff have the necessary knowledge and skills to be deemed fit to practise (Scottish Office 1998a, Scottish Executive 1999).

The professions themselves play a key role in assuring the quality of clinical practice. The Acute Services Review (Scottish Office 1998b) gives the following examples. The Royal Colleges provide accreditation for training of doctors by particular hospitals and almost one-third of Scottish GP practices undergo regular assessment and approval for GP vocational training. For individual doctors, the Colleges accredit satisfactory completion of specialist training and increasingly, the maintenance of professional skills through continuing medical education (CME) programmes. Furthermore, the General Medical Council has introduced new procedures for regulating medical practice while the UKCC and the Council for the Professions Supplementary to Medicine have responsibility for nurses and therapists respectively.

Finally, Learning Together, a strategy for education and training for all staff working in the health service, sets out major challenges to enable its staff to be competent to practise and provide high-quality care to patients (Scottish Executive 1999). It encompasses the following sections:

- quality care
- access and opportunity
- learning organisation
- lifelong learning
- careers.

Providing a quality service requires investment and commitment at all levels within an organisation. At the heart of a quality service is the transaction which takes place between practitioner and patient; that private trusting relationship within which is power and knowledge waiting to be given or taken. The practitioner, accountable for her decisions and actions, relies on providing care within a framework which facilitates, supports and recognises quality care. Ultimately a strategy is needed to provide clear direction for the organisation and the individuals within it. The organisational aspects will be addressed in the final section of the chapter.

AUDIT AND CLINICAL EFFECTIVENESS

Nursing has a long history of developing patient-focused standards of care, monitoring standards and using the development of standards to improve practice (Marr & Giebing 1994, RCN 1990). As the quality agenda has unfolded over time, these origins have prepared nurses well for audit and for the implementation of the key principles of clinical governance.

When audit became a nationally driven requirement, nursing embraced it as part of its strategy to improve patient care. Natural developments from early standard-setting initiatives had ensured that the review process of standards took account of best practice. Using the Dynamic Standard Setting System (DySSSy) (RCN 1990) framework, standards were written with a patient outcome focus and where there were implications for other disciplines, they were included if possible. Furthermore, one of the fundamental principles was ownership and involvement in the process. Where previously much of the work was based on personal commitment and goodwill, the clinical governance agenda

Box 13.13	Commonly used terms	
Evidence-based practice	*Clinical effectiveness*	*Audit*
Seek/identify the evidence	Appraise literature/ inform	[Set standard]
		Collect data
Appraise		
	Change	
Act		Compare
		Make changes
Evaluate	Monitor	Evaluate

brings with it accountability and strategy at the highest level.

As previously stated, terminology can be confusing but if you take a closer look at some of the most commonly used terms and processes, comparisons can be drawn (Box 13.13).

All approaches begin by identifying good practice, either in the form of the evidence from the literature or from a critical review where the literature has already been searched systematically or where the good practice is already identified and developed into a standard. All approaches have a stage which requires changing or taking action and finally a stage that checks that the change has taken place (Adams 1999, Adams 2000).

It is useful at the outset to clarify the nature of evidence as this is often overlooked in the literature surrounding this topic (Walsh 1998). Stetler et al (1998) put forward the following summary definition modelled after the work of the Evidence-Based Medicine Working Group (1992).

Evidence-based nursing de-emphasises ritual, isolated and unsystematic clinical experiences, ungrounded opinions and tradition as a basis for nursing practices ... and stresses instead the use of research findings and, as appropriate, quality improvement data, other operational and evaluation data, the consensus of recognised experts and affirmed experience to substantiate practice.

Evidence-based nursing originates from the view that to make clinical decision making more effective, more and better evidence is needed. However, the need for evidence to support day-to-day district nursing practice far outweighs the amount of available research. District nurses need to give careful consideration to what constitutes evidence before blindly being led down a path they do not wish to follow. Evidence-based nursing is based on the writings of evidence-based medicine but medicine has a more scientific base than nursing which is based on the humanities. Nursing is as much about 'caring' as 'curing'. Sackett et al (1996, 1997) and Cullum et al (1998) write that decision making should be informed by best practice research, clinical expertise and patient preferences. Stetler et al (1998) take a pragmatic view when defining evidence-based nursing and state that not all practice in a health profession can or should be based on science. They propose a model which identifies four potential bases for nursing practice:

- evidence-based practice
- philosophical/conceptual basis for practice
- regulatory basis for practice
- traditional basis for practice.

Finding the evidence which justifies why nurses do what they do is on the district nursing agenda but it is time consuming. There is now a wealth of literature listing sources to make this task easier (Adams 1999b). Finding the evidence is only the first step in this process; having found it, practitioners need to be able to critically appraise the evidence by determining its validity and applicability to their practice. Kitson (1997) and McSherry & Haddock (1999) challenge the nursing profession to make evidence-based practice a reality by becoming equipped with the knowledge and skills to critically appraise and evaluate the true benefits of their actions in the light of patient outcomes.

Thomson & Cullum (1999) describe a strategy which assists in this process and a hierarchy of evidence is put forward to assist in the critical appraisal process. Adams (1999c), in addition to giving guidance on sources of evidence, also gives guidance on interpreting evidence. The following Box 13.14 shows the classification system used by the Scottish Intercollegiate Guidelines Network to indicate the quality of evidence.

In promoting the journal *Evidence-Based Nursing* jointly published by the BMJ and the

Box 13.14	Grade Type of evidence (Sign 1999)
Ia	Evidence obtained from meta-analysis of randomised controlled trials
Ib	Evidence obtained from at least one randomised controlled trial
IIa	Evidence from at least one controlled study without randomisation
IIb	Evidence from at least one other type of quasiexperimental study
III	Evidence from non-experimental descriptive studies
IV	Evidence from experts and/or clinical experience

Vignette 13.3   Experiences of audit and quality improvement

In recounting some audit and quality improvement experiences in the community ... one audit which set out to be multidisciplinary ran into problems ... I think it was because our agendas were different ... the GPs wanted more staff and we wanted to improve care.

Another experience of audit recounted was an audit of incontinence pads usage. This topic was of interest to district nurses as it had a major impact on their day-to-day work ... but the rest of the multidisciplinary team had seemed to lack interest. Again, the agenda or motive appeared to be different: 'the others seemed to be budget minded'.

RCN, Cullum et al (1997) hope that the journal 'will make a major contribution to nursing and, ultimately, to patient care by bringing the findings of rigorous research to the attention of nurses, by promoting critical appraisal of research and by fostering implementation.'

The drive for clinical effectiveness is both national and local. Putting evidence into practice, however, remains a considerable challenge (Cullum et al 1998, Adams 1999d). One approach introduced to improve care has been the audit process.

Audit

Formal audit began within discrete disciplines with medical audit attracting large amounts of government funding following the requirement in the White Paper *Working for patients* (DoH 1990), for medical and financial audit to be undertaken. The support structure was set up both nationally and locally at that time. Nursing audit, along with paramedical audit, attracted some funding but had developed primarily because of practitioners' goodwill and their desire to achieve the highest standards of care for patients. The nursing profession had been involved in setting and monitoring standards for some time and had developed expertise in using the standard-setting process to improve care. While nurses had developed their approach, the medical profession undertook case reviews and peer reviews as ways to check out and improve practice. According to Crombie et al (1993):

Medical or clinical audit is now an expected part of routine practice and the work of all clinicians. Its introduction was broadly welcomed but its implementation has caused some bewilderment and confusion. Concern for the care of individual patients has always been an objective of practitioners; the difference that audit brings is that it requires a systematic and critical analysis of valid measures of the quality of care so that changes can be made to improve care.

Within 2 years of each discipline being involved in undertaking their own audits, it became clear that the systematic review and improvement of patient care could not be artificially divided among disciplines and the interdependency of professionals was apparent. If audit was concerned with improving patient care then it needed to be patient focused and therefore multidisciplinary (clinical) audit needed to be undertaken. Vignette 13.3 illustrates illustrates this

Unidisciplinary standards and audit are likely to continue as single professions put their own houses in order as shown in vignette 13.4 and strive for continued professionalism but increasingly, funded audit will be patient focused and therefore the standards will involve a range of contributing disciplines. With patient-focused standards, patient outcomes will be stated and though the routes to their achievement may differ these routes will cross over where collaboration takes place. Auditing of these standards will require multidisciplinary involvement, not least for 'taking action' when cooperation and collaboration

---

Box 13.15 Common types of audit (Kober 1995)
• Case presentation • Peer review • Adverse events and sentinel events • Criteria-based audit • Generic audit

from all contributing professional groups will be necessary to achieve improvement.

Kober (1995) found criteria-based audits to be by far the most common method, followed by surveys, case presentations and peer review, and least common were adverse and/or sentinel events (Box 13.15). These are outlined below.

Case presentation

This involves the review of individual cases with presentation to a group of peers or a clinical supervisor. Kober (1995) suggests that case presentation is a means of addressing complex moral issues that can be overlooked with quantitative audit methods.

Adverse and sentinel events

This provides the opportunity to explore poor outcomes, identify what went wrong and explore ways of minimising future risk.

Criteria-based audit

This approach offers a narrow focus with depth. Good practice is defined and can then be compared to actual practice. For example, for audit of patients' records, a checklist was developed which identified good record keeping. On a regular basis, managers then random sample patient-held records to compare actual practice against the checklist. Documented feedback is then given to the nursing team on the quality of record keeping.

Generic audits

This approach provides a snapshot of a service or an organisation, giving breadth with limited

---

Vignette 13.4 Fife Leg Ulcer Audit

The first community audit of leg ulcer management was conducted in 1996 led by a local district nursing sister. The audit identified:

- 20 patients in hospital and 247 in the community with leg ulcers
- a number of variations in the management of patients with leg ulcers

and made the following recommendations:

- introduction of a protocol
- introduction of a link nurse scheme for the development of best practice in leg ulcer management
- introduction of education and training programmes for nurses
- initiation of the development of health education material
- easy access for all community nurses to equipment for assessment, i.e. hand-held Doppler
- appointment of a tissue viability nurse to address the above recommendations and other wound management issues
- reaudit 12 months after protocol is in practice.

An outline of activity following distribution of the audit report is given below.

- A small steering group developed a protocol with a view to standardising management of patients with leg ulcers.
- Community nurses with special interest were identified and trained as link nurses.
- Relevant training was cascaded by link nurses; 35 workshops were conducted over a 3-month period (it was identified that staff new to the trust did not receive this workshop opportunity).
- Reaudit was conducted over a 2-month period.

Key findings of the reaudit:

- 68 nurses were involved
- 223 patients in the community and five in hospital
- 96% had access to a link nurse
- 81% had been given a Doppler assessment (nurses from two bases did not have easy access to a Doppler)

Vignette 13.5 The Monitor experience

A group of community nurses discussed their feelings, experiences and reactions when their service undertook an audit exercise using District Nursing Monitor.

'My reaction was HELP' said one, while another said 'It was a first and I was apprehensive'. For many district nurses the Monitor exercise was seen as 'criticising their work' rather than one which could improve care and consequently often created fear, apprehension, defensiveness and vulnerability.

Looking back, they identified that some of the standards within the audit document were unrealistic … and of course 'there were the ifs and buts – a full documented assessment was not always required' and on the other hand 'decisions about care cannot always be made based on two visits'.

On reflection much was learned from the exercise. It certainly 'improved patient documentation and record keeping'. It highlighted great variation in the standard of record keeping across the community and it came to light during the discussion and reflection time that some of the staff had remained unaware of the variation. Feedback had been given to the relevant staff and documentation had improved as a result but knowledge of this was limited.

The auditors themselves stated how they had needed a lot of support and met daily to plan and support each other. 'Going in and looking at colleagues' practice and paperwork was stressful and what right have I to do this?'

The overall feeling was that it would be less painful to undertake if there was to be a next time and they would understand that it was not a threatening exercise but one which would benefit patients and staff.

Some key points to note
Community nurses work independently and often in isolation. Opportunities to observe other colleagues at work and discuss and review practice and perform case reviews and peer reviews are few. It may therefore be difficult for a district nurse to be prompted to examine her current practice.

The fear and threat of the audit both for auditor and the audited was apparent.

In discussion, most district nurses talked about their experience of auditing patient documentation. One of the most interesting and important issues which was repeatedly identified was the large variations in the standard of documentation. Most were unaware of this and were shocked to find out about the differences which they described as 'frightening'.

---

depth. An example of this is Monitor for District Nursing which is one in a series of audit documents which examines nursing practice and documentation. This is highlighted in vignette 13.5.

The prime function of audit is to have a positive impact on the quality and effectiveness of care delivered to patients and clients, whether its focus is on clinical interventions or, as a secondary but important consideration, on the organisation of the service within which these interventions take place. (Robinson 1995)

Experience has shown, however, that the weakest stages in the audit cycle are implementing change and evaluating that the change has been made (closing the loop).

Implementing change means that not only problems need to be identified but also the causes of these problems. According to Crombie et al (1993), in their work on medical audit, 'identification of underlying reasons for failure to meet standards' is a missing component of the audit cycle. If you do not identify why standards are not met, how do you know what action to take to rectify this?

Audit should be an educational activity which is part of the everyday work of the district nurse and activities should be a mix of nursing audit and clinical audit as practices are explored and improved. For some, past audit activity has been synonymous with a judgemental fault-finding exercise, box ticking and something which takes practitioners away from patient care.

Øvretveit (1992) states that 'systematic and effective audit is unfamiliar and threatening to many practitioners. Even within a single professional group there are differences in views about the criteria of good practice and outcome, and a feeling that others do not properly understand or value an individual's approaches'. He goes on to say that he has found it even more difficult to introduce audit in multidisciplinary groups, where these differences in view are compounded by different professional cultures, suspicions and jealousies.

Given Øvretveit's and others' experiences, audit has perhaps been unsuccessful in achieving what it set out to do. The overall goal of improvement in care or effectiveness has often been lost along the way, giving rise to audit being an end in itself rather than a means to an end. The end product of audit should surely be best practice identified, implemented and shared as widely as possible within health care to ensure consistency of standards, equity and cost effectiveness.

Audit, both uni- and multiprofessional, should be an everyday part of the practitioner's role and the identification and implementation of best practice, evidence-based practice, is a necessity. The question remains as to how practitioners will find the time and develop the skills, where necessary, not only to remain up to date and deliver research-derived practice but also to access the relevant research. At the same time they need to be confident in their own experience and the work of colleagues in areas where little research has taken place to date.

One of the developments from Scottish national audit work has been the production of national and local clinical guidelines. For a time the local adaptation of a national guideline was known as a *protocol* but this has since changed to *local guideline*. *Protocol* was found to be a prescriptive term which limited flexibility and clinical judgement. Guidelines are written by a group of representatives of all people involved in an aspect of care, patients and professionals. One method for clinical guideline development is as shown in Box 13.16.

Nine desirable attributes of a guideline, adapted from American work, are outlined below (Grimshaw & Russell 1993).

1. Validity
2. Reproducibility
3. Reliability
4. Representative
5. Clinical applicability
6. Clinical flexibility

Box 13.16 Development of a guideline

- Identify the topic or formulate the question (this could be based on a known variation in this aspect of care or the frequency of the condition or procedure, implications of current practice or potential health gain).
- Undertake a systematic review of current literature. The review involves the retrieval of both published and unpublished material.
- Development of recommendations for practice from the evidence.
- Consultation with colleagues to augment the research findings.
- Achieve consensus.
- Develop the clinical guideline which describes mandatory and optional elements of care and categorises the evidence.
- Pilot the guideline.

Vignette 13.6 Audit experience

An interesting example of an audit was given recently by a practice nurse who had undertaken an audit in collaboration with one of the general practitioners to look at particular aspects of care advice and investigation of patients with coronary heart disease. The patients' records were used as the source of data and were examined to identify whether specific routine blood tests had been undertaken and whether advice on smoking, alcohol consumption and diet had been given.

On listening to the audit presentation I had categorised this audit as a retrospective record audit which would benefit future patients but not those involved in the audit. However, because patients' records were used and the audit undertaken locally, their care was rectified. In the short term a clinic was set up to 'fill the gap', take the tests and provide the advice. In the longer term measures were taken to enable routine blood tests to be taken when patients were attending for some other aspect of care and not to expect a visit simply to

take blood. The intention is to repeat the audit in the future.

The standards identified for the audit were as follows:

- 95% should have a recorded cholesterol level (random or fasting) within the last year
- 100% of patients should have received dietary advice if their cholesterol levels were 5.0 mmol or higher
- 100% of patients should have received advice about alcohol consumption
- 90% of patients should have stopped smoking
- 85% of patients should be taking aspirin daily if there are no contraindications
- 85% of patients should receive lipid-lowering therapy where appropriate (where there are no contraindications) if their cholesterol levels remain greater than 5.0 mmol despite adherence to a cholesterol-lowering diet
- 100% of patients should have their kidney and liver function tested prior to commencing and at regular intervals during lipid-lowering therapy.

---

7. Clarity
8. Meticulous
9. Scheduled review

In some instances, nurses are unaware of the existence of SIGN guidelines while for others the disease orientation and strong medical flavour of many reduce their relevance and applicability to practice. For this to change, nurses need to be involved in the initial identification of the guideline topic and have representation on the guideline development group. A good example where this was achieved was in the SIGN leg ulcer guideline development group where membership included;

- consultant vascular surgeon
- district nurse
- consultant dermatologist
- consultant plastic surgeon
- consultant rheumatologist
- two general practitioners
- lecturer in general practice
- liaison district nurse and leg ulcer specialist
- patient representative
- pharmacist
- physiotherapist
- practice nurse
- senior registrar in vascular surgery.

The results or outcomes of care interventions have been given a high priority as indicators of quality. Donabedian (1992) makes some cautionary statements when considering their use as shown in Box 13.17.

Nurses are committed to being able to justify their practice both from a professional point of view and in being accountable to their patients and clients. Providing nursing for patients is a service which has a high human element. Both provider and receiver of care are unique individuals meeting to identify health needs and subsequently plan, deliver and evaluate care. The provision of care depends on the communication between the parties to get it right. Furthermore, it is likely that more than one discipline is involved in providing care at any given time. Partnerships with other disciplines, services, agencies and with patients and the public now necessitate working together. This does not just happen by chance but requires careful planning, effective communication, respect, trust and appreciation of roles and presents many challenges.

Examining the histories of quality and audit from nursing, paramedical and medical perspectives, it is clear that each group can learn much from each other. Experiences, approaches, attitudes and motives have been very different,

---

Box 13.17 Some attributes of outcomes as indicators for quality (reproduced from Donabedian 1992 with permission)

Outcomes do not directly assess quality of performance. They only permit an inference about the quality of the process and structure of care.

The degree of confidence in that inference depends on the strength of the predetermined causal relationship between process and outcome (and structure and process).

Because that causal relationship is modified by factors other than health care, corrections must be made for the effects of these factors, by case-mix standardisation, or other means, so that like can be compared with like.

Because the relationship between process and outcome is a probability, it is necessary to collect an appropriately large number of cases before one can infer if care is better or worse or meets specified standards.

But poor outcomes can identify a set of cases that merit analysis of the process (and structure) of care in search for possible causes for the poor outcomes.

Outcomes have the important advantage of being 'integrative'. They reflect the contributions of all those who provide care, including the contributions of patients to their own care. Outcomes also reflect skill in execution as well as appropriateness of choice of a strategy of care.

The integrative property of outcomes is necessarily accompanied by an inability to isolate with certainty the specific errors or virtues that have contributed to bad or good outcomes. First process analysis and then structure analysis are needed for that.

Outcome measurement requires specification of the appropriate 'time window', which is the time when outcome differences caused by degrees of quality in health care are most manifest.

The varying time windows of specific outcomes determines the manner and degree of their usefulness in assessments. Immediate outcomes can be used for concurrent monitoring of care, so modifications in care can be made accordingly. Delayed outcomes are useful for retrospective monitoring, leading to improvements in future care.

Outcomes, if poor, indicate damage already done.

Outcomes as indicators of quality are more comprehensible to patients and the public at large than are indicators of the process of technical (but not interpersonal) care. But outcomes are also open to misrepresentation and misunderstanding by the public if the problem of multiple causation is not understood.

As in all evaluational activities, the availability of information, its completeness, its accuracy, its susceptibility to manipulation, and the cost of its acquisition are important considerations. Information about delayed outcomes (after the patient is discharged) is often difficult to get but some outcomes are susceptible to direct verification by an outside observer, in addition to being experienced and reported by patients.

Health-care professionals are less willing or able to establish valid normative standards for outcomes as compared to process.

---

however often complementary. The stereotypes of the nurse, doctor and paramedical member of staff have often prevented partnerships and collaborative working. Vignette 13.6 illustrates how collaboration can work in practice.

Within the participating professions there are different cultures, even different worlds, with each discipline sharing its own common identity and values, common goals and a common language of its own. Often, professional interests have been put before patients' interests and priorities. Indeed, the service provided often demonstrates decisions and actions which are based on the professionals' interests, understanding and expectations rather than the patient's.

Malby (1995) states that clinical audit is concerned with what happens to the patient rather than what the various professionals involved in care do. Wheeler (1995) identifies collaborative

Box 13.18 Different terminology

	Medical	*Nursing*
Standard	Precise quantitative measure	Broad [summary statement]
Criterion	Indicator written without a value	Precise [indicator with a value attached]

initiatives, including multidisciplinary care planning, teamwork and clinical audit, and highlights some of the key aspects which need to be addressed if progress is to be made in this increasingly important area. A lack of understanding of each others' language and terminology has often inhibited effective collaborative audit activity. Even simple and frequently used words such as standards, criteria and assessment have different meanings attached to them by different professionals. Box 13.18 shows an example.

Although nurses are committed to providing care which is effective, barriers often remain in the way. Turning evidence into everyday practice is a major challenge (Dunning et al 1998). Time needs to be taken to examine these and look for strategies to reduce these barriers. A few are mentioned below:

- time
- accessing evidence
- checking its validity and applicability in the clinical situation
- non-challenging cultures
- blame cultures.

Griffiths & Luker (1994) identify the non-challenging culture of district nursing teams. They identified ways in which district nurses avoid conflict with their colleagues in the name of 'teamwork' and their varying easing behaviours. In a study in 1997 Griffiths & Luker summarised that district nurses challenging a colleague on a treatment or care decision would depend on:

- whether the colleague in question was from her own or another team
- the personality of the colleague or relationship with the colleague
- whether the district nurse believed her own practice to be up to date

- the patient's unknown case history
- the patient's personality
- whether challenging would damage the nurse–patient relationship
- stress level of the substituting nurse
- perceived seriousness of the situation
- balance between patient advocacy and respect for a colleague's autonomy.

Improving processes

Having systems in place which facilitate 'getting it right first time' is an important aspect of continuous quality improvement. It is important for all professionals to define quality in the form of standards, guidelines or protocols and to conform to these standards. It is equally important to have systems in place to monitor the standards, share any good practice identified, take action when standards have not been met and ensure the standards are up to date and evidence-based. A culture needs to be nurtured which invests in constantly looking for opportunities to improve processes.

In order to facilitate change and problem solve it is necessary to examine the many complex processes undertaken when delivering care. A number of tools and techniques exist to assist in examining and improving processes. These are described in Box 13.19.

Box 13.19   Tools and techniques for improving processes

- Flow charting – a pictorial representation of the steps or activities in any process
- Fishbone (Ishikawa) cause and effect diagram – a tool used to identify causes of problems. After the desired or problem outcome has been identified, possible categories of possible causes are identified. Categories for a health-care issue may include people (manpower), machines (equipment), materials, methods (processes/procedures), policies, patients
- Brainstorming – a group activity to promote creativity and explore the maximum number of issues in a short time. It can be used to identify problems, solutions, ideas, strategies. Lists are generated from the group without stopping to critique any ideas until all the ideas have been gathered
- Brainstilling – a group activity which promotes individual reflection prior to sharing ideas

- Nominal group technique – a group activity used to gather ideas by each member stating their idea worked out in response to the question
- Force field analysis – a tool to assist in the identification of driving and restraining forces
- Gantt chart – a tool used to manage the planning and implementation of projects, it identifies timescales and priorities
- Simple statistical process control – data gathered over time and trends displayed are used to 'control' processes. Limits of 'control' are set based on current data and analysis and actions are undertaken if data gathered fall outside the control limits
- Pareto principle – a chart used to rank issues or problems. It is used to differentiate 'the vital few from the trivial many'

Box 13.20 Management quality (Øvreitveit 1992)

The most efficient and productive use of resources, within limits and directives set by higher authorities/purchasers. This refers to designing the service and implementing it without waste, duplication and mistakes (Øvretveit 1992).

Improving processes is an important aspect of continuous quality improvement. Other fundamental principles of a continuous improvement approach are outlined in the next section.

SERVICE EXCELLENCE IN DISTRICT NURSING

This final section puts forward a model for service quality in district nursing, addresses some organisational issues, including some examples of accreditation, and relates the principles of continuous quality improvement to the principles of clinical governance. Many clinical governance issues will relate to the organisation and management of clinical services rather than to individual clinical decisions.

Prior to the clinical governance agenda, trusts did not have integrated strategies for quality, audit, risk management, clinical effectiveness and research and development. Few links were found in health-care provider trusts between clinical audit and quality assurance departments (Packwood & Kober 1995).

Quality and audit activity was often based on goodwill by the professionals while effort was put in at a strategic level to measure cost, volume and activity. Furthermore, while quality activities were on the management agenda, audit was a professional issue and to a great extent was unprofessional.

With the advent of clinical governance, chief executives are accountable for quality. This new era will require a new management style which involves honest introspection and the courage to rise to the challenge to improve the quality of care and service (Box 13.20). Chief executives will be required to ensure that information about clinical activity and outcomes is thoroughly

---

Box 13.21 Cost of quality analysis

Activities can be categorised into:
- prevention – the cost of taking the time to 'get it right first time', e.g. accessing information; accurate, comprehensive assessment; training; fit to do the job; supervising till competent
- appraisal – the cost of checking that the right thing was done and met the required outcome, e.g. extended supervision, checking, audit activity which only maintains the status quo
- failure – the cost of discovering that the right thing was not done, e.g. requesting it be done again or repeating it yourself; non-compliance; inappropriate referrals
- non-measurable costs – the cost of low staff morale; reputation of service

---

analysed and perceived flaws in clinical procedures and standards will have to be confronted.

Clinical governance can only thrive when an organisation creates a working environment where ideas and good practice are shared, where education and research are valued and where the blame culture is eliminated. Clinical governance places the responsibility for quality of care jointly on organisations and individuals and recognises that providing a quality service requires investment and commitment at all levels within an organisation. The district nurse, while accountable for her decisions and actions, relies on the provision of a framework which facilitates, supports and recognises quality care. Ultimately, a strategy is needed to provide clear direction for the organisation and the individuals within the organisation.

Time is money and consideration of cost effectiveness is vital to the service to make best possible use of resources. It may be helpful to consider the analysis shown in Box 13.21 when undertaking and managing care on a day-to-day basis.

Accreditation

Accreditation has been used in industry and commerce to demonstrate and communicate the continuing achievement of a certain standard. This external mark of its achievement often successfully markets the organisation. The most usual standards achieved include ISO 9000 series (formerly BS5750), Investors in People, EFQM (European Foundation Quality Model, Business Excellence Model).

A similar approach has been adapted for health-care provision and accreditation standards include:

- King's Fund organisational audit
- Investors in People
- hospital accreditation
- laboratory accreditation
- Chartermark
- CASPE for community hospitals
- RCGP accreditation.

Many of the initial attempts to measure service quality were modelled on methods of measuring product quality, including Deming's and Juran's process control methodologies (Oakland 1993). Service quality has been defined as meeting or exceeding what customers expect from a service. A customer's evaluation, whether service purchaser or service user, is of paramount importance and their resulting level of satisfaction is thought to determine the likelihood of repurchase or reuse which impacts on reputation and ultimately on measures of success. Zeithaml et al (1990) state that 'Judgements of high and low service quality depend on how customers perceive the actual service performance in the context of what they expected. Therefore service quality can be defined as the extent of discrepancy between customers' expectations or desires and their perceptions'.

The SERVQUAL model

The SERVQUAL model (Zeithaml et al 1990) has been used for evaluating service quality in a number of differing services. The authors identified 10 dimensions which were important to service quality (Box 13.22), and following further research, reduced these to five dimensions (Box 13.23) by using qualitative and quantitative approaches in the form of focus group discussions and customer surveys.

The model identifies the five gaps where discrepancies may be found in perceptions and expectations of both providers and customers.

The key to delivering high-quality service is to balance expectations and perceptions and close any gap between the two.

Good-quality health care delivered consistently and to a high standard must be a key objective of the NHS. It is a shared responsibility of everyone working in the NHS, and covers all aspects of health care including the effectiveness of clinical practice, the environment in which it is delivered, and responsiveness to the needs of patients. One of the key components in continuously improving is managing change. To promote a strategy for continuous quality improvement, the managing and embracing of change needs to be at the heart of the organisation and individuals need to be committed to constant change. This demands trust, flexibility, creativity and risk taking and clear direction and commitment from the top of the organisation. The key principles within a continuous improvement approach outlined in Box 13.24 (Gilbert 1992, Koch 1992, Schroeder 1993) can be found in the vision for the new health service (Scottish Office 1997).

In examining organisational approaches, responsibilities and frameworks, the picture would be incomplete without looking at the national scene. Clinical governance has brought a number of new national organisations and systems to set and monitor standards and many of these are described in the literature. These organisations include:

- National Institute for Clinical Excellence (NICE) (not Scotland)
- Clinical Resource and Audit Group (CRAG)

Box 13.22 Original 10 SERVQUAL dimensions for evaluating service quality (Zeithaml et al 1990)

Tangibles
Reliability
Responsiveness
Competence
Courtesy
Credibility
Security
Access
Communication
Understanding the customer

Box 13.23 The five SERVQUAL dimensions related to district nursing Boxes 13.22 and 13.23 Reproduced from Zeithaml 1990 with permission of The Pree Press, a division of Simon & Schuscer Inc.

These have been applied to the district nurse's caring role and some examples are given. The dimensions could be applied to other aspects of her role, e.g. teaching students.

Tangibles: Appearance of communication materials and ease of understanding
- Care planning documentation
- Patient education written materials
- District nurse's appearance/uniform
- Appearance of surgery/health centre

Reliability: Ability to perform the promised service, stated or implied, dependably and accurately
- Adherence to care plan
- Sincere interest in solving problems and queries
- Service performed right first time
- Service performed at the time/frequency promised

Responsiveness: Willingness to help patients and provide prompt service
- Tell when service will be performed
- Visits take place in a planned and regular way
- Always perceived as 'willing to help' and never too busy

Assurance: Knowledge and courtesy of the district nurse and her ability to convey trust and confidence
- Credibility of district nurse instilling confidence
- Patients/families feel safe in the relationship
- Mechanisms for feedback from patients and families
- District nurse responds to feedback on her performance
- Regarding patient care
- Consistently courteous
- Knowledge to deal with questions and queries from patients and families

Empathy: Caring individualised attention which arises from the effort to know patients/families and their needs
- Adequacy of time
- Times when service is offered are convenient to patients/families
- Personal attention and patients'/families' best interests at heart
- Understand specific needs of patients/families
- Unmet needs are identified and met within reason
- User friendliness of documentation used
- Communication and relationship between district nurse and patients/families with knowledge and appreciation of commitments and responsibilities
- Ease of access to district nurse

Box 13.24 Principles of continuous quality improvement (Schroeder 1993)

- Clear focus on organisational mission – known, valued underpinning and guides
- Continuous improvement – means every aspect can always be improved upon
- Customer orientation – internal and external
- Leadership commitment
- Empowerment
- Crossfunctional collaboration
- Focus on processes
- Focus on data and statistical thinking

- Commission for Health Improvement (CHI) (not Scotland)
- Clinical Standards Board for Scotland (CSBS)
- Scottish Health Technology Assessment Centre (SHTAC)

CONCLUSION

Much has been said and written about the implementation of quality and clinical effectiveness. There are structures at national and local levels with clear accountability – individual, collective and organisational – so it is time to turn rhetoric into reality.

Acknowledgements

For providing precious time and information for the vignettes, the following are acknowledged: district nurses and managers from Argyll and Clyde, Fife; Dr. Milne, GP, and Irene McDonald, J. practice nurse, Fife. I would also like to thank Professor Donabedian, who took the time to write personally.

REFERENCES

Adams C 1999a Clinical effectiveness: a practical guide. Community Practitioner 72(5): 125–127
Adams C 1999b Clinical effectiveness: part two – finding the best evidence. Community Practitioner 72(7): 205–211

Adams C 1999c Clinical effectiveness: part three – interpreting the evidence. Community Practitioner 72(9): 289–292
Adams C 1999d Clinical effectiveness: part four – putting evidence into practice. Community Practitioner 72(11): 354–357

Adams C 2000 Clinical effectiveness: part five – evaluating clinical change. Community Practitioner 73(1): 435–438

Astedt-Kurki P, Haggman-Laitila A 1992 Good nursing practice as perceived by clients: a starting point for the development of professional nursing. Journal of Advanced Nursing 17: 1195–1199

British Standard, Institute 1994 BS EN 9000-1 Quality management and quality assurance standards: Guidelines for selection and rule. British Standards Institute, Milton Keynes.

Butterworth T, Woods D 1998 Clinical governance and clinical supervision; working together to ensure safe and accountable practice. A briefing paper. University of Manchester, Manchester

Clarke J B, Wheeler S J 1992 A view of the phenomenon of caring in nursing practice. Journal of Advanced Nursing 17: 1283–1290

Cook R 1999 Clinical governance: the role of community practitioners. Community Practitioner 7(4): 83–85

Crombie I K, Davies H T O, Abraham S C S, Florey C du V 1993 The audit handbook improving health care through clinical audit. John Wiley, Chichester

Crosby P B 1980 Quality is free: the art of making quality certain. McGraw-Hill, New York

Crosby P B 1989 Let's talk quality. McGraw-Hill, New York

Cullum N, DiCenso A, Ciliska D 1997 Evidence-based nursing: an introduction. Nursing Standard 11(28): 32–33

Cullum N, DiCenso A, Ciliska D 1998 Implementing evidence-based nursing: some misconceptions. Evidence-based Medicine 1(2): 38–40

Davy M 1998 Patients' views of the care given by district nurses. Professional Nurse 13(8): 498–502

Deming W E 1986 Out of the crisis. Massachusetts Institute of Technology, Centre for Advanced Engineering Studies, Cambridge, Massachusetts

Department of Health 1990 Working for patients. HMSO, London

Department of Health 1992 The patient's charter. HMSO, London

Department of Health 1993 A vision for the future. HMSO, London

Department of Health 1997 The new NHS: modern, dependable. HMSO, London

Donabedian A 1966 Evaluating the quality of medical care. Millbank Memorial Fund Quarterly 44: 166–203

Donabedian A 1970 Patient care evaluation. Hospitals 44(7): 131–136

Donabedian A 1972 Models for organising the delivery of personal health services and criteria for evaluating them. Millbank Memorial Fund Quarterly 50: 103–153

Donabedian A 1980 The definition of quality and approaches to its assessment, vol. I. Health Administration Press, Michigan:

Donabedian A 1982 Explorations in quality assessment and monitoring: the criteria and standards of quality. Health Administration Press, Michigan:

Donabedian A 1985 The methods and findings of quality assessment and monitoring: an illustrated analysis, vol III. Health Administration Press, Michigan:

Donabedian A 1992 Lecture outlines and illustrative materials for the seminar on quality assessment and assurance. Brasenose College, University of Oxford

Dunning M, Abi-Aad G, Gilbert D, Gillam S, Livett H 1998 Turning evidence into everyday practice. King's Fund, London

Evidence-Based Medicine Working Group 1992 Evidence-based medicine: a new approach to teaching the practice of medicine. JAMA 268 (17): 2420

Ford J S 1990 Caring encounters. Scandinavian Journal of Caring Sciences 4(4): 157–162

Fosbinder D 1994 Patient perceptions of nursing care: an emerging theory of interpersonal competence. Journal of Advanced Nursing 20: 1085–1093

Gilbert J 1992 How to eat an elephant: a slice by slice guide to total quality management. Tudor Business Press, Sevenoaks

Griffiths J M, Luker K A 1994 Intraprofessional teamwork in district nursing: in whose interest? Journal of Advanced Nursing 20: 1038–1045

Griffiths J M, Luker K A 1997 A barrier to clinical effectiveness: the etiquette of district nursing. Clinical Effectiveness in Nursing 1: 121–130

Grimshaw J M, Russell I T 1993 Achieving health gain through clinical guidelines I: developing scientifically valid guidelines. Quality in Health Care 2: 243–248.

Joss R, Kogan M 1995 Advancing quality: total quality management in the National Health Service. Open University Press, Buckingham

Juran J M 1988 Juran on planning for quality. Free Press, New York

Kitson A L 1997 Using evidence to demonstrate the value of nursing. Nursing Standard 11(28): 34–39

Koch H 1992 Implementing and sustaining total quality management in health care. Longman, Harlow

Kober A 1995 The nature of clinical audit and progress made. In: Kogan M, Redfern S (eds) Making use of clinical audit. Open University Press, Buckingham

Malby R (ed) 1995 Clinical audit for nurses and therapists. Scutari Press, Harrow

Marr H, Giebing H 1994 Quality assurance in nursing. Concepts, methods and case studies. Campion Press, Edinburgh

Maxwell R J 1984 Quality assessment in health. British Medical Journal 288: 1470–1472

Morgan C, Murgatroyd S 1994 Total quality management in the public sector. Open University Press, Buckingham

McSherry R, Haddock J 1999 Evidence-based health care: its place within clinical governance. British Journal of Nursing 8(2): 113–117

NHS Executive 1998 Achieving effective practice – a clinical effectiveness and research information pack for nurses, midwives and health visitors. Leeds: NHS Executive

Norman I J, Redfern S J 1993 The quality of nursing. Nursing Times 89(27): 40–43

Oakland J 1993 Total quality management: the route to improving performance, 2nd edn. Butterworth-Heinemann, Oxford

Øvretveit J 1992 Health service quality. An introduction to quality methods for health services. Blackwell Scientific Publications, Oxford

Packwood T, Kober A 1995 Clinical audit and its relationship to other forms of quality assurance and knowledge generation. In: Kogan M, Redfern S (eds) Making use of clinical audit. Open University Press, Buckingham

Robinson S 1995 The benefits of and constraints on clinical audit. In: Kogan M, Redfern S (eds) Making use of clinical audit. Open University Press, Buckingham

Royal College of General Practitioners (Scotland) 1999 Practice Accreditation, A college system of quality team development version 1. RCGP, Edinburgh

Royal College of Nursing 1990 Standards of care: district nursing. RCN, London

Royal College of Nursing 1998 Guidance for nurses on clinical governance. RCN, London

Sackett D L, Rosenberg W M C, Gray J A M, Haynes R D, Richardson W S 1996 Evidence-based medicine: what it is and what it isn't (editorial). British Medical Journal 312(7073): 71–72

Sackett DL, Scott Richardson W, Rosenberg WMC 1997 Evidence-based medicine. How to practice and teach EBM. Churchill Livingstone, Edinburgh

Schroeder P 1993 Improving quality and performance concepts, Programs and techniques Mosby, St Louis

Scottish Executive 1999 Learning together: a strategy for education, training and lifelong learning for all staff in the National Health Service in Scotland. Scottish Executive, Edinburgh

Scottish Office 1997 Designed to care: renewing the National Health Service in Scotland. Stationery Office, Edinburgh

Scottish Office 1998a Guidance on clinical governance. NHS MEL (1998) 75. Stationery Office, Edinburgh

Scottish Office 1998b Acute services review report. Stationery Office, Edinburgh

SIGN 1999 SIGN guidelines: an introduction to SIGN methodology for the development of evidence-based clinical guidelines. Scottish Intercollegiate Guidelines Network, Edinburgh

Sines D 1997 Preface. In: Mason C (ed) Achieving quality in community health care nursing. Macmillan, London

Stetler C B, Brunell M, Giuliano K K, Morsi D, Prince L, Newell-Stokes V 1998 Evidence-based practice and the role of nursing leadership. Journal of Nursing Administration 28(7/8): 45–53

1996 Guidelines for professional practice. UKCC, London

United Kingdom Central Council for Nursing, Midwifery and Health Visiting

Thompson C, Cullum N 1999 Examining evidence: an overview. Nursing Times Learning curve 3(1) 7-9

Walsh M P 1998 What is evidence? A critical view of nursing. Clinical Effectiveness in Nursing 2: 86–93

Walton M 1989 The Deming management method. Management Books 2000, Didcot

Wheeler D 1995 Breaking down professional boundaries. In: Malby R (ed) Clinical audit for nurses and therapists. Scutari Press, Harrow

Williamson C 1992 Whose standards? Consumer and professional standards in health care. Open University Press, Buckingham

Zeithaml V A, Parasuraman A, Berry L L 1990 Delivering quality service: balancing customer perceptions and expectations. Free Press, New York

FURTHER READING

Bendell T 1990 The quality gurus: what can they do for your company? Department of Trade and Industry, London

Chambers R 1998 Clinical effectiveness made easy: first thoughts on clinical governance. Radcliffe Medical Press, Oxford

Collard R 1993 Total quality success through people. Institute of Personnel Management, London

Lilley R 1999 Making sense of clinical governance. A workbook for NHS doctors, nurses and managers. Radcliffe Medical Press, Oxford

Øvretveit J 1993 Coordinating community care. Multidisciplinary teams and care management. Open University Press, Buckingham

Øvretveit J, Mathias P, Thompson T (eds) 1994 Interprofessional working for health and social care. Macmillan, London

Parsley K, Corrigan P 1999 Quality improvement in health care 2e. Stanley Thornes (Publishers) Ltd, Cheltenham

Pietroni P, Pietroni C 1996 Innovation in community care and primary health. The Marylebone experiment, Churchill Livingstone, Edinburgh

Royal College of Nursing 2000 Clinical Governance: how nurses can get involved. RCN, London

Sale D 1996 Quality assurance for nurses and other members of the healthcare tea, 2nd edn. Macmillan, Basingstoke

Tingle J 1998 Clinical governance and record keeping: legal issues. British Journal of Community Nursing 3(8): 382–384

Walshe K, Walsh N, Schofield T, Blakeway-Phillips C 1999 Accreditation in primary care. Radcliffe Medical Press, Oxford

Wright C, Whittington D 1992 Quality assurance: an introduction for health care professionals. Churchill Livingstone, Edinburgh

Zwaneberg T, van Harrison J (eds) 2000 clinical governance in primary care. Radcliffe Medical Press, Oxford

14

Economic evaluation

Emma McIntosh   Mandy Ryan

Key points

- Costing
- Benefit assessment
- Economic evaluation

INTRODUCTION

Nurses command a strong and influential position in guiding the health service in cost-effective practice (Lessner et al 1994). Recent changes in the provision of primary care services (DoH 1997, Scottish Office 1997), an increasingly elderly population and the move towards community care will have implications for the role of the district nurse. It is therefore important that this role is evaluated.

Economic evaluation provides a framework for evaluating the services provided by district nurses. Within the context of health care, this framework is concerned with identifying, measuring and valuing the costs and benefits of alternative health-care interventions. Costs and benefits are then compared and decisions made regarding the efficient allocation of scarce health-care resources. Within the context of district nursing, the costs and benefits of the service need to be identified. Wilson-Barnett (1992) proposes five nursing functions which are useful in thinking about such costs and benefits (Box 14.1). The challenge is to identify, measure and value the resources and benefits involved in achieving these functions. Only then can efficient decisions be made.

In the next section issues arising in the identification, measurement and valuation of costs are

---

Box 14.1   Five nursing functions (Wilson-Barnett 1992)

Wilson-Barnett (1992) suggests that of prime importance in nursing are those functions which:
1. relate to resolving clearly identified patient problems
2. are requested and/or appreciated by consumers, including family
3. are demonstrated as effective in aiding adjustment to illness or recovery, independence and self-care
4. are demonstrated as effective in preventing health problems or in promoting better health
5. are the most cost-effective way to achieve intended goals.

Box 14.2   Costs to be included in an economic evaluation of district nursing

Direct costs
1. Health-care resources
   • staffing, e.g. district nurse time
   • consumables, e.g. drugs
   • overheads, e.g. administration and laundry
   • capital, e.g. buildings and equipment

2. Related services
   • community services, e.g. district nurse specialising in the care of people with diabetes
   • ambulance services, e.g. for accident and emergency
   • voluntary services, e.g. voluntary workers in residential hostels for people with mental health problems

3. Costs to patients and their families/friends
   • extra expenses incurred through treatments, e.g. over-the-counter drugs or medical aids and adaptations
   • additional costs of being in hospital/at GP, e.g. childminding expenses
   • travel costs to and from GP/hospital/leg ulcer clinic

Indirect costs
Time lost from work, e.g. attending leg ulcer clinic
Costs external to health and welfare services

---

considered (related to function 5 in Box 14.1). Attention will then turn to benefit assessment (functions 1–4). Two issues are discussed: what is it we are trying to measure and how can we measure such factors? Box 14.1 suggests that benefit assessment should take a broad approach, considering health outcomes and broader aspects of care which may be valued by users of the service (and their families). Having considered issues raised in valuing costs and benefits, the reader is introduced to alternative frameworks for conducting an economic evaluation (i.e. bringing costs and benefits together).

ISSUES IN COSTING

Opportunity cost

The economic concept of cost is 'opportunity cost'. This concept takes as its starting point the premise that resources are scarce. Therefore, every time we choose to use resources in one way, we give up the 'opportunity' of using them in other beneficial activities. The opportunity cost of any health-care intervention is defined as the benefit foregone by *not* using that resource in its best alternative use. Only if a resource has a next-best use does it have an opportunity cost. The concept of opportunity cost embodies the crucial notion of sacrifice – in economics, something only has 'value' if a sacrifice has been made or is being made for it.

Using this definition of cost, items to be included on the cost side of an economic evaluation are any 'resources' which have an alternative use.

Often, costs (and benefits) are misclassified within economic evaluations (Donaldson & Shackley 1997). For example, anxiety has often been counted as a 'cost' and cost savings as 'benefits'. However, anxiety per se does not have an opportunity cost – it is not a resource which could be used in some other activity. Anxiety is a negative effect on health or well-being and should be accounted for as a dis-benefit on the benefit side of an evaluation. Likewise, 'cost savings' are negative costs and should be accounted for on the cost side.

Categorising resources to be included within economic evaluations

Box 14.2 provides guidance on costs to be included in an economic evaluation involving district nursing.

Staffing costs often comprise the largest component of health-care resources. This is likely to be the case with the labour-intensive community service which district nurses provide. There will only be an opportunity cost of staff time if time released could be used in an alternative way (Ratcliffe et al 1996). The opportunity cost is the value of the benefits forgone. This may be illustrated by thinking about the introduction of district nurse care for a service previously provided by general practitioners (GPs). The value of the cost savings will depend on the alternative use to which the GPs' time is put. If released GP time is used to do something of equal value (i.e. treat another patient) then the cost savings can be valued at the GPs' market value, i.e. their salary plus on-costs (such as National Insurance and Superannuation). However, if the alternative use of their time is leisure or some combination of leisure and paid work, the opportunity cost should be valued accordingly (see below for information on valuing leisure time). If there are uncertainties regarding the alternative use of GP time, sensitivity analysis may be used (see below).

Consumables are items which are used for or on behalf of each patient such as drugs, dressings and disposable equipment. Consumables are replaced on a regular basis, hence within a costing exercise, actual monetary costs are both appropriate as well as readily available.

Overhead costs are those costs shared by more than one programme, e.g. heat and light, laundry, cleaning and administration. These services are provided centrally and costs are apportioned amongst the various sectors using various means. The most favoured technique is marginal analysis (see below). Here an attempt is made to see which costs, if any, would change if a given service or provision were introduced or removed from the overall activity. Thus, it may be concluded that overhead costs are zero for a proposed health-care intervention if such costs will not change as a service increases or decreases. An alternative, and possibly easier, technique to take account of overhead costs is to calculate per diem or average overhead costs, i.e. total overhead costs divided by total patient utilisation. For a description of the various methods of overhead allocation, see Drummond et al (1987).

Capital items include land and building as well as large items of equipment. Despite an initial outlay, the opportunity costs of capital are spread over time. This is accounted for by spreading the opportunity cost of capital assets over the number of years of life judged relevant. One way of doing this is to calculate an equivalent annual cost (EAC). Using this method, the initial outlay on a capital asset is converted to an annual sum which, when paid over the estimated lifespan of the equipment, would equal the resources invested plus their opportunity cost. This EAC takes account of the fact that the resources invested to purchase the capital equipment could have earned a certain rate of interest if invested, i.e. it takes account of their opportunity cost, the forgone benefits of their next-best use. EACs are readily available (Appendix 1). If an item of surgical equipment cost £1000 and has a lifespan of 5 years, and assuming a discount rate of 6% (see below for information on discounting), this would be 'equivalent' to five annual payments of £237.40. This higher total cost of £1187 (5 × £237.40) reflects the opportunity cost of capital (the extra amount reflecting the 'cost' of tying resources up in capital goods and not having these resources available for other uses).

The cost of other related services includes staffing, supplies, overheads and capital costs associated with ambulance, voluntary and other community services. For example, the closing down or downsizing of a rheumatoid arthritis outpatient clinic may seem efficient from the hospital resource perspective. However, this may give rise to an increase in the number of district nurse visits in the community. It would then be important to include this cost within an evaluation of outpatient rheumatoid arthritis clinics, as the additional cost of the nurse visits may offset the predicted savings accrued through reduction of outpatient clinics. These related services are valued as described above for staffing, consumables, overheads and capital costs.

Voluntary services are often excluded from costing studies. The argument against their inclusion is based on the reasoning that such services are provided 'free of charge' and therefore incur no costs. However, despite not having a monetary cost, such services have an associated opportunity cost if the time spent doing voluntary work had an alternative use, whether that alternative be paid work, unpaid work or leisure.

Depending on the perspective of the study, costs (savings) to patients, their families and their friends may also require inclusion in an evaluation. Such costs may relate to both time and money. For example, time and money costs may be incurred in travelling to and from rheumatoid arthritis clinic appointments. Childminding costs may be incurred when staying in hospital or attending such arthritis clinics. When a relative or friend is required to care for an ill patient there is an associated opportunity cost as they may do so at the expense of a paid job or some leisure activity. Money costs incurred should be valued at the actual amount.

Indirect costs, or production gains, consist of time lost from work and costs external to health and welfare services. For example, when comparing drug therapy with surgical treatment for a condition, the calculation of indirect costs would be important if the drug therapy meant the patient could continue to work while the surgical treatment required absence from work. The opportunity cost of time depends on the alternative use of the resource – if this is paid employment then the value can be proxied as the average wage rate. For unpaid labour the value is currently proxied at 54% of the average wage rate and for leisure time the value is taken as 43% of the average wage rate (Department of Transport 1989). Often indirect costs are excluded from economic evaluations of health-care programmes because they are difficult to identify and are often negligible (Donaldson & Shackley 1997, Drummond et al 1987, Ratcliffe 1995). There is an ongoing debate in the literature regarding the inclusion of productivity gains in economic evaluation (Brouwer et al 1997, Gold et al 1996, Johannesson & Karlsson 1997, Koopmanschap et al 1995, Liljas 1998).

It is clear from Box 14.2 that there are numerous types of costs to include in an economic evaluation. Collecting such information may be both time-consuming and expensive. A shortcut

method, known as reduced list costing, may be used to generate research economies. Knapp & Beecham (1993) showed that by identifying a reduced list of services which accounts for the greater part of the total cost of care in mental health and by concentrating on these key services, the majority of costs can be predicted. However, Whynes & Walker (1995) show that whilst use of a reduced list is likely to generate substantial research economies, it may do so at the expense of accuracy.

Care should be taken to avoid double counting when collecting costing data. For example, suppose a costing exercise is taking place for a leg ulcer clinic and this clinic involves the nurse's time, the GP's time and the consumables. The researcher may collect detailed estimates of nurse time and supplies used for a typical consultation as well as an average cost of a consultation for the GP from GP accounts. Care must then be taken to ensure that the data available from the GP accounts for GP time do not include costs for consumables and nurse time (which have already been accounted for).

Finally, costs occurring at different points in time should be adjusted for inflation and reported in the same base year. This can be done by using a retail price index or hospital and health services price index.

The following section introduces some refinements to costing exercises. Whilst they are included within this costing section, they are also relevant to benefit assessment.

The importance of the margin

An important concept in costing (and benefit) exercises is that of the margin. The margin is concerned with change. The marginal cost is the cost/saving of producing one unit more/less of a programme. Decisions concerning the allocation of scarce health-care resources are usually concerned not with whether to introduce a service but rather whether to expand or reduce a service. For example, with regard to district nursing, the question may be one of whether to expand the current service and increase the number of community visits to, say, the elderly diabetic patients

Table 14.1   The importance of discounting and removing the effects of inflation in costing

Alternatives	Year 0	Year 1	Year 2	Year 3	Total costs
Old operation	**£2500**	**£0**	**£0**	**£0**	**£2500**
New operation + re-treatments					
• Undiscounted and includes inflation at 3%	£1050	£515	£530.45	£546.36	£2641.81
• Undiscounted and inflationary effects removed	£1050	£500	£500	£500	£2550
• Inflationary effects removed and costs discounted	**£1050**	**£471.70**	**£445**	**£419.80**	**£2386.50**

rather than whether to provide district nursing at all. Given this, costing studies should be mainly concerned with measuring marginal costs, not the generally more accessible, but often inappropriate, average costs.

Discounting

Costs (and benefits) of health-care interventions can occur at different times. For example, in prevention programmes costs are incurred early in the scheme whereas the benefits may stretch years into the future. Individuals generally prefer to incur costs in the future (and receive benefits sooner). Given this preference, costs that are incurred in the future should be given less weight, i.e. be discounted. The greater the preference for costs to occur in the future, the higher the discount rate (%). Currently, the UK Treasury recommends a discount rate of 6%. Discounting formulae and tables are readily available in the literature (HM Treasury 1994).

Using a discount rate of 6% and the table in Appendix 1, £1 spent in year 0 (i.e. those costs occurring now) is worth £1, £1 spent in year 1 is worth £0.94 pence (i.e. a 6% discount rate gives a weight of 0.94 in year 1), £1 spent in year 2 is worth £0.89 pence (or has a weight of 0.89) and so on. It is clear to see that the further into the future costs occur, the less weight they are given. Their lower weight in the future is a reflection of the value then as opposed to their value today. Namely we have a greater need for funds today to invest in beneficial activities than in the future when we may have more resources at our disposal.

Table 14.1 shows the effects of discounting at 6% and removing the effects of inflation. Imagine a new type of operation is being introduced which is less costly at the outset but gives rise to a number of re-treatments. Undiscounted and including annual inflation at 3%, the new operation appears more expensive – £2641.81. Removing the effects of inflation but remaining undiscounted, the new operation is still more expensive – £2550. However, it is only by removing the effects of inflation as well as discounting the future re-treatment costs that the true costs are displayed and it shows the new operation to be less expensive – £2386.50. Further examples of discounting benefits are provided in the section on 'Benefit Assessment'.

Sensitivity analysis

Every evaluation will contain some degree of uncertainty, imprecision or methodological controversy and as a result assumptions will have to be made (Drummond et al 1987). Assumptions are often made about both the costs and benefits of interventions. What would be the effect on costs if length of hospital stay was three days instead of two? What would be the effect on costs and leg ulcer healing rates if the community ulcer clinics were held twice a month rather than once a month? Would a drug still be as cost-effective if it improved pain scores by only 20% instead of 40%? What would be the effect on costs if a GP used her released time for leisure activities? Sensitivity analysis allows the testing of the sensitivity of the results to the assumptions made. For a comprehensive summary of the main types of uncertainty and the corresponding role of sensitivity analysis in addressing this, see Briggs et al (1994).

Costing and district nursing

As is clear from above, before carrying out any costing exercise it is important to first identify which elements of a service actually incur costs. Olver & Buckingham (1997) identified those conditions accounting for the largest proportion of district nurse time. The main conditions included diabetes, leg ulcers, senility, urinary symptoms, osteoarthritis, rheumatoid arthritis and multiple sclerosis. Ruta et al (1997) identified the key work patterns of district nurses in terms of the patients they see, where the consultations occur and what their main duties are. They show that almost all contacts occur in the patient's home with elderly people and that the majority of tasks relate to aspects of care such as changing dressings, bathing patients, washing and dressing patients, assessing needs, caring for leg ulcers, observation and teaching and counselling. This suggests that if a reduced list costing exercise was carried out, consideration would be given to the value of district nurses' time. A detailed summary is provided in Netten et al (1999) of how to cost a district nurse's time. Other resources used include consumables, overheads from clinics and travel costs. Such detailed workload analysis is useful as a starting point in costing exercises.

There are some costing exercises available in the area of district nursing, mainly concerned with treating leg ulcers in the community (Bosanquet et al 1993, Freak et al 1995, Simon et al 1996). Bosanquet et al (1993) showed that the costs of district nurse visits were the greatest component of annual cost in the treatment of venous ulcers, with patients with long-term ulcers having 36 district nurse visits per year at a unit cost of £18.90 per visit (1993 costs), a total annual district nurse cost of £680.40 per patient per year. Freak et al (1995) found that staff costs were by far the greatest proportion of cost in the treatment of leg ulcers. Simon et al (1996) also carried out a detailed costing study of leg ulcer clinics and found that staff costs were by far the greatest cost, followed by the cost of hospital inpatient stay. The cost of consumables in the form of dressing materials, bandages and topical applications was also a major contributor to the high cost of leg ulcer care. These studies will be returned to later in the section on 'Economic Evaluation', where the costs reported in the studies will be considered alongside the health benefits from the district nurse interventions.

If almost all district nurse contacts are in the patient's home, as Ruta et al (1997) suggest, and staff costs make up the majority of costs, then achieving the correct skill mix is crucial. Lightfoot et al (1992) note that achieving an appropriate mix of staff in district nursing is crucial to optimisation of cost-effectiveness: 'A key stage in effective establishment of design is to mix the range of relevant skills and experience of staff to produce the optimum level of care within the resource constraints of finance and supply of such staff. The results of this process are likely to be significant in terms of the quality and outcomes of community nursing'. Carlisle (1992) revealed some direct association between the growth of skill mix and the cost of community nursing services. Sines (1995) notes that the most important challenge to the district nursing profession relates to the redefinition of skill mix and it is within this framework that today's district nurse must redevelop her role and demonstrate skilled proficiency and diversity. With continual changes in legislation (Kelly & Oleary 1992, RCN 1992), it is unclear what the optimum skill mix in district nursing is. What is important, however, is that evaluation of the relevant skill mix alternatives is carried out in order to maximise the benefit to patients within the available resources.

BENEFIT ASSESSMENT

Robison & Exworthy (1995) note that, whilst measuring the impact of nursing interventions is not a new idea, little progress has been made in developing outcome measures for nursing interventions in the community. In developing such outcome measures, the crucial question is: what are the benefits from district nursing? Given the nature of care provided by district nurses, consideration must be given not only to improvements in health outcomes but also to the value of non-health outcomes (e.g. counselling, reassurance, provision of information) and the process of treatment (e.g. receiving treatment at home rather than in a clinic, attitudes of nurses, continuity of care). The following section outlines the methods of benefit assessment used in health economics, beginning with unidimensional health outcomes measures and concluding with broader measures of benefit which allow for consideration of health outcomes, non-health outcomes and process attributes.

Clinical measures of outcome

Initial attempts to measure benefits in health economics were very narrow. The outcome measure was clinical in nature and unidimensional, e.g. life-years gained; pain reduction; cases detected; disability days avoided; and cholesterol reduction. A common measure of clinical outcome in district nursing is 'healing rates' (Bosanquet et al 1993, Franks et al 1992, Simon et al 1996).

Quality-adjusted life-years (QALYs)

Quality-adjusted life-years (QALYs) were developed to take account of the fact that an individual may be concerned with the quality of their life as well as the quantity of life (Williams 1985). To estimate QALYs, expected life-years gained from given health-care interventions are estimated (usually by either the results of randomised controlled trials or health-care professionals) and combined with information on the quality of these life-years (via the estimation of quality weights usually by patients in the condition or the community). For example, if a health-care intervention results in a health state with a quality weight of 0.85, on a scale of 0 to 1, and the individual would be in this health state for the remainder of life, say 10 years, then the number of (undiscounted) QALYs would be 8.5. If the number of QALYs without the intervention were 4, then the QALYs gained from the intervention would be 4.5 (8.5 – 4 = 4.5). The QALYs gained from one health-care intervention may be compared with QALYs obtained from alternative health-care interventions, as well as from doing nothing. There are two main steps in the QALY framework: deciding what dimensions of health outcomes to value and thereafter attaching quality weights to these outcomes. These two stages will be considered in turn.

Dimensions in the QALY framework

Generic health outcome measures are designed to measure general dimensions of health outcome that can be relevant to many types of illnesses and diseases. Hence, generic outcomes can be compared across many different specialities. The original generic QALY proposed two dimensions of health outcome: distress and disability (Williams 1985). More recently, a European quality of life instrument, the EuroQol, has been developed (EuroQol 1990, Kind et al 1994, Williams 1995). This takes a broader, more multidimensional approach than the Rosser matrix, with five dimensions: mobility; self-care; usual activities; pain/discomfort; and anxiety/depression (Box 14.3). The Short Form 36 (SF-36) is a generic measure of health status widely used in health service research (Ware & Sherbourne 1992). It consists of eight dimensions of health: physical functioning; physical role functioning; bodily pain; general health; vitality; social functioning; emotional role functioning; and mental health.

Generic measures of health outcome, by their very nature, may be criticised for being too narrow and insensitive to the outcomes of specific conditions and condition specific measures may be more appropriate (Donaldson et al 1988). Examples of condition-specific measures include the Arthritis Impact Measuring Scale (AIMS) (Meenan et al 1980) which was developed to assess the physical, emotional and social well-being of patients with rheumatic conditions; the Functional Living Index for Cancer (FLIC) (Schipper et al 1984); and the QL Index (Spitzer et al 1981) which were developed specifically for use with cancer patients. For more details on specific health status measures, see Walker & Rosser (1993).

Box 14.3 The EuroQol descriptive system (reproduced from Dolan P, Guder C, Kina P, Williams 1998 A CHE Discussion Paper no 138, with permission)

Mobility
1. No problems in walking about
2. Some problems in walking about
3. Confined to bed

Self-care
1. No problems with self-care
2. Some problems washing or dressing self
3. Unable to wash or dress self

Usual activities
1. No problems with performing usual activities (e.g. work, study, housework, family or leisure activities)
2. Some problems with performing usual activities
3. Unable to perform usual activities

Pain/discomfort
1. No pain or discomfort

2. Moderate pain or discomfort
3. Extreme pain or discomfort

Anxiety/depression
1. Not anxious or depressed
2. Moderately anxious or depressed
3. Extremely anxious or depressed

Note: For convenience each composite health state has a five-digit code number relating to the relevant level of each dimension, with the dimension always listed in the order given above. Thus, 11223 means:

1 No problems in walking about
1 No problems with self-care
2 Some problems with performing usual activities
2 Moderate pain or discomfort
3 Extremely anxious or depressed

Attaching quality weights to these outcomes

Once important dimensions have been identified, quality weights need to be attached to the various possible outcomes (whether a generic or programme-specific health outcome measure is used). The three most common methods of establishing weights are: visual analogue; standard gamble; and time trade-off.

Using the visual analogue scale (VAS), respondents are presented with possible outcomes of a health-care intervention and asked to place these along a physical line such that their placing reflects their relative ranking (Nord 1991). The relative distance between their placing is also meant to reflect respondents' relative preferences for the outcomes. Zero is usually taken to be the worst outcome (death) and 1 the best (full health). The quality weight is taken as the point at which the outcome is placed on the line. This method is not popular with economists since it does not incorporate any notion of sacrifice.

The standard gamble (SG) embodies the notion of sacrifice by asking respondents to sacrifice 'certainty' in valuing a health outcome (Torrance 1986). Quality weights are estimated by presenting an individual with a number of choices in which they must choose between a certain outcome (B) or a gamble which may result in either a better outcome (A) than the certain outcome (with a probability *p*) or a worse outcome (C) than the

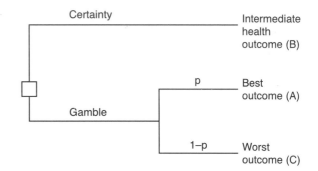

Figure 14.1 Example of a standard gamble question.

certain outcome (with a probability 1-*p*). The certain outcome is always an intermediate outcome in the sense that the better outcome is always preferred to it and the worse outcome is less preferred to it. The probability of the best outcome is varied until the individual is indifferent between the certain intermediate outcome and the gamble. This probability is the quality weight for the certain outcome (McNeil et al 1981). This technique is repeated for all intermediate outcomes.

Figure 14.1 shows the standard gamble format. It is clear that if the certain outcome (B) is undesirable then the individual will be willing to take a treatment gamble even if the probability of the preferred outcome is very low. Thus, the quality weight score for outcome (B) would also be very low. Hence, using the standard gamble technique, the more undesirable an outcome (B), the higher the likelihood that the individual will accept the gamble even with a low probability of success and the lower the quality weight for the undesirable outcome. This approach was used by Brazier et al (1998) in devising quality weights for the generic health outcomes defined in the SF-36.

The time trade-off (TTO) technique was developed as an alternative, and easier, method than SG for estimating quality weights (Torrance et al 1972). It is favoured by economists over the VAS as it embodies a notion of sacrifice, namely 'time'. The approach involves presenting individuals with a choice between living for a period t in a specified but less than perfect state (outcome B) versus having a healthier life (outcome A) for a time period h where $h<t$. Time h is varied until the respondent is indifferent between the alternatives. The quality weight given to the less than perfect state is then h/t. Using the TTO technique, the more undesirable outcome B (the outcome being assessed), the more years of life an individual would be willing to give up to be in the best outcome (A) and the lower the ratio h/t and in turn, the lower the quality weight for outcome B. Figure 14.2 shows the time trade-off technique. This approach was used by Dolan et al (1996) in devising quality weights for the generic health outcomes within the EuroQol instrument.

Using quality weights to estimate QALYs

Once quality weights have been estimated on a scale between 0 and 1, using the techniques outlined above, QALYs are obtained by multiplying the quality weight for a given health state by the length of time spent in that state. The process of estimating QALYs can be explained with a hypothetical example of evaluating the introduction of district nursing care.

Imagine an elderly patient with diabetes has a relatively poor health state which is valued by the EuroQol descriptive system, in Box 14.3, as 22222, i.e. some problems walking about, some problems washing or dressing, some problems with performing usual activities, moderate pain or discomfort and moderately anxious or depressed.

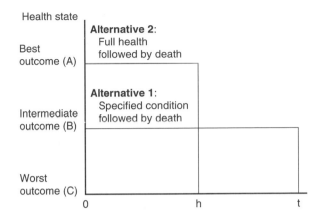

Figure 14.2 Example of a time trade-off question.

The introduction of district nurse-led care, and the support, education and advice provided, helps the patient improve her ability to care for herself. She now has no problems with self-care or pain and discomfort resulting in less anxiety and depression. The improved health state would be classified as 21211 on the EuroQol system. The improvement in health state from 22222 to 21211 is equivalent to moving from a health state valuation of 0.52 to 0.81 (with these quality weights being taken from the generic quality weights matrix, which has estimated weights for all health outcomes derived from EuroQoL). If this improvement lasted for 10 years, the (undiscounted) gain from the district nurse services would be 2.9 QALYs (10 years × 0.29). The discounted gain in QALYs would be 2.13 (Table 14.2). The discounting of future health benefits using this example clearly shows that, with a positive time preference (i.e. a preference for benefits now rather than later), benefits occurring in the later years, e.g. year 10 (0.16), have less value attached to them than benefits occurring in year 1 (0.27).

Willingness to pay

The technique of willingness to pay (WTP) as a benefit measurement tool is based on the premise that the maximum amount of money an individual is willing to pay (sacrifice) for a commodity is an indicator of the utility or satisfaction to him of that commodity. Further, when an individual considers their maximum WTP they will take

Table 14.2 Estimating QALYs from EuroQol

Year	No district nurse support		District nurse support		Improvement in quality of life from nursing support	Discounted improvement in quality of life from nursing support
	EuroQol description	Quality weight	EuroQol description	Quality weight		
1	22222	0.52	21211	0.81	0.29	0.27
2	22222	0.52	21211	0.81	0.29	0.26
3	22222	0.52	21211	0.81	0.29	0.24
4	22222	0.52	21211	0.81	0.29	0.23
5	22222	0.52	21211	0.81	0.29	0.22
6	22222	0.52	21211	0.81	0.29	0.20
7	22222	0.52	21211	0.81	0.29	0.19
8	22222	0.52	21211	0.81	0.29	0.18
9	22222	0.52	21211	0.81	0.29	0.17
10	22222	0.52	21211	0.81	0.29	0.16
				QALYs gained =	2.19	2.13

account of all the attributes of the service of importance to them, not just health gains (Ryan 1996a, Ryan et al 1997). Given this, WTP is likely to be suitable for valuing the benefits of district nurse care. For a review of the WTP technique in health, see Diener et al (1998).

Three main techniques have been used in health care to elicit maximum WTP: open ended; payment card; and closed ended. Using the open-ended technique, respondents are asked directly what is the maximum amount of money they would be prepared to pay for a commodity. Using the payment card technique, respondents are presented with a range of bids and asked to circle the amount that represents the most they would be willing to pay. The individual's true maximum WTP will lie somewhere in the interval between the circled amount and the next highest option. The closed-ended approach asks individuals whether they would pay a specified amount for a given commodity, with possible responses being 'yes' or 'no'. The bid amount is varied across respondents. Figures 14.3–14.5 provide examples of such questions within the context of a policy question concerning the provision of maternity services. For more information on these techniques, see Mitchell & Carson (1989).

Whilst no WTP studies were identified in the literature which assessed the value of district nurses, a number of studies were identified

> One way of measuring the value to you of care in the midwives unit is to ask you what you would be prepared to give up to receive this care instead of care in the labour ward. The easiest way to ask this is to see what is the most you would be willing to pay to receive care in the midwives unit instead of care in the labour ward. Of course, both types of care are free on the NHS and will stay free. We also believe that people should not have to pay for health care. This is simply a way of measuring how strongly you feel about having midwives unit care instead of the labour ward. So, imagine that you do have to pay.
>
> There are no right or wrong answers. The amount you say could be large or small. We are interested in your view.
>
> What is the maximum amount of money you would be prepared to pay to receive midwives unit care instead of labour ward care? (*Please write your answer in £s in the space below. One way to think of this is to imagine you are at an auction at which the most you would pay for any item shows the importance you place on that item. How far are you prepared to go?*)
>
> £_____

Figure 14.3 Example of an open-ended WTP question (Donaldson et al 1998).

which demonstrate the potential use of the instrument in this area. Thompson et al (1984) used WTP to assess the value of a cure for arthritis. They found that patients with this condition were willing, on average, to pay 17% of their family income for such a cure. Donaldson et al (1998) used WTP to assess women's preferences for midwife-managed care versus consultant-led care in

Please consider whether you would be willing to pay each of the following amounts for midwife-managed care instead of labour ward care. *Remember that any money you spend on midwife care will not be available for you to spend on other things.*

Willing to pay?

Amount	YES	NO
£0		
£30		
£50		
£100		
£150		
£200		
£250		
£300		
£350		
£400		
£500		
£600		
£700		
£800		
£900		
£1000		

Please tick (✓) YES if you are sure you would be willing to pay the amount

Please tick (✓) NO if you are sure you would not be willing to pay the amount

Please CIRCLE the maximum amount you would be willing to pay

If above, you were willing to pay at least £1000, please state the **maximum** amount of money you would be willing to pay.

£ _____

Figure 14.4 Example of payment card WTP question.

Please consider whether you would be willing to pay £350 for midwife-managed care instead of labour ward care. *Remember that any money you spend on midwife care will not be available for you to spend on other things.*

So would you be willing to pay £350*?

Yes

No

*Bid amount varies across respondents.

Figure 14.5 Example of closed-ended WTP question.

the provision of maternity care. Whilst most women expressed a preference for care in a midwives unit, strength of preference, as reflected by WTP, was greater among those who expressed a preference for care in a consultant-led ward. Walraven (1996) estimated WTP for district hospital services in rural Tanzania, showing that patients and households were willing to pay large amounts for this service. Johannesson et al (1997) measured WTP for a reduction in the number of micturitions and urinary leakages in patients with urge incontinence and found that patients with this condition would pay substantial amounts.

Conjoint analysis

Conjoint analysis (CA) can be used to estimate utilities (for health outcomes, non-health outcomes and process attributes) and WTP indirectly. The technique is well established in the market research literature and is widely used in transport economics and environmental economics. It is now only beginning to be used in health economics (Bryan et al 1998, Propper 1995, Ryan

	Clinic A	Clinic B
Medical staff you see	Specialist nurse	Junior doctor
Time in waiting area	Up to 10 minutes	Up to 20 minutes
Continuity of contact with same staff	Yes	No
Change in 'pain' between appointments	Small reduction	No reduction
Phone-in/advice line service	No	No
Length of consultation	25 minutes	25 minutes

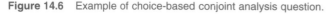

Which clinic would you prefer (*tick one box only*)?

Prefer Clinic A ☐   Prefer Clinic B ☐

Figure 14.6   Example of choice-based conjoint analysis question.

1996b, 1999). Its increased use in health economics can be partly explained by the desire for a technique that can take account of more than health outcomes.

The initial stages of a CA study are similar to that of the QALY approach, i.e. establish what dimensions are important and what levels to give to them. The technique differs from the QALY framework in the way preferences are elicited. Using CA, preferences may be elicited using ranking, rating or discrete choices. Economists have favoured the latter approach, partly because the approach incorporates sacrifice and also because it is based in a branch of economic theory known as random utility theory. Individuals are asked to make numerous choices between two options, A and B, which vary with regard to the attributes of interest (which may be health, non-health attributes and process attributes, or any combination of these). Regression techniques are used to analyse the responses. From this, it is possible to establish the following: the relative importance of different attributes in the provision of the good or service; how individuals trade between these attributes; benefit scores for different configurations of goods or services; and WTP for both individual attributes and configurations of attributes if cost is included as an attribute.

Ryan (1999) provides a review of the application of conjoint analysis in health care. Whilst no studies were identified which assessed the value of district nursing, Bate & Ryan (1998) examined patient preferences for a specialist nurse in the provision of rheumatology services.

The type of choices respondents faced in this study is shown in Figure 14.6. The results indicated that whilst patients would prefer to see a junior doctor, they would be willing to see a specialist nurse for improvements in other aspects of care (time in waiting area, continuity of contact with same staff, length of consultation, pain levels).

ECONOMIC EVALUATION

This section examines how the costs and benefits discussed in the previous sections can be brought together within the framework of an economic evaluation. The three principal economic evaluation techniques are: cost-effectiveness analysis (CEA); cost-utility analysis (CUA) and cost-benefit analysis (CBA).

The technique(s) chosen will be determined by both the question being addressed (allocative efficiency or technical efficiency) and the benefits to be measured (health outcomes, non-health outcomes and/or process attributes). An allocative efficiency question is concerned with whether or not to allocate resources to a given programme. Diverse health-care programmes compete for the limited resources, i.e. asthma clinics versus diabetes clinics versus district nurse-led community leg ulcer clinics versus rheumatology nurse practice services. An allocative efficiency question would be: should there be a community leg ulcer clinic or an asthma clinic? In contrast, technical efficiency is concerned with 'within programme' efficiency, i.e. how best to provide a given service. The resources or budget allocated to a programme are taken as given and the issue is simply 'how best' to provide that service. A technical efficiency question would be: when providing care for patients with leg ulcers, is it best to provide specialised district nurse-led community leg ulcer clinics or traditional care? Or, when providing rheumatology clinics, is it best to provide a nurse practitioner service or a consultant-based service? The following section examines the methods of economic evaluation with specific examples in district nursing.

Cost-effectiveness analysis

Cost-effectiveness analysis (CEA) can only be used to address questions of technical efficiency. It examines the effects of at least two competing alternatives 'within a fixed budget'. A ratio for each alternative is provided, the numerator being cost and the denominator the health effect. Such effects are measured in unidimensional terms, i.e. life-years saved, heart attacks prevented, percentage reduction in cholesterol concentration or improvement in limb function, healing rates. The cost-effectiveness ratio produced is therefore a measure of 'cost per unit of effect'. The alternative with the lowest cost-effectiveness ratio, is the preferred choice. (An alternative form of CEA is cost-minimisation analysis (CMA). This is the same as CEA except the units of effect have been shown to be identical and hence all that the evaluator is concerned with is the alternative with the least cost.

A number of studies were identified which applied a cost-effectiveness type approach to evaluate the role of district nurses in treating leg ulcers. The need for such work was identified from reports showing leg ulcer treatment in Britain to be ineffective (Negus & Friedgood 1983, Ryan 1987). Studies which showed improved success rates tended to be centred in specialist clinics and hospitals. However, treatments based at hospitals are only likely to reach a minority of the large numbers of elderly patients in the community who have leg ulcers (Bosanquet et al 1993).

A study on community leg ulcers investigated the cost-effectiveness of a new service provided by community leg ulcer clinics, staffed by district nurses, and compared it with treatment in existing hospital-based venous ulcer care clinics (Bosanquet et al 1993). Data were provided prospectively from district nurses and retrospectively from patients. The project aimed to treat all patients with current leg ulcers within the Riverside District Health Authority (DHA). Full coverage was achieved for all current and known patients. Patients were initially reviewed using a comprehensive questionnaire covering social background, quality of life and use of health services for the previous 2 years. Information was gathered on patient utilisation of inpatient hospital treatment, outpatient visits, GP consultations, district nursing services, frequency of bandaging, district nurse physiotherapy and social services (Franks et al 1992). Each patient contact with any aspect of NHS service was then costed using information provided by the DHA about local treatment costs. Costs of the new service were based on data collected directly from the six clinics involved, covering staffing levels and other resources. At each clinic detailed records were kept of the number of patients attending and the number of patients seen at home. The results showed that the new community clinics gave rise to healing rates of 80% within 12 weeks, this healing being maintained at 48 weeks. These results contrast with the healing rate of 20–22% at 12 weeks achieved by the old methods of treatment in the community. In addition to this, the cost of the new clinics was much less, proving to be a clearly cost-effective alternative to the old method.

A study carried out by Simon et al (1996) evaluated the costs and outcomes of community leg ulcer clinics staffed by district nurses and supported by specialist nurses. The study compared the impact of five community clinics on leg ulcer healing and the cost of the service with the natural evolution of care in a clinic where no coordinated attempt was made to change current practice. The main outcome measure was the proportion of ulcerated limbs completely healed within 3 months and the total cost of leg ulcer care. As in the study above, the results of this

---

Box 14.4   Cost-effectiveness study of community leg ulcer clinics (Simon et al 1996)

Objective
To compare the outcome and cost of care for leg ulcers in community leg ulcer clinics in Stockport DHA with Trafford DHA as a control.

Main outcome measures
The proportion of ulcerated limbs completely healed within 3 months and total cost of leg ulcer care.

Results
The introduction of community clinics in Stockport improved healing of leg ulcers from 26% in 1993 to 42% in 1994, compared with Trafford, where 23% healed in 1993 and only 20% in 1994. This improved result in

Stockport was achieved while the annual expenditure on care of leg ulcers was reduced from £409 991 to £253 371. In the same year the cost of leg ulcer care in Trafford increased from £556 039 to £673 318.

Conclusion
The introduction of district nurse-led community leg ulcer clinics in Stockport improved care and lowered costs compared to the traditional approach the clinics replaced. The major improvements in healing and reductions in costs shown in Stockport were a direct result of the introduction of coordinated community leg ulcer clinics.

---

study provide a clear case where economic evaluation is crucial in the area of district nursing, namely where district nurse care led to improved care as well as less cost. The study is summarised in Box 14.4.

The results of both studies showed that the new community clinics gave rise to cost savings and improved healing rates. These are very clear cases for implementation of the proposed clinics. However, a more common situation is where both benefits and costs are greater. A judgement is then required as to whether the extra benefits, e.g. improved healing rates, are 'worth' the extra costs.

The main limitation of CEA is that the unit of health effect must be undimensional. Thus, only interventions with the same goal can be compared (hence, the technique can only be used to address technical efficiency). Further, important effects may be excluded from analyses. For example, in some cancer therapies, while years of remaining life are an important outcome measure, the quality of those remaining years may also be important. Similarly, non-health outcomes and process attributes may be important. For example, within a consultation between a district nurse and an elderly person concerning leg ulcers, in addition to an improved healing rate, the elderly person may also value the information, advice and support obtained from the nurse and general patient care.

In CEA, the phrase 'within a given budget' is of crucial importance. Often authors produce a ratio of *extra* costs per *extra* unit of health effect

of one intervention over another, calling this an incremental cost-effectiveness ratio (ICER) (Kuntz et al 1996, Michel et al 1996). Such ratios are not cost-effectiveness analyses. CEA, by definition, assumes that health effects should be maximised 'within a given budget' and that alternatives with the lowest cost per unit of effect should be chosen. An ICER assumes that there are additional benefits for additional costs and this suggests that, since they are 'additional', these costs will come from outwith the fixed budget. Hence, given limited resources, some judgement is required as to whether such extra costs are worth incurring as they will have to be taken from some other programme. This takes us back to the broader issues of allocative efficiency, i.e. whether to allocate, not how to allocate. CEA cannot address such a question.

Cost-utility analysis

Cost-utility analysis (CUA) has become synonymous with using the QALY as its benefit measure. CUA can be seen as an improvement on CEA as it attempts to combine more than one outcome measure and takes account of both quality and quantity of life. One reason for the development of the QALY framework was that cost-per-QALY comparisons could be made across health-care interventions, i.e. so that allocative efficiency questions could be addressed. Such comparisons can only be made when generic QALYs are used, such that alternative health-care interventions are compared on the same dimensions. Using QALYs for questions of allocative efficiency, marginal cost per additional QALY league tables are constructed. The number of QALYs achieved from a health-care budget will be maximised by allocating resources to those interventions with the lowest cost per QALY ratio.

Returning to the example of QALYs discussed earlier (Table 14.2), 2.13 additional QALYs were achieved from district nurse support. This can be combined with the cost of district nurse care within a CUA framework. If the patient had spent a total of 10 hours with the district nurse and the cost per hour was £46 (Netten et al 1999), the cost per QALY for nurse care would be £216 (£460/2.13). This cost per QALY can be used to assess technical efficiency, comparing it to a cost per QALY for an alternative method of providing support to patients with diabetes. Alternatively, this could be used within an allocative efficiency framework and compared to the cost per QALY gained from using district nurse time in another beneficial activity.

A CUA of the community psychiatric nurse (CPN) in primary care was carried out by Gournay & Brooking (1995). They estimated the cost per QALY of the CPN treating less serious mental health problems compared with that for treating the seriously mentally ill. Quality weights were obtained using the Rosser–Kind generic matrix (Williams 1985). The cost per QALY for the former group was several times more than for the latter group, suggesting little justification for CPNs to continue working in the former area.

The use of QALYs to address allocative efficiency have been criticised on a number of grounds (Gerard & Mooney 1993). Three main problems have been identified:

1. the relevant measure of cost in QALY league tables is restricted to health service resource use
2. the measure of benefit is restricted to health outcomes
3. the legitimacy of transferring marginal costs and benefits to different settings is debatable.

Expanding on this last point, Donaldson & Shackley (1997) question whether the original context of the study allows the results to be transferred to the local context of the decision maker as each item in the league table has a different comparator. The cost per QALY gained of programme A may have been produced by comparing programme A with programme B. However, if B is inefficient to begin with, A may be inefficient too. Yet, even if A is inefficient, it may still look good because it was compared with B (another inefficient programme).

Whilst CUA has become synonymous with QALYs, the technique can be broadened to include measures of utility that take account of health outcomes, non-health outcomes and process attributes. Rather than estimate a cost per QALY, a cost per 'util' would be estimated. Utilities could be estimated using CA (Farrar et al 2000, Ryan et al 2000). However, this approach is still in its infancy and further research is needed to look at how utility scores estimated from CA studies can be used to address both technical efficiency and allocative efficiency questions. On the issue of allocative efficiency, Hakim & Pathak (1999) used CA to calculate preference scores for EuroQol health states. Such use of CA within a generic health measurement tool represents a step towards using the method within an allocative framework in health care.

Cost-benefit analysis

In a cost-benefit analysis (CBA) costs and benefits are measured in commensurate units, normally money. Willingness to pay may be used to estimate the monetary benefit. Within a CBA, costs are compared to benefits and the provision of the good encouraged when the benefits outweigh the costs. However, such a decision rule is not sufficient when deciding on the provision of a publicly provided commodity, such as health care, within a fixed budget context. This is because too many interventions may pass this criterion (Hoehn & Randall 1989, Pauly 1995). If the project being considered is from a given public budget, the crucial question is not just whether the benefits outweigh the costs but also whether other projects, where benefits outweigh costs, are valued less. One way to overcome this would be to elicit respondents' WTP for a group of health-care interventions all competing for limited resources. This approach was adopted by Olsen & Donaldson (1998). Here respondents were asked their WTP in increased earmarked taxation for three different health-care programmes: a helicopter ambulance service, more heart operations and more hip replacements.

CBA may be used to address both technical efficiency and allocative efficiency questions. Indeed, it is not constrained to comparing programmes within health care but can be used to inform resource allocation decisions both within and between sectors of the economy (Drummond & Stoddart 1995). It can also be used to value health outcomes, non-health outcomes and process attributes.

There have been relatively few CBA studies in the literature. Zarnke et al (1997) found that 60% of studies claiming to be CBAs were actually cost comparisons where no attempt had been made to value benefits in monetary terms. However, it is clear that the CBA framework may be suitable to evaluate the costs alongside the health, non-health and process benefits of district nursing. An example of a relevant policy question within this context would be an evaluation of district nursing care for terminally ill cancer patients. Since the district nurse cannot provide a 'cure' per se, the 'health' oriented measures of CUA and CEA would not reflect any 'value' of the district nurse. However, in these situations the district nurse provides invaluable support, counselling and general nursing care to patients and relatives. A CBA would compare the costs of the district nurse making such home visits with the monetary value of these visits to the patients and possibly relatives.

Whilst CBA is potentially very appealing, since benefits and costs can be directly compared and the benefit measure takes account of everything that is important to the respondent, the issue of valuing benefits in monetary terms raises a number of points. Two potential problems with this approach are that respondents may object to being asked WTP for health care and WTP is related to ability to pay (with higher income individuals having a higher WTP). Studies from health care have shown that whilst some individuals do object to answering WTP questions, others respond in a theoretically valid way (Diener et al 1998). The issue of ability to pay is only a problem if preferences are related to income, e.g. if two health-care interventions are being compared, A and B, and lower income groups prefer A and higher income groups B, then WTP for B will be higher because of the income distribution. This can be dealt with by weighting WTP values (issues remain of how to estimate these weights). However, if low and high income groups have the same preference structure, ability to pay will not be a problem.

The balance sheet approach (McIntosh et al 1999) is an alternative form of CBA which overcomes the potential problem of placing monetary valuation on benefits. Rather than requiring all costs and benefits to be valued in monetary terms, the balance sheet approach requires all costs and benefits to be measured in physical units. Available monetary values can then be augmented by other measures of costs and benefits. These may include measures of quantity (e.g. numbers of referrals) and time (e.g. time spent waiting for a consultation). Such an adaptation of CBA highlights the technique's role as an aid to decision making (Sugden & Williams 1978). It also supports Culyer (1985) who, while realising the imperfections of CBA in practice, also recognised its importance as a framework for decision making:

A good CBA will: identify relevant options for consideration; enumerate all costs and benefits to various relevant social groups; quantify as many as can be sensibly quantified; *not* assume the unquantified is unimportant; use discounting where relevant to derive present values; use sensitivity analysis to test the response of net benefits to changes in assumptions; and look at the distributive impact of the options.

CONCLUSION

This chapter has provided an introduction to the issues surrounding economic evaluation in health care, with specific reference to district nursing. The methods for identifying, measuring and valuing costs and benefits have been outlined and the techniques for bringing together costs and benefits within an economic evaluation technique described. Few studies have evaluated the role of the district nurse and what work is available has tended to assume that only health outcomes matter. Given the 'holistic' nature of the role of the district nurse, broader outcomes are likely to be important. Depending on the type of question asked, CEA, CUA (possible going beyond QALYs) and CBA all appear potentially useful for evaluating district nursing.

Finally, economic evaluation should be seen as a framework which will aid the decision-making process. Such a framework helps to make more informed decisions by rendering the costs and benefits of any intervention or service explicit. In doing so, more informed decisions can be made about the allocation of resources to various programmes. The outcome or benefit measure chosen will decide the 'type' of economic evaluation carried out; if a number of outcome measures are chosen, a variety of economic evaluations may be performed.

Acknowledgements

The authors are funded by the Medical Research Council (MRC). The Health Economics Research Unit is funded by the Chief Scientist Office of the Scottish Executive Health Department (SEHD). The views expressed in this chapter are those of the authors, not the MRC or SEHD. The authors are grateful to Steve Morris from the Department of Economics at City University, London, for his useful advice.

REFERENCES

Bate A, Ryan M 1998 Using conjoint analysis to evaluate the extended role of the nurse: an application to the rheumatology specialist nurse. Discussion paper no. 05/98. Health Economics Research Unit, University of Aberdeen

Bosanquet N, Franks P, Moffatt C et al 1993 Community leg ulcer clinics: cost-effectiveness. Health Trends 25(4): 146–148

Brazier J, Usherwood T, Harper R, Thomas K 1998 Deriving a preference-based single index from the UK SF-36 Health Survey. Journal of Clinical Epidemiology 51(11): 1115–28

Briggs A, Sculpher M, Buxton M 1994 Uncertainty in the economic evaluation of health care technologies: the role of sensitivity analysis. Health Economics 3: 95–104

Brouwer W B F, Koopmanschap M A, Rutten F F H 1997 Productivity costs measurement through quality of life? A response to the recommendation of the Washington Panel. Health Economics 6: 253–259

Bryan S, Buxton M, Sheldon R, Grant A 1998 Magnetic resonance imaging for the investigation of knee injuries: an investigation of preferences. Health Economics 7: 595–603

Carlisle D 1992 Nurses last? Nursing Times 88: 18

Culyer A J 1985 Economics. Blackwell, Oxford

Department of Health 1997 The new NHS: modern, dependable. Stationery Office, London

Department of Transport 1989 Values of time and vehicle operating costs for 1989. COBA 9 Manual, Annex II, section 8.2.8.3–8.10. Department of Transport, London

Diener A, O'Brien B, Gafni A 1998 Health care contingent valuation studies: a review and classification of the literature. Health Economics 7: 313–326

Dolan P, Gudex C, Kind P, Williams A 1995 A social tariff for EuroQol: results from a UK general population survey.

Discussion paper no.138. Centre for Health Economics, University of York, York

Dolan P, Gudex C, Kind P, Williams A 1996 The time trade-off method: results from a general population study. Health Economics 5: 141–154

Donaldson C, Shackley P 1997 Economic evaluation. In: Detels R, Holland W, McEwan J, Omenn G (eds) Oxford textbook of public health, 3rd edn. Oxford University Press, Oxford.

Donaldson C, Atkinson A, Bond J 1988 Should QALYs be programme specific? Journal of Health Economics 7: 239–257

Donaldson C, Hundlay V, Mapp T 1998 Willingness to pay: a method for measuring preferences for maternity care? Birth 25: 32–39

Drummond M F, Stoddart G L 1995 Economic evaluation of health-producing technologies across different sectors: can valid methods be developed? Health Policy 33: 219–231

Drummond M F, Stoddart G L, Torrance W 1987 Methods for the economic evaluation of health care programmes. Oxford University Press, Oxford

EuroQol 1990 EuroQol – a new facility for the measurement of health-related quality of life. Health Policy 16: 199–208

Farrar S, Ryan M, Ross D, Ludbrook A 2000 Using discrete choice modelling in priority setting: an application to clinical service developments. Social Science and Medicine 50: 63–75

Franks P J, Wright D D I, Fletcher A E et al 1992 A questionnaire to assess risk factors, quality of life and use of health resources in patients with venous disease. European Journal of Surgery 158: 149–155

Freak L, Simon D, Kinsella A, McCollum C, Walsh J, Lane C 1995 Leg ulcer care: an audit of cost-effectiveness. Health Trends 27(4): 133–136

Gerard K, Mooney G 1993 QALY league tables: handle with care. Health Economics 2: 59–64

Gold M R, Siegel J E, Russell L B et al 1996 Cost-effectiveness in health and medicine. Oxford University Press, Oxford

Gournay K, Brooking J 1995 The community psychiatric nurse in primary care: an economic analysis. Journal of Advanced Nursing 22: 769–778

Hakim Z, Pathak D S 1999 Modelling the EuroQol data: a comparison of discrete choice conjoint and conditional preference modelling. Health Economics 8: 103–116

H M Treasury 1994 Economic appraisal in central government. A technical guide for government departments. HMSO, London

Hoehn J, Randall A 1989 Too many proposals pass the benefit cost test. American Economic Review 79: 544–551

Johannesson M, Karlsson G 1997 The friction cost method: a comment. Journal of Health Economics 16: 249–255

Johannesson M, O'Connor R M, Kobelt-Nguyen G, Mattiasson A 1997 Willingness to pay for reduced incontinence symptoms. British Journal of Urology 80: 557–562

Kelly T A, Oleary M 1992 The nursing skill mix in the district nursing service. NHS Management Executive, Value for Money Unit. HMSO, London

Kind P, Dolan P, Gudex C, Williams A 1994 Practical and methodological issues in the development of the EuroQol: the York experience. Advances in Medical Sociology 5: 219–253

Knapp M, Beecham J 1993 Reduced list costings: examination of an informed short cut in mental health research. Health Economics 2: 313–322

Koopmanschap M A, Rutten F F H, van Ineveld et al 1995 The friction cost method for measuring indirect costs of disease. Journal of Health Economics 14: 171–189

Kuntz K M, Tsevat J, Goldman L et al 1996 Cost-effectiveness of routine coronary angiography after acute myocardial infarction. Circulation 94: 957–965

Lessner M W, Organek N S, Shah H S, Williams C A, Bruttomesso K A 1994 Orienting nursing students in cost-effective clinical practice. Nursing and Health Care 15: 458–462

Lightfoot J, Baldwin S, Wright K 1992 Community Nursing Study Stage One. Report on a study of establishment setting and review for district nursing and health visiting services. Social Policy Research Unit, DH 947 6.92 JL. University of York, York

Liljas B 1998 How to calculate indirect costs in economic evaluations. Pharmacoeconomics 13: 1–7

McIntosh E, Donaldson C, Ryan M 1999 Recent advances in the methods of cost-benefit analysis: matching the art to the science. Pharmacoeconomics 15: 357–367

McNeil B, Weichselbaum R, Stephen G, Pauker G 1981 Speech and survival. New England Journal of Medicine 305: 982–987

Meenan R F, Gertman P M, Mason J H 1980 Measuring health status in arthritis: evidence for the sensitivity of a health status measure. Arthritis and Rheumatism 23: 146–152

Michel B C, Seerden R J, Rutten F F H et al 1996 The cost effectiveness of diagnostic strategies in patients with suspected pulmonary embolism. Health Economics 5: 307–318

Mitchell R C, Carson R T 1989 Using surveys to value public goods. Resources for the Future, Washington DC

Negus D, Friedgood A 1983 The effective management of venous ulceration. British Journal of Surgery 70: 623–627

Netten A, Dennet J, Knight J 1999 Unit costs of health and social care. Personal Social Services Research Unit, University of Kent at Canterbury

Nord E 1991 The validity of a visual analogue scale in determining social utility weight for health states. International Journal of Health Planning and Management 6: 234–242

Olsen J A, Donaldson C 1998 Helicopters, hearts and hips: using willingness to pay to set priorities for public sector health care programme. Social Science and Medicine 46: 1–12

Olver L, Buckingham K 1997 Analysis of the district nurse workload in the community. British Journal of Community Health Nursing 2: 127–134

Pauly M 1995 Valuing health benefits in monetary terrs. In: Sloan F (ed) Valuing health care: costs, benefits and effectiveness of pharmaceuticals and other medical technologies. Cambridge University Press, Cambridge

Propper C 1995 The disutility of time spent on the United Kingdom's National Health Service waiting lists. Journal of Human Resources 30: 677–700

Ratcliffe J 1995 The measurement of indirect costs in economic evaluation: a critical review. Project Appraisal 10: 13–18

Ratcliffe J, Ryan M, Tucker J 1996 The costs of alternative types of routine antenatal care for low risk women: shared care versus care by general practitioners and community midwives. Journal of Health Services Research and Policy 1: 135–140

Robison J, Exworthy M 1995 Primary care nursing: approaches and opportunities. Primary Care Management 5: 11–14

Royal College of Nursing 1992 Skill mix and reprofiling: a guide for RCN members. RCN London

Ruta D A, Duffy M C, Farquharson A, Young A M, Gilmour F B, McElduff S P 1997 Determining priorities for change in primary care: the value of practice-based needs assessment. British Journal of General Practice 47: 353–357

Ryan M 1996a Using willingness to pay to assess the benefits of assisted reproductive techniques. Health Economics 5: 543–558

Ryan M 1996b Using consumer preferences in health care decision making: the application of conjoint analysis. Office of Health Economics, London

Ryan M 1999 Measuring benefits in health care: the role of discrete choice conjoint analysis. Paper presented at International Health Economics Association, Rotterdam, June

Ryan M, Ratcliffe J, Tucker J 1997 Using willingness to pay to value alternative models of antenatal care. Social Science and Medicine 44: 371–380

Ryan M, McIntosh E, Dean T, Old P 2000 Trade offs between location and waiting times in the provision of health care: the case of elective surgery on the Isle of Wight. Journal of Public Health Medicine (in press)

Ryan T J 1987 The management of leg ulcers, 2nd edn. Oxford University Press, Oxford

Schipper H, Clinch J, McMurray A et al 1984 Measuring the quality of life of cancer patients. The Functional Living Index – Cancer: development and validation. Journal of Clinical Oncology 2: 472–483

Scottish Office 1997 Designed to care: renewing the National Health Service in Scotland. Scottish Office Department of Health, CM 3811. Stationery Office, Edinburgh

Simon D A, Freak L, Kinsella A et al 1996 Community leg ulcer clinics: a comparative study in two health authorities. British Medical Journal 312: 1648–1651

Sines D 1995 Community health care nursing. Blackwell Science, Oxford

Spitzer W O, Dobson A J, Hall J et al 1981 Measuring the quality of life of cancer patients. Journal of Chronic Disorders 34: 595–597

Sugden R, Williams A 1978 The principles of practical cost-benefit analysis. Oxford University Press, Oxford

Thompson M S, Read J L, Liang M 1984 Feasibility of willingness-to-pay measurement in chronic arthritis. Medical Decision Making 4(2): 195–215

Torrance G 1986 Measurement of health-state utilities for economic appraisal: a review. Journal of Health Economics 5: 1–30

Torrance G, Thomas W, Sackett D 1972 A utility maximization model for evaluation of health care programs. Health Services Research 7: 118–133

Walker S, Rosser R 1993 Quality of life assessment: key issues in the 1990s. Kluwer Academic Publishers, Dardrecht

Walraven G 1996 Willingness to pay for district hospital services in rural Tanzania. Health Policy and Planning 11: 428–437

Ware J, Sherbourne C 1992 The SF-36 short-form health status survey 1. Conceptual framework and item selection. Medical Care 30: 473–483

Whynes D K, Walker A R 1995 On approximations in treatment costing. Health Economics 4: 31–39

Williams A 1985 Economics of coronary artery bypass grafting. British Medical Journal 291: 326–329

Williams A 1995 The role of the EuroQol instrument in QALY calculations. Centre for Health Economics, York

Wilson-Barnett J 1992 Priorities in allocating nursing resources. Journal of Advanced Nursing 17: 645–646

Zarnke K B, Levine M A H, O'Brien B J 1997 Cost benefit analysis in the health care literature: don't judge a study by its label. Journal of Clinical Epidemiology 50: 813–822

FURTHER READING

McGuire A, Henderson J, Mooney G 1992 The economics of health care. An introductory text. Routledge, London

Morris S 1997 The economics of nursing. In: Morris S (ed) Health economics for nurses: an introductory guide. Prentice Hall, Hemel Hempstead

Appendix 1   Discount factors and equivalent annual costs of £1 per year for a discount rate of 6% (base year = year 0)

Year(s)	Equivalent annual cost of £1	Discount factor (= present value of £1)
1	1.0600	0.9434
2	0.5454	0.8900
3	0.3741	0.8396
4	0.2886	0.7921
5	0.2374	0.7473
6	0.2034	0.7050
7	0.1791	0.6651
8	0.1610	0.6274
9	0.1470	0.5919
10	0.1359	0.5584
11	0.1268	0.5268
12	0.1193	0.4970
13	0.1130	0.4688
14	0.1076	0.4423
15	0.1030	0.4173
16	0.0989	0.3936
17	0.0954	0.3714
18	0.0924	0.3503
19	0.0896	0.3305
20	0.0872	0.3118
21	0.0850	0.2942
22	0.0830	0.2775
23	0.0813	0.2618
24	0.0797	0.2470
25	0.0782	0.2330
26	0.0769	0.2198
27	0.0757	0.2074
28	0.0746	0.1956
29	0.0736	0.1846
30	0.0726	0.1741
31	0.0718	0.1643
32	0.0710	0.1550
33	0.0703	0.1561
34	0.0696	0.1379
35	0.0690	0.1301
36	0.0684	0.1227
37	0.0679	0.1158
38	0.0674	0.1092
39	0.0670	0.1031
40	0.0665	0.0972
41	0.0661	0.0917
42	0.0657	0.0865
43	0.0653	0.0816
44	0.0650	0.0770
45	0.0647	0.0727
46	0.0644	0.0685
47	0.0641	0.0647
48	0.0639	0.0610
49	0.0637	0.0575
50	0.0634	0.0543

15

Information management and the use of technology

Val Baker

The challenge is for the NHS to harness the information revolution and use it to benefit patients. (Tony Blair, Prime Minister, 2 July 1998)

In attempting to arrive at the truth, I have applied everywhere for information, but in scarcely an instance have I been able to obtain hospital records fit for any purpose of comparison. If they could be obtained ... they would show subscribers how their money was being spent, what amount of good was really being done with it, or whether the money was not doing medical mischief rather than good. (Florence Nightingale 1863)

Key points

- Information management and technology strategy
- The scope of information management and technology in the primary care setting
- Information systems for clinical benefit
- System integration
- User issues
- Security

INTRODUCTION

It is the responsibility of those in health service management to direct the way forward through the implementation of strategies. The information management and technology strategies (IM&T Strategy) for the health service are published following widespread consultation with key 'experts' and clinical staff across all aspects of health care. They generally are focused to respond to the direction detailed by government health-care strategies.

Each country within the United Kingdom has its own IM&T strategy but all reflect the same ideology: that technology should support care. It is the intention of the national strategies that health authorities and health boards must then develop local IM&T strategies to meet the national direction. Trusts will then develop IM&T strategies for local use. These should be developed in collaboration with business and operational plans, health improvement plans (HIP) and trust implementation plans (TIP). Although each of these has a different emphasis on detail, all aim for a common goal. This is primarily to implement and use patient-based systems that support clinical care and to introduce relevant technology to support the clinical process, including access to other appropriate systems. Strategies will focus at a high level on items which provide improvements to current systems or intention to change; communication networks such as email and NHSnet connectivity; linkage to other agencies, standards and protocols for use of technology; information management; data protection and adherence to security rules.

Strategies should reflect the organisational strategic plan, fit the situation and be feasible, acceptable and affordable. Local strategies must meet the ideals and direction of national strategies, thereby ensuring that there is consistency throughout the NHS. Often there is funding provided with a national strategy launch and application criteria for funding will be set by the strategy. So, for example, if the NHS is to implement clinically based systems, initiatives reflecting implementation for clinical benefit are likely to be given priority.

SCOPE OF IM&T IN THE PRIMARY CARE SETTING

Information management and technology is a growth industry. It is all around us every day and we have become so accustomed to it that we accept it as the norm. This is the case whether we are booking an airline ticket; banking over the phone, scanning our groceries in the supermarket, paying bills with plastic cards, directly dialling Uncle Jim in Sydney or chattering on the Internet. However, we tend to have a different perception of IM&T in health care.

Until recently, the power of IT to transform health-care delivery processes was largely underestimated. The availability of virtually unlimited computing power, data storage and communication bandwidth has opened up new opportunities for change. This will have a major influence on long-term strategic thinking.

To many people technology on its own means the highly advanced technical medical equipment that monitors and maintains life and supports surgical procedures. This is fully accepted as value for money. The difficulty arising in relation to computers may be partly due to the historic use of large legacy systems that chiefly collected patient administrative details and offered little in return to clinicians and nurses. Along with major advances in easy-to-use computer technology and developing network infrastructures have come vastly changed perceptions in the use of information. We have reached an exciting period of information communications development and clearly this is of specific importance to community nursing at a time when primary care is very much the focus of government health strategy.

Since 1988 there have been a number of government documents published, both White and Green Papers, which have emphasised care in the community. The most significant of these are as follows.

1988 *Community care – agenda for action* (DoH) (the second Griffiths Report) which proposed a change in the assessment and delivery of care in the community.
1989 *Working for patients* (White Paper) (DoH). The 'internal market', offering efficient and effective services provided like a business. This paper proposed a programme of action intended to secure a better choice of services through increasing competition.
1989 *Caring for people* (White Paper) (DoH). Community care in the next decade. This document complemented *Working for patients* and set out proposals for improving community care.
1990 The GP Contract (DoH). This contract explicitly specified services GPs are to provide and increased the flow of information for monitoring the delivery of services to meet local needs.

1990 National Health Service and Community Care Act. *Working for patients* and *Caring for people* became law (DoH).

1991 *Towards a primary care led NHS*. A government executive letter outlining changes in GP fundholding.

1997 *Designed to care* (White Paper, Scottish Office) *The new NHS* (White Paper, England and Wales) (DoH)

There has been a wind of change leading to the 1997 papers with emphasis on reducing bureaucracy and the demise of the internal market and a focus on clinical effectiveness.

The most recent government papers focus on cooperation between services and integrated planning of health care. There is an emphasis on a patient-centred and seamless service based on a partnership approach and a commitment to clinical effectiveness, which is responsive to the needs and wishes of patients, coordination and reliability of care through the use of technology and information. There is also a fundamental shift towards primary care groups (DoH 1997a) and primary care trusts (Scottish Office 1997). This offers the opportunity for community staff to become more closely involved in local decisions relating to the delivery of health care.

In order to identify health needs and monitor effective and valued outcomes, the right information must be collected and managed appropriately. During the Heathrow debate in May 1993 (DoH 1994) led by the chief nursing officers for England, Wales, Scotland and Northern Ireland, challenges were laid down for the nursing profession to lead the way into the 21st century. A fundamental point raised was that nurses, along with every other supplier of services across the health and social care sector, must ensure that wherever possible they should clarify what works in clinical practice and disseminate this information to those in the clinical areas, who should implement it. It was pointed out that effectiveness will increasingly be the key to recognition and that research-based knowledge must underpin and inform nursing practice. To enable this process to take place it is essential that nurses recognise the full potential of information technology and to this end IM&T

strategies have been published in order to direct and lead the health service in ways which support the current White Papers.

The most recent IM&T strategies (DoH 1998) aim to increase technology in the clinical support arena. The emphasis is on use of technology in order to support the clinician in the search for accurate, useful information which will inform decision making, highlight clinical effectiveness and support clinical governance initiatives.

Information management

Information is the fundamental linchpin of health care. All our decisions are based on effective use of information whether it is on the best treatment to offer, the best location to provide the care, the most useful equipment to provide, the relevant member of staff to provide care. Information management is about the use and interpretation of data and the best combinations for use in clinical practice as well as analysis, research, audit and other organisational requirements.

Numbers or measurements, of themselves, have no significance until matched with context. For example, clinical evidence requires combinations of data and quality measurements. Numbers of people being treated for leg ulcers are not very significant on their own. The addition of a combination of data relating to age, sex, treatment and duration of treatment enables decisions to emerge in relation to care. Facts *do not* speak for themselves; background and contextual information are necessary to enable judgement. This is information management.

Although in district nursing practice on a daily basis, much of the management of information

Box 15.1	Use of information in the nursing process
Assess	Practice notes, previous nursing notes, referral letter, nursing knowledge supported by information gained
Plan	How, where, when, what, why, who
Implement	Client interaction, discussion, observation and documentation of continual assessment and care plans
Evaluate	Evidence, result and evaluation of aim of care

takes place in discussion, at a certain level there will be a need to analyse the information for wider use (Box 15.1). At this stage, technology is useful. Computer applications are commonly used for analysis; this does not remove the need for interpretation but, indeed, increases the requirement for clinical evaluation of the facts based on knowledge of circumstance. Information management is becoming increasingly important for the measurement of the health service and this should start with greater emphasis on the use of information in daily practice.

Data collection for information in community nursing

Community nurses are in the habit of submitting data to their service management for information purposes. Most of the information is, by necessity, related to numbers: numbers of people seen perhaps within age bands, client groupings or other formats; numbers of treatments given; numbers of clinic attendances and so on. This is the most useful information for resource management. However, information most useful to the health-care professional is normally that written in the care plan, case record or other clinical notes. Other information may be held by other professionals involved in the care of the patient. This could be electronic, as in a GP computer system, or manual, as in case records, and the district nurse will access the information in the best way possible. Collecting information must be seen to be of value to district nurses or their motivation to collect it will be minimal.

A dataset is a group of items relating to specific information which can be coded (Box 15.2). A series of datasets need to be aggregated for

---

Box 15.2   A typical dataset

Name, date of birth, address, unique identifying number (NHS number, Community Health Index (CHI) number, case record number), source of referral, date of first contact, professional involved, contact type, location of contact, discharge reason, date of discharge, etc.

---

national statistical returns which become the basis for resource allocation in the health service. Datasets for community nurses have historically suffered from lack of development. The result is that most existing datasets relate to tasks. This is not necessarily very meaningful or useful to the district nurse. Unfortunately, at the time of writing, there is no official dataset which adequately describes the provision and measurement of community health care in the district nursing services. There are a number of very good local developments but these are not widely used. If they are to be of any use for widescale audit and research these datasets must be made consistent in order to enable comparative study.

The new NHS (DoH 1997a) White Paper suggests there is a need for information that relates to 'specific groups or clients' and this should be reflected in central data requirements. This is supported by the fact that planning and monitoring of health care involve analysis, interpretation and prediction of the relationships between:

- populations and/or patient groups who are at risk of developing an illness/disability or have an illness or disability which requires care or treatment
- services, care or treatments required by or provided for these populations or patient groups
- expected or actual outcomes as a result of receiving these services, care or treatments.

Baker (1998) recommends the review of early work on care description datasets which reflect provision of care to particular client/patient groups. Categorising of care in this fashion is meaningful to nurses and enables useful analysis at practice level as well as for business purposes.

Use of information

District nurses must learn to question data. They need to ask why. They need to question the relevance and use of the data, identify information requirements and learn the power of information by using it to analyse, enhance and change practice. Data collected on a routine basis must be useful and can be employed in a number of ways.

To review care practice

The *Strategic guidance on the effective use of information to support the management and delivery of nursing and midwifery care* (NHS Executive 1995) suggests that a process designed to review care practice in order to suggest improvements will be supported and enabled by the use of quality information (Box 15.8). The process needs to be built into an overall model, which facilitates:

- *learning and personal development* – changes in care practice which will benefit not only this patient but others
- *application of learning* – ensuring that the lessons learned from analysing information are carried through and become part of regular care practice.

To measure outcome of care

- Which processes result in better patient outcome?
- Monitor complaints.
- What are the current levels of pressure sores, infections, wound breakdown? Is this acceptable? Which patient group does this relate to?
- Measure healing against evidence, e.g. leg ulcer healing rates.
- Rate of hospital readmission.

Resource management

- Skill mix.
- Dependency levels within descriptive profiles of patient care.
- Most suitable time and place for treatment.
- Number of evening visits.

Communication

- Health-care summaries.
- Discharge/referral notes.
- Shared records.
- Electronic transfer of requests, etc. enhance speedy accurate communication.
- Patient-held record.

Box 15.3 Care practice for patients with permanent vegetative state

Wanted: Information on permanent vegetative state to help deliver care for this type of resident in a nursing home, drawing up guidelines with the health authority. Information would have an impact on:
- initial assessment (all sorts of different aspects of care for this type of patient)
- monitoring of care/care administration/audit or standards of care (taking up new ideas, would try to incorporate into what is being done at the home, would help to provide the most cost-effective care)
- improved quality of life to patient and/or family (helps with greater involvement with family)
- legal or ethical issues (big debate over non-treatment; patient advocacy always an issue with people who cannot speak for themselves).

IT in the primary care setting

The patient administration system

The vast majority of GP surgeries have computers. These are primarily patient administration systems and link GPs within a practice through terminals on their desks. These systems enable the GP to access patient administrative detail, (name, date of birth, address and so on), add encounter details (notes about the contact with the patient although these may vary according to the system used), prescription details and appointments. GPs use their systems to varying degrees; some only use them for prescribing and others, having reduced the manual record to the bare minimum, rely on their computer for the majority of their information needs. Practice nurses may have access to the GP system on a regular basis in order to check details or add information.

If information about individual patients is to be shared among relevant professionals then it follows that general practitioners are the key to ensuring accurate basic information is available from their systems.

Community information systems

Many trusts operate community information systems for the collection of community service activity data. These vary enormously across the country, as does the requirement for their use.

They are mostly used for statistical returns based on the number of contacts made by the district nursing service. The result is that most community systems are seen as data collection tools rather than patient information systems.

Results of a study of the uptake and application of community information systems in England and Wales in 1997 concluded that the primary driver of most trusts using a community information system is to allow clinicians to improve the way they carry out their work by providing them with easier access to better information. The second most important objective was fulfilling the information requirements of health commissioners and GPs (Audit Commission 1997).

Community systems usually form a network with a central trust database of some sort and in some areas staff can also access the information at their base. In a number of rural areas, laptop computers are available to staff who can then access information from a remote base.

Community information systems will develop so that information can be shared with general practice and other relevant professionals.

Office applications

Office applications are those that facilitate word-processing and other software applications used in the local setting, usually on personal computers. Examples are the Microsoft suite of applications, analysis packages such as SPSS and desktop publishing packages for the creation of leaflets and books.

Intranet

The need for communication is a basic human requirement. We are very used to using the telephone to communicate verbally over a distance. Electronic written communication can be enabled through the use of a facsimile machine linked to the telephone line or a data network. A network is a complex set of technical connections between computers allowing them to transfer data in such a way that the links can interpret and act on the data.

An intranet is a term which describes a local area network (LAN). A LAN will cover a restricted area such as a building or a number of buildings on a campus. The intranet enables an identified group of people to communicate with each other and share information. Most commonly for district nurses, their use of an intranet will be either within the practice or surgery base where they work or within the trust area. Electronic mail (email) is the most common use of this network communication. It is used for unstructured messages, not data transfer, although file attachments containing limited data and documents can be transferred relatively easily.

It is useful at this point to mention some drawbacks of the use of email. It is an interesting psychological fact that email brings out the worst in people. The lack of face-to-face contact combined with the simple coldness of communicating via the computer can turn many well-mannered and polite people into bad-tempered, angry respondents. A common term for this is 'flame-mail'. It is important to train staff to use email effectively and to read their message clearly before sending it. Using email effectively may involve change in practice and should be carefully thought out.

Besides email, the LAN will allow for agreed use of particular network files. These can be for shared documents, spreadsheets, newsletters, journals and so on, monitored and maintained by those administering the network.

NHSnet

There are over 1 billion messages now exchanged annually in the NHS and a national electronic network now exists so that these can be passed efficiently. The NHS net is a wide area network restricted to the NHS user. It provides a wide range of telecommunications facilities under managed service framework agreements between the NHS Executive and the suppliers. Its purpose is to enable an integrated approach to interorganisational communications across the NHS.

The government IT strategy is to ensure all health-care agencies and institutions are linked to the NHSnet, thereby opening up the development of electronic transfer of information across a wide area. There are, of course, strict protocols and guidelines for use and access will be controlled by secure gateways (firewalls) in order to maintain confidentiality.

Internet

Put simply, the Internet is a very large network of networks and computers spanning the globe. Millions of computers are linked together by telephone lines, fibreoptic cables, satellite and microwave links. For the majority of ordinary users, access to the Internet is from a personal computer, a modem and an account with a service provider, of which there are many.

More and more health centres, surgeries and clinics are allowing staff to access the Internet for journals and other health-related information held either locally or worldwide. The NHS has responded to demand for Internet access by developing Web pages, which offer information and services designed for NHS purposes, including electronic books, library services, bulletin boards, statistical databases and so on. The health service in Scotland has, for example, developed a Website entitled SHOW (Scottish Health On the Web) which can be accessed by professionals, managers and also, for most areas, the public as well. The SHOW site contains a number of pages each relating to current health issues (see vignette 15.1). Web page and email addresses are commonly printed at the end of articles or other documentation.

Vignette 15.1   Scottish Health on the Web

Jimmy Brown was moving to Inverness from Singapore. He logged onto the Internet and was able to access the SHOW (Scottish Health On the Web) Website. He typed Inverness in the search space and was shown a list of health-related information sources in that town. He wanted to register with a GP in a specific part of Inverness and, if possible, where there was specialist expertise in asthma because he was a sufferer and was midway through a planned programme of treatment in Singapore. By searching the available information on all practices in Inverness, he was able to confirm all his requirements and also let the practice know who he was and that he wished to register. By connecting to the practice via the SHOW Website, many of his details could be automatically transferred.

In some areas patients have access through specially developed information banks which are based on access to the Internet. Health Education pages, for example, are available with information such as advice on smoking or the availability of local services.

If the GP practice is accessing the Internet from the LAN within the building, it has to pass through a 'gateway' in the NHSnet. The practice address will be a NHS address whereas 'stand-alone' access will be supplied through a service provider address; examples include Compuserve, AOL and One Line.

Telemedicine

The EC Directorate responsible for information technology has provided the following definition of telemedicine:

This is that area of medical activity focused upon the investigation, monitoring, and management of patients and the education of patients and clinical staff, using systems which allow ready access to expert advice no matter where the patient (or expert) is located.

It should be stressed that the predominant focus of telemedicine is on established and emerging technologies since the above definition could easily describe a phone call between the district nurse and a patient. Used effectively, it means that patients could be monitored at home. To date, there is not enough evidence to show that telemedicine is cost effective and needs driven rather than technology led; however, there is no doubt that it can be a useful tool in rural areas and areas where specialisms are now concentrated in 'centres of excellence'. Although telemedicine is more common in the United States, it is growing here in the UK and, in particular, some community staff may have been involved in telemedicine initiatives for midwifery.

Teleconferencing

Teleconferencing is the generic term for meeting at a distance using an electronic communication medium. This could be three people in three rooms using the internal telephone system or it could also be by use of the computer or video.

Teleconferencing has been common in many areas of the British Isles for some time and particularly in education. A widely used videoconference network is LIVENET in the University of London where campuses, including some operating theatres, are linked by fibreoptic cables. The system is used for multisite lectures and tutorials.

INFORMATION SYSTEMS FOR CLINICAL BENEFIT

How often have you heard or even said, 'Describe to me the benefits of your system in relation to patient care'? This has to be one of the most difficult questions to answer because the expectations are high and the realisation of benefits is slow. Implementing a computerised system is a painstaking process, involving much research into clinical processes which have to be translated and specified into logical models for the software developer. The amount of time and resource expended, along with the frustrating delays and turnarounds, can irritate users to such an extent that they are no longer motivated to use the system.

Once a system has been developed, it is not easy to change so it is important to plan carefully before starting. Following the development, the system has to be tested in practice before 'roll-out'. Training and follow-up training are fundamental but above all, the users must believe in the system or it is not going to work for them.

With good-quality information going into a system, the benefits to the nursing team should be fairly evident (Box 15.4). Patients, too, will benefit from more accurate information collection and hopefully less need to repeat details. Better communication between those involved in the care will increase patient confidence. However, this is all academic if the information is not of use to the district nurse in practice. Information collected must support clinical decisions, be easy to collect and be available as and when required. It should enable the delivery of integrated and effective care, help in the prioritisation of need and leave the nurse more time to spend with the patient (Box 15.5).

Coombs (1998) indicates that human and organisational issues such as those above are considered the most important factors in terms of success of an information system. An example of good practice in this area is illustrated by vignette 15.2.

As already described, community information historically reflects activity rather than patient-based information. During the 1990s a number of initiatives were set up to develop descriptive datasets for community health-care professionals. The project team at the Information Management Group of the NHS (IMG), which was responsible for the information aspects of *Working for patients* (DHSS 1989), recommended the adoption of nationally agreed minimum datasets in England and Wales. At the same time a Scotland-wide project was being set up to develop a common dataset for the community nursing and paramedical services. Both these projects concluded with a suggested minimum

---

Box 15.4 Specific examples of benefits of a health-care IT investment (taken from the NHS Management Executive Investment Appraisal Guide 1994)

- Reduction of monotonous and repetitive tasks
- Less routine work
- Better planning and control of services
- Greater range of information for the individual
- Scope for more self-supervision
- Tidier environment
- Less fear of making mistakes
- Extension of work relations beyond local area
- More time for creative and specialised work
- Better communication between work areas
- Interdisciplinary cooperation
- Enhanced scope to identify inefficiencies
- Information for audit and research
- More reliable information
- More accurate and timely information

Vignette 15.2 Example of good practice

Community nursing staff in Edinburgh Health-care NHS Trust have been using a community information system designed by them for their own use. The system has now been in operation since 1995 and up to 750 staff have been trained to use palmtop computers. The information collected is based on the core community dataset (CCDS) which was developed by community staff in Scotland during 1993–94. The system is not networked and therefore supports the philosophy that the information is owned by the health-care professionals and management information is a byproduct. Caseload information is carried on the palmtop and contact data are entered onto screens designed to look like records. Data are uploaded into the database back at the surgery or clinic, thereby updating a common database for all professionals working from that site. Data are downloaded at the same time so that information relating to the last few contacts is available to nurses as and when they want it. When asked what is useful for them, staff will normally say that it is having accurate information such as phone numbers, alerts, previous contact details, etc. at their fingertips. Reports for business administration are extracted monthly.

Nursing staff took some time to come to terms with the ownership of the data and therefore were unsure of what they could do with the information. However, there is now evidence across the service of information use to support practice. This has included local audit of use of terminology, development of care aim standards, reflective analysis of source of referral in particular care groupings, development of a dependency scale based on more accurate duration of contacts, resource analysis to support a vacancy in a small team, prediction of workload based on trend analysis and general contact reporting in various forms.

Box 15.5 Principles important in the design of computerised clinical support systems (Hajioff 1998)

Acceptability:	the system should be acceptable to patient and clinician. This is a complex principle and impinges upon the others. It also involves broader issues such as clinical freedom, electronic patient data confidentiality and system safety and stability.
Currency:	the knowledge base of the system should be accurate and up to date.
Validity:	any clinical inferences drawn by the system should be based upon evidence. This may include statistical evidence from clinical trials, expert opinion or agreed best practice.
Relevance:	the system should be relevant to the context in which it is to be used. Software designed for a tertiary care environment may have limited applicability to primary care and vice versa.
Transparency:	the system of inference should be transparent to the user with reasons and background information readily available.
Accessibility:	the system should be accessible and easy to use. If this is not the case, it is likely to remain underused.
Non-intrusiveness:	the system should not destructively intrude into the clinician – patient interaction.

Box 15.6 Minimum dataset in relation to describing care provision for each patient

Scotland:	Care description (or package); care aim; reason for care
England/Wales:	Care programme; care objective; reason for care

dataset which was slightly different in content and terminology but very similar in concept: care description rather than number crunching (see Box 15.6).

The aim at the time was to enable more effective descriptions for purchasers. Neither project conclusion has been fully accepted for national implementation to date. However, reviews were undertaken during 1988–89 (Secta 1998) and the results are awaited. Although the focus is no longer on purchasing, the need to describe community care provision still exists and will become more necessary with the current emphasis on clinical effectiveness and clinical governance. The datasets reflect care packages and care objectives with a renewed emphasis on clinical outcome.

Vignette 15.3 A health visitor

When I worked for a community trust we had two baby clinics – one in the morning and one in the afternoon. In rationalising the service it was decided that both clinics should be in the morning. I had an intuitive feeling that those attending in the afternoon had the greatest health need, for all sorts of reasons. The parents were unemployed and were more likely to lie in in the morning, but wanted something to do in the afternoon. I was concerned that the change would mean we would not

meet the health needs of those who required our help most. I tried to substantiate my gut feeling with analysis. I looked back over clinic attendances and demonstrated that it was families of social class III and IV who generally attended in the afternoon. When i presented my data and demonstrated that this change would mean that those who had the greatest need would not get any service, it was decided to leave the clinics as they were.

Box 15.7   Useful information

Information should be: good, accurate, useful, accessible, auditable, searchable and legible.

The national IM&T strategies actively encourage the development of systems that support clinical care. The systems should be person based and management information should be a byproduct of clinical data. Community nurses should ensure they are in a position to influence the development of information systems by becoming involved in the analysis and use of information in practice.

Useful information will vary depending on circumstances. In daily care useful information is related to the patient as an individual. As well as demographic details, nurses will want to know about diagnosis, treatments, medication, allergies and so on. They will also want to know things like GP telephone number, perhaps next of kin or if there is a problem in the domestic situation.

Circumstances where information is useful include sharing information in a team or wider context, information to support evidence-based practice, resource management, outcome measurements, quality targets, standards, profiling and trend analysis; information to support care delivery and professional development (Vignette 15.3). Information for the monitoring of clinical performance is a requirement of recent government White Papers (DoH 1997a, Scottish Office 1997).

For NHS policy makers and in health authority/board management terms, useful information relates to the amount of care, type of care, location of care provision and how much resource it requires.

Information requirements are therefore complex and in relation to describing the clinical encounter, datasets must be useful as well as meaningful at a variety of levels (Box 15.7).

SYSTEM INTEGRATION

One of the key principles of the national IM&T strategies is that information should be collected once and once only. This requires integration of systems which 'speak' to each other so that information is shared. For example, integrating the GP system with the community information system would enable a person's name, address and date of birth to be entered only once. The common data are perceived as being held in one place; this may be one physical place, such as the GP database, or it may be 'virtual'. A virtual database is a technical facility which enables data to be gathered from a number of interconnected databases.

The integration process must support common language. This is easier said than done. For example, patients can be 'clients' and contacts can be 'encounters' depending on the health-care profession. Diagnosis is coded in ICD10 in hospital systems but READ clinical terms are used in GP systems. READ clinical terms are the result of a project initially led by Dr James Read to develop a comprehensive thesaurus of common clinical terms and phrases. The clinical description must be carefully defined so that it is understood by all those who require to use it. Discipline-based terms may differ from each other, even in dialect. The READ thesaurus endeavours to cope with language and even dialect variation in some areas of practice. Software developed must also adhere to common technical standards and protocols as outlined by both European and other international guidelines (NHS Executive 1996).

If systems are to be integrated, issues relating to monitoring the transfer of large quantities of data must be considered. Who is in charge and who will assess the data quality, for instance?

Electronic transfer

One of the most useful items of information is the discharge summary. The development of an electronic discharge summary based on common core datasets is one of the first steps towards passing of accurate, clear, concise, patient-based information via the NHSnet. Electronic transfer of information between general practice and some local hospitals is commonplace but only recently has there been suggestion of a common format which could be transferred between any two agents electronically. Referral letters, health record summaries, lab reports, test results and prescriptions are all examples of items which can be electronically transferred. Many GPs consider the electronic transfer of case records a priority.

Issues relating to transfer are mainly to do with signature, coding and matching of patient details at each end and the development of suitable quality assurance processes. Some practices will have PCs linked to the network which will store and either print off the document for filing or send it to the patient administration system electronically. All these issues require careful debate.

The introduction of electronic direct booking of outpatient appointments is an aim of the Labour government (DoH 1997a, Scottish Office 1997) (Vignette 15.4). Technology exists to support such a concept but as with most systems implementation, there are a variety of important 'people issues' to address first. Having said that, there are many places where it already happens

---

Vignette 15.4   Direct online booking for outpatient appointments

If a GP has on-line access to information about the length of time a patient will have to wait, he can see the state of all consultants' lists and may decide not to refer to his 'favourite' consultant but to the one with the shortest waiting time. Where this happened in one hospital, it resulted in a reduction of a popular consultant's list from 18 months to 12 weeks in a period of 1 year.

---

to a degree. Where clinicians have worked together to develop referral criteria for particular conditions, they have been able to offer evidence to show that there is an increase in appropriate referral and reduction in non-attendees.

The electronic patient record

The electronic patient record (EPR) concept is a description of one patient record held electronically. A central database in a trust enables the user to access any other record held on the data server at appropriate levels. The data on the server will come from a variety of patient-based computer systems in the organisation and link the patient record by using a unique patient identifier. This then appears to the user as a single record. For example, a charge nurse in a medical ward may wish to know the results of blood tests, any previous medication or social work assessments. In the past, all of this may have been held on individual case note inserts but has since been computerised, thus enabling access wherever and whenever required.

To date, most effort in the development of the EPR has been in the acute setting but there is no technical reason why such a record could not be developed for community services and, indeed, across the spectrum of services (Vignette 15.5). The introduction of a smart card is a step towards that concept and already exists in some other countries. In the main, this concept has been faster to develop when supported by the health insurance business. Usually, however, the smart card gives only very limited although accurate information about who the patient is whereas the EPR is the whole health record.

Vignette 15.5 Multidisciplinary records

Following a case study presentation given by a GP at the Nursing Specialist Group Conference in 1998, a nurse asked: 'I wondered what, in your practice, is the present state of play with the multidisciplinary record? Do you all share the same data or do you all hold on to your own data in different parts of the computer?'. The GP replied: 'everybody uses the computer now (1997), it is in one database. We had our neuroses at first; we kept records like a lot of people. It is a maturing process. It may well

be that the nurses do the same. Basically there is one record. We have a diabetic service which the nurses run. We only get involved when there are problems, so the audit of our diabetic care is really an audit of nursing care. The computer is a common database so the social manager uses it too. It is a common database for a lot of personnel. The practice computer produces community activity data which we ship off to the community trust'.

Knowledge-based systems

There are two major distinctions of importance to district nursing in relation to knowledge-based systems. First, there are knowledge-based systems which support the nurse in practice and second, there are those providing access for the general public to information on health, lifestyles, diseases, medicines, 'experts' and much more. The move towards knowledge-based health care requires that:

- clinical, managerial and policy decisions are based on sound information about research findings and scientific developments
- the sharing of information actually occurs.

Knowledge-based systems for the district nurse are those that support decision making. Protocols based on care pathways, evidence-based research, prescribing information, journals and research-based extracts may be made available to the community nurse on a local intranet or certainly at Internet access points such as libraries. 'Intelligent' or 'expert' systems will provide automatic guidance based on protocols and indicators. For example, when entering data relating to a particular screening assessment, the system would guide the nurse to the most appropriate treatment by forcing answers to questions already agreed and mapped out as an integrated pathway or treatment protocol (Box 15.8). The most obvious application for use is within the area of prescribing. However, evidence-based practice is a key driver in primary care and more guidelines and protocols, such as diabetic management and treatment of leg ulcers, are becoming available electronically.

Box 15.8 Benefits of the new generation of knowledge-based systems (Pritchard 1995)

- Timely access to relevant knowledge
- Easy-to-use guidelines for a very large range of patient-specific tasks
- Helping the health-care professional to rank the decision options
- Reminding of potential dangers in a clinical situation
- Evaluating the process of conforming to guidelines
- Evaluating the outcomes

The Cochrane database is an electronic library which is put together by a network of health-care providers and others collaborating to maintain and disseminate up-to-date reviews, by specialty, of relevant randomised controlled trials of health care. This and other databases such as Medline are available on the Internet and local communication networks. Rogers (1998) states that the public is about to be massively empowered through on-line access to information on health, lifestyle, medicines and much more. Information is power and this is shifting to the public through access to the vast resources available through the Internet.

In order that the information available remains of value and will not be harmful to the public, there is a responsibility for telematics and informatics professionals to ensure accreditation takes place. Doctors and nurses will need to accept challenges from patients who are becoming increasingly knowledgeable about their health problems. By using the Internet, the user is all of a sudden catapulted into a community of thousands and therefore there is potential for an incredibly rich exchange of knowledge. The problem is that on the Internet anyone can wear a white coat and there is no way of judging the quality of the information. The 1998 IM&T strategies acknowledge this issue with the intention to set up access to accredited information by going through 'national gateway' sites.

USER ISSUES

Training

Training in IT skills is fundamental. Strachan (1997) noted that probably the most important issue in terms of human resources is investment in training. Results detailing the issues for the successful use of nursing information systems showed that in 16 of the 68 issues mentioned by respondents, training and support of some kind were highlighted; eight had 100% consensus and two were 'top ten' priorities. It is essential that training starts in colleges and universities to encourage computer literacy. However, individual system training is quite different and has to be supported by trusts and training departments. Just as it is important to have a strategic approach to system implementation, so it is important to have a strategic approach to IM&T training. Training programmes need to be developed which fully support the needs of the healthcare organisation. This must include training in the use of the information and should span all levels of user. Systems will not be used beneficially if inadequate training is offered. People need to believe in the information systems and want to use them. Information must be perceived to be a priority asset.

IT training is provided in a variety of settings. There are national programmes that exist in the NHS as well as recommended national contracts for training. Also, computer-assisted learning packages are useful at a local level once initial training has been established.

Finally, it is essential that IM&T staff possess all the skills and knowledge required of the IM&T function in the trust so that they can adequately support staff.

Attitude

Health-care professionals, like many others, have been slow to realise the full potential of computerisation. Ball & Hannah (1994) identified major sources of resistance to change. First, there has been vast oversell by the suppliers. Computer companies knew little about the health-care industry during the early development of medical systems and made some unrealistic claims. Computers were presented as the panacea for all organisational and management problems. Second, clinical staff have not until recently been involved in procurement of systems for their own use and therefore left the task to those who understood the technology but not the clinical processes. The result was a breakdown in communication that led to either inappropriate design or underutilisation of systems. Third, according to Ball & Hannah (1994), nurses saw computers as a threat that challenged their traditional roles of ethics and confidentiality.

Another cause of resistance has been lack of consultation during the design and implementation stage of system development. Systems have been introduced without any consideration of the anxiety felt by many individuals. There is little evidence to suggest that these findings have changed (Table 15.1). This is especially true in district nursing where the computer resource has historically been considerably underfunded.

When nurses are not encouraged to see the potential of the new technology by effective teaching then barriers are very quickly built. Nurses are less likely to use the system to its full potential. Nurses working against the technology and not with it are more likely to enter data that are the most convenient and often inaccurate. Consequently, information extracted is poor or wrong, thereby supporting the feeling of uselessness.

Systems can fail in a variety of ways if user needs are not considered. The Health Systems Division of the NHS in Scotland undertook a review of human–computer interaction (Health Systems Division 1995) and highlighted the following issues.

- *Information systems must be safe to use.* If computers and peripheral equipment are awkwardly placed, staff feel less incentive to use them.

Table 15.1 Practice nurses' opinions on computer use (from postal questionnaire survey of 77 practice nurses in Portsmouth and Worcester area, 1997. (Miller A, Jeffcote R 1997)

The use of computers by nurses in general practice in my opinion ...	Strongly agree (%)	Agree (%)	Don't know (%)	Disagree (%)	Strongly disagree (%)	Did not answer (%)
Is administratively essential	19	57	3	16	1	4
Acts as a barrier to the patient–nurse relationship	1	16	12	61	8	3
Provides an effective way of recording information	31	60	3	3	0	3
Has improved the quality of my work	8	32	21	32	4	3
Is better for patient record management than paper files	14	55	9	19	0	3
Leads to less time being available for patient care	2	29	9	46	10	4
Promotes a closer relationship with patients	1	9	27	56	3	3
Makes good clinical sense	19	61	6	9	0	5

- *Poor interaction impacts on users.* When systems fail to support users in their work, then that work may not be done or users may have to work around the system, resulting in extra work and frustration. There may even be overall rejection of the system.
- *Early emphasis on user issues will avoid problems later.*

The EVINCE (*Establishing the Value of Information to Continuing Nursing Education*) Project (Davies et al 1997) examined the impact of information on the clinical practice and knowledge of nurses, midwives and health visitors. Conclusions from this report are presented in Box 15.9

The EVINCE research also identified that nurses' competence in the use of computers had a major impact on the information-seeking pattern.

User involvement

The extent to which patients seek information and play an active role in the treatment of their illnesses is growing and being encouraged more and more. Recent government documents have highlighted the need for patients to be fully involved in decisions about not just personal care but health services for a locality. District nurses are in a unique position to offer advice

---

Box 15.9 The EVINCE project conclusions

- Nursing professionals seek information from the sources most immediately available: base/ward, colleagues and personal collections.
- Colleagues are mainly used as sources of information for informal updating and patient care queries concerning drug therapy or treatment.
- Libraries and other computer-based resources such as CD-ROM are used mainly for course work and updating knowledge.
- The Internet has yet to make an impact on information seeking by nursing professionals.
- Nursing professionals prefer making personal visits to a library and particularly value access to journals for browsing and CD-ROM databases.
- Often, more than one source is tried to satisfy a query. Problems concern time constraints both in locating the information and waiting for identified information to arrive.

---

and guidance to patients looking for the best information to support their needs. Besides access to the Internet, the nurse must be aware of all information sources and act as an advocate for patients by being fully prepared to interpret the information for the patient.

Second, patients have a right to know about information held in relation to their care. It is therefore important that all documentation, computerised or otherwise, is accurate, meaningful and concise. In many areas, highly developed

---

Vignette 15.6   Patient-held multidisciplinary records: an example in practice

Patients are cared for by a variety of professionals from the community trust, general practice, acute hospitals and social services. To support these complex arrangements, staff within Cornwall Healthcare Trust developed a multidisciplinary patient record.
The record contains:
- advice for the patient on how it will be used
- key patient information
- details of the health teams caring for the patient and contact telephone numbers
- patient assessments
- care plans and evaluations
- investigations
- medication

- referrals
- discharge information.
The record is set up by the lead professional (usually the district nurse) but owned by the patient who keeps the record with him if he is admitted to hospital. It is updated by all nurses and professions allied to medicine (PAMS).
The benefits of the multidisciplinary record include:
- better coordination of care
- increased communication between professionals
- consistent and complete social and care history is available
- empowerment of the patient
- less duplication of records and record keeping.
(Audit Commission 1997)

---

patient-held records are becoming widely used (see vignette 15.6). This involves patients in all aspects of their care. However, until we are a highly automated nation of technocrats with digital computers which link to the surgery database or each of us holds a smart card which can be swiped through the community nurse's laptop database, these are likely to remain manual records.

There is little doubt that over the next decade we will move into an era where the patient will have a more influential say in both the type of care given and the information collected and used.

SECURITY

Computerised information systems are now used to support most NHS activities, including the treatment of patients. The security of the data held in these systems is of vital concern (Box 15.10).

The degree to which confidentiality, integrity and availability are preserved in the face of threats is a measure of the security of a system. Security strategies lay down procedures whereby security is implemented and measured across a trust or organisation. There is usually a named individual responsible for IT security who works alongside users and system administrators to ensure appropriate security measures are taken. Levels of access, such as log-on passwords, will be implemented according to the need of the individual using the system. Hoy (1997) suggests

Box 15.10   Security of health-care data

- *Confidentiality.* No unauthorised person, NHS staff or outsider, should have access to health-care data or other data used for supporting functions.
- *Integrity.* It should be possible to trust the information generated by the system. It must be certain, for instance, that data used for patient treatment are not only present but are accurate and fit for purpose in every detail.
- *Availability.* The system should be able to provide information when and where it is needed.

three approaches to data protection: hardware, software and organisational.

The hardware approach

Controls over access might include physical barriers such as doors, special locks, locks on individual machines, locking data storage, using storage media which are not easily removable and control over the use of communication links to the system. Smart card, finger print and voice control mechanisms have all been developed.

The software approach

The most common method of control is the password or PIN (personal identification number).

Encryption is a technique used to scramble data in the system so that they are incomprehensible unless the 'key' to unscrambling is known.

Box 15.11 Legislative documents which govern security

- Data Protection Act 1984, revised and updated 1998
- Computer Misuse Act 1990
- Disclosure of Personal Health Information
- Formal Security Standards Access Modification (Health) Order 1987
- Access to Health Records Act 1990
- Access to Health Records (Northern Ireland) Order 1993

The organisational approach

A system's security is only as strong as its weakest link. The organisation needs to carefully plan siting of terminals, printers and data storage and the disposal of unwanted information such as printouts. Decisions should be made relating to access and the convenience of users should be balanced against the requirements of confidentiality and the law (see Box 15.11).

During the 1990s the exchange of information electronically between organisations really exploded and the concern of the BMA and others for the confidentiality and security of data greatly increased. In response, the Chief Medical Officer asked Dame Fiona Caldicott to set up a group to consider and report on the NHS handling of confidential patient-identifiable information. This related to a guidance paper produced by the Department of Health (1996), *The protection and use of patient information*, and was to advise on relevant improvements. Subsequently the Caldicott Report was published (DoH 1997b) which sets out six principles on which dataflow should be tested:

1. justify the purpose
2. do not use patient-identifiable data unless it is absolutely necessary
3. use the minimum necessary patient-identifiable data
4. access to patient-identifiable data should be restricted on a 'need-to-know' basis
5. everyone accessing this information must be aware of their responsibilities
6. understand and comply with the registration.

Professional guidance for records and record keeping

The UKCC is extremely concerned with all types of information and how it is recorded, so much so that it produced *Guidelines for records and record keeping* (UKCC 1998) which was issued to all registered nurses.

The UKCC expects that students from the very beginning of their educational programmes should recognise the importance of accurate, comprehensive and up-to-date records and their role and responsibility in record keeping in the interests of patient care. The council document clearly states 'the important activity of making and keeping records is essential and an integral part of care and not a distraction from its provision'.

The 1998 guidelines offer support to community nurses using computers. The document highlights the advantages of computer records, saying that they tend to be easier to read, less bulky, reduce the need for duplication and can increase communication across the interprofessional health-care team. At the same time, nurses remain accountable for the information they enter onto the computer and must ensure adequate security is in place.

CONCLUSION

Information management and technology is daunting. The world of technology changes very quickly and what seems like a struggle today will be a matter of course very soon. There seems to be no end to advances in the speed of computers and the reliability of communication networks. However, it is still a costly business and even more so due to these advances which are often forced upon us in order to 'keep up'.

Nowhere is there more scrutiny on purchase and use of IT than in the health service. What is required is adequate technology to support clinical need. Nurses must be aware of the sensible use of computerisation to support their work and be vocal in its implementation. The nursing profession is in a position to recognise the importance of IT which enables collection and management of meaningful information and the use of that information to monitor, evaluate and improve practice. Nurses will be in the forefront of teams that introduce patient information systems and must recognise that technology is not necessarily the limiting factor to successful implementation. We must learn to work with the technology and not against it, understand how it changes practice and how nursing can benefit. Success depends on real and shared agendas for change.

REFERENCES

Audit Commission 1997 Comparing notes. A study of information management in community trusts. Audit Commission Publications, Oxford

Baker V 1998 Assessing the information needs and IM&T requirements for primary care trusts. Unpublished report

Ball M J, Hannah K J 1994 Introduction to nursing informatics. Springer-Verlag, New York

Coombs C 1998 The factors determining the success of a CIS. Information Technology in Nursing 10(3): 9–15

Davies R, Urquart C J, Smith J et al 1997 Establishing the value of information to nursing continuing education: report of the EVINCE Project. British Library Research and Innovation Centre, West Yorkshire

Department of Health 1988 Community care-agenda for action. HMSO, London

Department of Health 1989 Caring for people: Community care in the next decade and beyond. HMSO, London.

Department of Health 1990 National Health Service and Community Care Act. HMSO, London

Department of Health 1994 The challenges for nursing and midwifery in the 21st century. HMSO, London

Department of Health 1996 The protection and use of patient information. HMSO, London

Department of Health 1997a The new NHS: modern, dependable. HMSO, London

Department of Health 1997b Caldicott Committee. Report on the review of patient-identifiable information. HMSO, London

Department of Health 1998 Information for health. HMSO, London

Department of Health and Social Security 1989 Working for patients. HMSO, London

Hajioff S 1998 Computerised decision support systems – an overview. Health Informatics Journal 4(1): 23–27

Health Systems Division 1995 Usability – the state of the art of information systems in the NHS in Scotland. HMSO, Edinburgh

Hoy D 1997 Protecting the individual: confidentiality, security and the growth of information systems. Informed Touch (1): 78–87

NHS Management Executive Investment Appraisal 1994 NHS Training Division, Bristol

NHS Executive Information Management Group 1995 Strategic guidance on the effective use of information to support the management and delivery of nursing and midwifery care. IMG, Birmingham

NHS Executive Information Management Group 1996 The NHS IT standards handbook, version 3. IMG, Birmingham

Miller A, Jeffcote R 1997 Practice Nurses opinions on computer use. Health Informatics Journal 3: 10-16

Pritchard P 1995 Decision support for GPs – towards a more certain future. Journal of Informatics in Primary Care (3): 3–5

Rogers R 1998 A global information society for health. British Journal of Healthcare Computing and Information Management 15 (5): 30–32

Scottish Office 1997 Designed to care – renewing the health service in Scotland. HMSO, Edinburgh

Secta for the NHS Executive 1998 The critical appraisal of the 1995 community minimum dataset proposals. IMG, Leeds

Strachan H 1997 Issues for the successful use of nursing information systems. Information Technology in Nursing 9(1): 4–6

1998 Guidelines for records and record keeping. UKCC United Kingdom Central Council for Nursing, Midwifery and Health Visiting

FURTHER READING

Abbott W, Bryant J R, Sotheran M K 1996 Aspects of informatics. HISG, Eastbourne

Department of Health 1993 New world, new opportunities. HMSO, London

Department of Health and Social Security 1989 Caring for people: community care in the next decade and beyond. HMSO, London

Department of Health 1998 Health services accreditation – a guide to the process. The Stationery Office, London

NHS Wales 1996 Getting the benefits: All Wales benefits realisation project. HMSO, London

NHS Executive and Greenhalgh B 1996 Using clinical information in integrated healthcare. HMSO, London

NHS Executive Information Management Group 1997 Benefits of using clinical information. IHCD, Bristol

NHS Executive 1996 IM&T security manual. HMSO, London

NHS Executive 1995 NHS-wide networking programme. HMSO, London

Olszewski D, Jones L 1998 Putting people in the picture. Scottish Association of Health Councils. HMSO, Edinburgh

Index